beauty therapy

Jane Hiscock
Frances Lovett

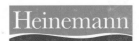

Heinemann Educational Publishers,
Halley Court, Jordan Hill, Oxford OX2 8EJ
Part of Harcourt Education

Heinemann is the registered trademark of
Harcourt Education Limited

© Fareham College 2002

First published 2002

2006 2005 2004 2003

10 9 8 7 6 5 4 3 2

A catalogue record for this book is available from the British
Library on request.

ISBN 0 435 45157 X

Page layout and illustrations by Hardlines, Charlbury, Oxon

Original illustrations © Heinemann Educational Publishers, 2002

Printed and bound in Great Britain by Bath Colour Books

Websites

Please note that the examples of websites suggested in this book
were up to date at the time of writing. It is essential for tutors to
preview each site before using it to ensure that the URL is still
accurate and the content is appropriate. We suggest that tutors
bookmark useful sites and consider enabling students to access
them through the school or college intranet.

Tel: 01865 888058 www.heinemann.co.uk

Contents

Acknowledgements

We are extremely grateful to so many people for their support and guidance in the development of this book – it has been an enjoyable challenge, but anyone who has ever put pen to paper will realise the huge amount of work that goes into a book – so, our heartfelt thanks go to:

In the first place, our husbands and children, who shouldered, above the call of duty, a good proportion of domestic duties, whilst we had our heads down. Thanks, guys!

The team at Heinemann for their professional, gentle, yet firm guidance – giving a caring hand when we needed it. Pen and Anna you are wonderful!

All our colleagues at Fareham College: the management team, Mary Mussell and Joan Champion, for their support; the Business Development Centre, headed by John Tomlinson, for the practical collaboration. Our fellow lecturers have been amazing, with contributions and positive stroking, when required. Their contributions have been invaluable to the success of the contents.

The professionals within the industry have also been very helpful, in providing high-quality products and photographs. Our thanks go to:

Angela Barbagelata, Fabes and the team at Carlton Professional, Lancing – for providing equipment

Cherry International

Jessica The Natural Nail Company – for super manicure products.

Charles Fox, London – for make-up products and brushes

Bellistas Ltd – for information

SBC (Europe) Ltd – for make-up products and photographs.

Our picture researcher Sally Smith came up trumps with the attractive skin disorders pictures, and our photographers Gareth and Tony were certainly more aware of the inside of a beauty salon than before the shoot started. The quality of the photographs is amazing, and we are delighted with the end results.

Tina Lawton and Sue Williams from Warrington College were of enormous help in the Key Skills development, and they were most generous for sharing good practice.

Finally, but by no means least, we would like to thank our awarding body, the Vocational Training Charitable Trust (VTCT) and the Federation of Holistic Therapies (FHT).

Jane Hiscock and Frances Lovett

Photo acknowledgements

Gareth Boden: pages 1, 11 (centre), 13, 23, 26, 29, 30, 45 (left), 54, 111 (left and centre), 128 (bottom), 129 (row 2, right), 145–149, 152, 157–158, 170, 172, 174, 176–177, 180–187, 189, 196, 210, 216–220, 222–227, 230–231, 234–236, 240, 249–251, 253, 255 (bottom), 256–258, 260, 263, 269, 280–288.

Corbis: page 120 (2nd right).

Federation of Holistic Therapists (FHT): page 151.

Grassé: pages 19, 60.

Mediphoto: page 121 (row 1, right).

Peter Morris: page 11 (row 1, left), 45 (right), 125, 128 (row 1), 129 (row 1; row 2, left and centre), 255 (top), 276–277.

SBC (Europe) Ltd: page 17.

Science Photo Library: page 28 (row 1, left; row 2, left), 116 (row 1, right; row 2, 2nd left), 117 (row 1, left), 120 (2nd left), 121 (row 2, left), 246 (bottom), 273 (top and bottom).

Science Photo Library / Biophoto Associates: page 28 (row 2, right).

Science Photo Library / Mike Devlin: page 272 (bottom).

Science Photo Library / Alain Dex, Publiphoto Diffusion: page 116 (row 1, left).

Science Photo Library / John Radcliffe Hospital: page 121 (row 2, right).

Science Photo Library / Dr P. Marazzi: page 28 (row 1, centre; row 2, centre; row 3), 116 (row 1, left; row 2, 2nd right), 117 (row 1, right; row 2, right), 118 (row 1, left and right; row 2, right), 119 (row 1, right; row 2, left), 120 (right), 121 (row 1, left; row 2, centre), 245 (top and bottom), 246 (top), 272 (top), 274.

Science Photo Library / David Parker: page 273 (centre).

Science Photo Library / Dr H. C. Robinson: page 119 (row 2, right).

Science Photo Library / Jane Shemilt: page 117 (row 2, left), 275.

Science Photo Library / St Bartholomew's Hospital: page 28 (row 1, right), 116 (row 1, centre), 118 (row 2, left), 119 (row 1, left).

Science Photo Library / James Stevenson: page 120 (left).

Science Photo Library / Western Ophthalmic Hospital: page 116 (row 2, right), 245 (centre).

Mike Wyndham: page 121 (row 1, centre).

INTRODUCTION

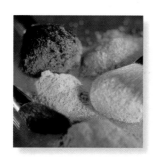 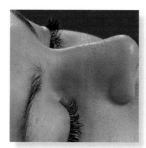 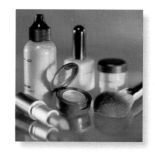

How to use this book

This book has been designed with *you* in mind. It has a dual purpose:

1   To lead you through the NVQ level 2 Beauty Therapy qualification, providing background, technical guidance with possible evidence collection and key skill information.

2   To provide a reference book that you will find useful to dip into, long after you have gained your qualification. The comprehensive cross mapping within the individual chapters will guide you through the NVQ units and indicate where the information applies – and should prevent repetition!

Each of the practical units contains the same essentials – the **Professional basics**. This has been presented as a separate section that should be worked through and adapted to the unit you are taking, at the time. The anatomy required for each unit has also been separated so that it can be accessed and referred to easily. As the anatomy is a constant theme through each unit, each anatomy topic shows exactly in which unit / element it is required as knowledge. Remember that you only have to learn it once and apply the knowledge to the practical area you are working through.

Back to basics

If you are familiar with the NVQ system and are confident about the background to this method of gaining a qualification, then skip this section, and move on! If you are new to the NVQ system then read on!

NVQ = National Vocational Qualification

This is a different, but highly successful method of gaining a qualification.

You may not have used it before, for example if you have come straight from school, or if you have not been in a training situation for some time.

What is an NVQ?

This is not an exam, with a pass or fail outcome. NVQ uses continual assessments, in each unit, building up to a qualification. It is a fairer option for those of us who freeze at the thought of an exam room!

There are several beauty therapy awarding bodies offering NVQs. Your training establishment will be able to guide you through the particular one they use, but the standards do not vary too much, and the information within this book should cover all eventualities.

How do I gain an NVQ?

The qualification is gained by showing lots of **evidence** within each unit and is practically based, so each student gets a very good grounding in all the skill areas.

This means that when you go into a salon, you have dealt with most client requests and have lots of confidence to perform the service, which after all is what the client is paying for.

How do I get my evidence?

Many forms of evidence are acceptable and your trainer / lecturer will be able to guide you through the best options for your individual learning programme. Each of the types of evidence is valid. These are:

- observed work
- witness statements
- assessment of prior learning and experience (APL)
- oral questions
- written questions and / or assignments
- other.

These will be recorded on **evidence sheets** provided and will form **a portfolio**. A portfolio is just a collection of all the evidence together. It should be **indexed** and easy to follow.

Why index?

An **assessor** will observe or guide you through the types of evidence listed above. This person will have had special training and a specific qualification designed to help you present your evidence in a format suitable for your awarding body.

For quality control and fairness across the subject areas, an **internal verifier** will check the assessor, and the portfolio instruction. This will be performed within your section / school at your place of training and should take place on a regular basis.

The awarding body also has an **external verifier** who will visit your training establishment regularly, and check that both assessors and internal verifiers are giving the correct information to you, the candidate. Then your portfolio can be accredited with a certificate. This can be achieved a unit at a time, or applied for all at once.

So, an organised portfolio is essential to present your work in an easy-to-view format.

What evidence do I need?

You should ask your assessor about the most suitable method for the work you are doing. Most portfolios have a mixture of evidence.

If you have **external previous evidence (APL)** or recent qualifications they can also be counted. For example, if you work in a shop, part-time, and have experience using the till, dealing with customers and complaints, then a **witness statement** from your employer, that is current, valid, signed and dated is very acceptable evidence.

This evidence would cover some of the reception units, as well as some communication units and the interpersonal skills required. It also covers some of the **ranges** required in your assessment books.

Other valid evidence could be photographs, project work, videotape or client record cards.

Standards

To give the overall picture we can look at what you are going to need to do. First, your training establishment will register you with its awarding body.

> The Crusty Loaf
> 12 High St
> Summertown
> Bedfordshire
> MK26 3YL
> 2nd September 2002
>
> To whom it may concern,
> Martine Angelou has been working for the Crusty Loaf for 15 months and is a trustworthy and honest employee. In the course of her duties she works the till, deals with cheques, credit cards and cash, and regularly cashes up. Martine has also had to deal with suppliers, with difficult customers and the odd complaint. I find her helpful, courteous and she works well with colleagues. She is able to take the initiative when required. I recommend her to you.
>
> Yours faithfully,
> Regina O'Farrell
> Manager

The awarding body will then issue you, the candidate, with your **assessment book**. Take care of it; treat it like gold, as it is very precious. It will become your only source of evidence for all your hard work.

Within your assessment book you will be given guidance on how to achieve each unit.

There are conditions and terms that you must follow.

Performance criteria

You must perform these in the course of your assessed treatment. They are numbered and your assessor will tick them off as they are observed. For example, Unit 6.3: performance criteria e.g. 'the skin is left clean and free of all traces of make up prior to further treatment'.

Ranges

These must be covered through the various methods of assessment previously discussed – observed performance, oral question or simulation, written question, project or through APL; for example, an eyebrow using hot wax for Unit 7.

Essential knowledge

Each unit is quite specific about the knowledge and understanding supporting the practical application.

Need to know may not be directly assessable but supports the essential knowledge. This may be in the form of an oral question. For example: a facial steaming treatment is not a range to be assessed within Unit 6, but you need to know about it and the effects it has in relation to pre-warming the skin. You may be shown a demonstration of how to use one, without being assessed upon it. You may be asked a question on it.

Need to understand provides the evidence and is directly assessable.

How this book is designed to help you

The purpose of this book is to inform and guide you through your NVQ level 2 Beauty Therapy qualification. To reinforce your learning process and get you thinking, there are several features to help you.

Reality checks

These are an important feature of the book. Each reality check gives you a chance to stop and think about your practice and the safest and most effective way to carry out your treatment. Many reality checks relate to performance criteria or essential achievement and your professionalism as a therapist.

Remember

Remember points can be found within each unit to highlight specific areas we feel you need to pay particular attention to.

In the salon

These scenarios are real-life situations that you may face in an actual salon! These are designed to highlight situations with circumstances that may need to be dealt with. For example, there may be a scenario about a customer complaint, which you have to relate to your knowledge of legislation and inter-personal skills. Scenarios help you to think ahead and give an indication of what may happen in a commercial salon.

Knowledge tests

These are put at the end of a topic to test your knowledge and understanding. They will not be valid as evidence for your portfolio unless they are carried out under assessment conditions, but they are very good revision – and fun!

Your questions answered

These bring up the 'what if' questions that you may think of during your work in the practical units.

Prompt

You will find these features at the end of certain topics. They are flow diagrams, which summarise the most important things to remember. An example is shown on the outside edge of this page – it is a summary of NVQs and their structure.

Why beauty therapy?

Every year, hundreds of students who have completed their NVQ level 2 in beauty therapy go on to have a happy and fulfilling career in beauty and hairdressing salons, cosmetic stores, spas and health farms, and on board cruise liners and aeroplanes. Others choose to 'go it alone', working from home, or on a mobile basis. Some will use their qualification on a part-time basis, while they continue with their existing day job, hoping to build up enough clients so that they can eventually take their therapy work full-time. However, many students use their NVQ level 2 as a stepping stone to go on to do further training so that they can broaden their career options or specialise in an area that is of particular interest.

This section takes a look at some of the varied job opportunities open to those who have completed their NVQ level 2.

Beauty therapist

This is the ideal role for those who complete their NVQ level 2 in beauty therapy but do not wish to go on to do further training. As a therapist, you would mainly be providing clients with facials, manicures, and pedicures. This could be in a number of settings, including a beauty or hairdressing salon, in a department or cosmetic store, or at a health farm. Good communication skills are important, particularly if you are working in a store, as you will be expected to encourage your clients to buy the beauty products you have demonstrated on them. Once you have proved yourself, your employer may offer you further training, but check if this training is well recognised in case you decide to move on. In terms of salary, you will probably receive a basic level of pay plus commission, which means the more experienced you become and the more treatments you do – the more money you are likely to receive. Your salary will also be added to by any commission you receive from selling products after a treatment, for example products for home use after a facial.

Beauty therapist (body treatments)

In order to become a beauty therapist who can offer body treatments, you will need to complete a beauty therapy NVQ level 3 qualification or equivalent, such as an International Beauty Therapists' Diploma. This will allow you to carry out mechanical and electrical body treatments to enhance body shape, electrical epilation (hair removal), and body massage, as well as facials, manicures and pedicures, etc. While studying, you can also take optional units in nail enhancement, aromatherapy, and specialist make-up techniques. Some courses also include figure diagnosis and spa treatment.

NVQ Beauty Therapy made up of ten units.

Each unit is a brick in the wall.

When the ten units are completed the wall is finished and your certificate can be applied for.

Each unit has performance criteria that you must do.

Ranges that you must cover.

Essential knowledge that you must learn to support your practical skills.

An assessor will help you to put together your evidence.

This is a file called a portfolio.

The assessor is helped by an internal verifier.

Who will make sure the portfolio has all the right information.

An external verifier comes to your college or training establishment to oversee the whole process and give information from the Awarding Body. The application forms for your qualification can then be signed and your certificate will arrive.

Having such a wide range of skills will make you more attractive to potential employers: they won't have to employ a therapist and an aromatherapist if you can perform all of these treatments yourself, and more. To be a successful beauty therapist you will need to be adaptable, a good communicator and happy to work largely on a one-to-one basis with your clients with little supervision. Obviously, you will have to feel comfortable handling other people's bodies, including the not-so-beautiful ones, and you'll also need the stamina to stay on your feet all day. Most beauty therapists working for a salon, health farm or similar will receive a basic wage plus either a performance-related bonus or commission on sales and treatment.

Make-up artist

For those who wish to specialise in make-up, there are many exciting and different job opportunities available. With the right personal skills and artistic flare, you could find yourself working on a wide range of clients. Further specialist training will allow you to work in the following areas: camouflaging scars on burns victims; retouching superstars for television; beautifying brides for their big day; or maybe even preparing the dead for the chapel of rest! Whichever of these routes you take, it is more than likely that you will need to have further training or contacts within your particular field of interest. Unfortunately, having the right vocational skills is often no longer enough when it comes to getting the job you want – it's also about being in the right place at the right time, and knowing the right people.

As a make-up artist, your wages may be varied and even unpredictable, depending on a number of factors, including whether you are self-employed or employed, who you are employed by, and the length of your contract of employment. Where you live is also a factor – freelance work, for example, will be more available in a city.

Holistic therapist

Many therapists go on to train in holistic therapies to diversify the range of skills they have to offer. A great number of clients who visit a therapist are not doing so simply to improve their looks on the outside. Taking time out from a busy schedule to visit an attentive therapist and be pampered for an hour or so can be very stress-relieving, and just as important as the beauty treatment itself. If you can carry out holistic therapies as part of your repertoire it means you have the opportunity to meet many of your client's needs with the appropriate treatments. There are many holistic therapies to choose from, with Swedish body massage, Indian head massage, aromatherapy and reflexology perhaps being the best known and most popular.

Holistic therapists require a good understanding of anatomy and physiology, and you will need to be comfortable about working on the client's whole body, whether they are young or old, male or female, smooth or hairy. Many holistic therapists now find themselves working alongside doctors and nurses in the healthcare setting: this could be in a GP clinic, in a home, hospital or hospice. Wages can vary according to whether you are self-employed or working for a salon, health farm, spa or other, and whether your employer is willing to pay commission.

Aromatherapist

Aromatherapists must have a recognized body massage qualification. Aromatherapy is a massage with a difference: after an in-depth consultation, the aromatherapist will blend together different essential oils that are carefully selected to meet the individual needs of the client. These oils are then added to a carrier oil, and a massage is performed on all or on parts of the body. Professional training is vital as essential oils are potentially dangerous to both the client and the therapist if not used correctly.

Reality Check!

Many beauty therapists are attracted to the prospect of working on cruise liners, and as they have a wide range of beauty and body massage skills, they make ideal candidates for the job. The benefits can be very inviting: many of the clients tip generously, your food and accommodation is paid for, and you get to travel the world. But there are some draw backs to the job as well, including long periods away from home, rough-weather trips, an extremely demanding schedule, and usually a very basic wage. But the job can be extremely rewarding. Remember, whatever you have in mind for the future, always try to speak to a therapist who has tried and tested the career path you are thinking of taking. If you are a member of a professional association, the association may be able to put you in touch with such a person, or perhaps your college lecturers could help. That way you will get to hear about all aspects of the job, the good and the bad, and not just a glorified version from your prospective employer(s).

If aromatherapy interests you, then there are two routes you can take:

- IIHHT Diploma – M17 Body massage + M27, M28 Aromatherapy
- NVQ Level 3 Beauty therapy Unit 17.

Masseuse/sports therapist

Many therapists who go on to qualify in body massage and/or sports massage often find work at health clubs, leisure centres, in salons or on cruise liners. Your primary role in any of these contexts would be to help clients rid themselves of life's stresses and strains or to return them to their exercise routine safely after a minor injury. After GP approval, an increasing number of therapists are now also working alongside physiotherapists or other health professionals in day centres, and even hospitals. And of course, there are those lucky few who get the opportunity to work for a football club or other sporting organisation, or become the personal masseur of someone rich and famous.

The pay will largely depend upon the prestige of clients and the environment in which you are working, and the amount of funding available for the type of treatments you provide.

Electrologist

Electrology is a highly specialised treatment that uses electrical current to remove unwanted hair permanently. You will need a well-recognised beauty qualification in order to gain the appropriate skills and professional insurance cover needed. Those who wish to do electrology generally go on to do a beauty therapy NVQ Level 3, although it can be gained as a separate unit. Naturally, this line of work will require you to be confident with needles, have a steady hand, good eyesight and to have an understanding of health and safety issues. As demand is high for this specialised treatment, the wages can be among the most generous on offer at those salons or clinics that provide this service. Often the client is referred to the clinic by her GP.

Depilationist

Waxing and sugaring are popular, non-permanent methods of hair removal. Although neither of these methods are as long lasting as electrolysis, the effects of the treatment can last for up to six weeks and large areas can be tackled in one sitting. Many therapists go on to specialise in this subject as it attracts a high number of regular clients which can prove lucrative for those therapists who are self-employed or receiving commission as part of their pay package. These are also good treatments for a mobile therapist to offer, especially at the beginning of the summer and at Christmas.

Demonstrator/retailer

A number of cosmetic companies, usually based in department stores, employ qualified therapists to provide make-up tips and promote beauty products to potential customers. In most instances, you will receive further training from the company you are employed by, with much emphasis being placed on sales techniques. You will need to be confident with people and have a well-groomed appearance to go far in this line of work.

The salary is likely to consist of a basic wage and a sales-related commission. There are also some cosmetic companies that work directly with therapists on a self-employed basis. Typically this would mean that your wages would be commission only, so how well you do depends entirely on the number and value of products that you sell at house parties, etc. Beware of companies that require you to buy their products up front, as you will be left holding the goods if you are unable to sell them any reason.

Nail technician

Nail bars are now popping up in just about every city centre as the demand for treatments, ranging from basic manicures to bejewelled extensions, are becoming increasingly popular. Whether you choose to work at a nail bar, at a beauty or hair salon, or as a mobile or home-based therapist, you will need to take further training if this is the area in which you would like to specialise in. Having completed your beauty therapy NVQ level 2 you will already have the manicure certificate that this work requires, but you will need to go on to take further units in nail enhancement and nail art if you wish to provide a full range of techniques.

Possible jobs – Profile 1: Wendy Chesswas (36) – Hamlin, Germany

I did my beauty therapy NVQ level 2 in July 2000, and just managed to complete a course in Indian head massage before the army posted my husband to Germany for three years. Having two children and being on the move all the time has always meant finding office work when and where I could, but now I have a career that I can start up without difficulty – whichever part of the world we're in. At the moment I am the only beauty therapist at our garrison, and with over 400 families here, I have plenty of regular clients! There are a number of beauty therapists and salons in the Hamlin area, but the army wives feel more comfortable having a facial or their legs waxed by someone from 'back home'. I work from a tranquil little room in our attic, which my clients love and see as a bit of a retreat! Although I don't make a fortune, I generally have appointments every day, and I've just bought myself a car with the money I make from my treatments. But I also just love meeting people, and having the luxury to fit my work around my personal and family commitments when necessary, rather than the other way round.

Possible jobs – Profile 2: Kate Raison (28) – Hampshire

I used to work full time as a sales consultant for a home furnishing company, but when my son Corey came along three years ago, I decided it was the ideal time to make a career change and so I went to college to study beauty therapy. I am now a counter manager for Lancôme at my local Boots store. My work involves giving consultations, showing customers how to apply make-up and products, monitoring and ordering stock, and managing the stand in general. Although I went on to complete an IHBC International Beauty Therapy Diploma, which covers things like electrical and mechanical beauty treatments, I believe it was my NVQ level 2 that gave me the relevant skills I needed for my current job. I'm also qualified in aromatherapy and body massage, and I've recently started a course in reflexology. I do enjoy my work at the moment, but I think I will eventually pursue a career in the field of holistic therapies. It's all quite addictive – once you've trained in one or two therapies, you find you want to do more and more!

Possible jobs – Profile 3: Emily Keighley (19) – Basingstoke

I completed my NVQ level 2 in July 2000, then went straight on to do my level 3 as I knew it would be difficult to get work in a salon in my area without having both. I now work in a busy salon with three other beauty therapists, a chiropodist, a chiropractor, a reflexologist, a masseuse, and the salon manager. I cover a whole range of beauty and holistic treatments, but I would say the most popular ones I do are waxing and manicures. A typical week for me would be Tuesday to Saturday, 9 to 5, but if the salon is particularly busy – especially in the summer – then I'm often required to work longer hours and/or an extra day. When I first started working at the salon, I used to fall asleep almost as soon as I got home in the evenings: I never imagined how busy and tiring the job would be! As a beauty therapist in a salon, most of your day involves standing on your feet, but no matter how tired you are, you have to remain cheerful and give each client your very best. I think it's an aspect of the job you just don't appreciate when you're at college, going backwards and forwards from the classroom to the salon, and having lots of breaks. Even now it's a relief to see I'm pencilled in to do a manicure as it means I get to sit down for half an hour! But the job is very rewarding, particularly when you build up a regular clientele of your own.

A day in the life of make-up artist Claire Williams

Claire is a mother of two and lives with her husband in Cardiff, Wales. She is a part-time lecturer in beauty therapy at Coleg Glan Hafren and a freelance make-up artist, specialising in film and television.

05.40

I give myself 20 minutes in the morning to have a quick shower, get dressed and be out of the door for just after 6.00am. No time for breakfast unless I want to get up earlier, so I'll try to grab something on location.

06.05

Leave the house with my map so that I can find the location where filming is taking place today. I have just started an eight-week contract, which is about average for a TV drama, and know that most of today's filming will be outside. It's pouring down!

06.50

Arrive at the mobile make-up truck and have about 10 to 15 minutes to get my work area prepared. By 7.00am my first actor, Actor A, arrives. He's a male, needing straight make-up and no wig, so it will take me about 15 minutes

07.25

A cup of coffee and a bacon sandwich arrives for me but I only get a few bites before Actor B arrives. This time it's a woman, so I have a 45-minute slot to do her hair and make-up. Have to check the photos in the Continuity File to make sure she looks exactly the same as when she was being filmed yesterday.

08.15

Actor C arrives, another female. Again, I have a 45-minute slot, but after half an hour, the Assistant Director arrives, wanting to hurry Actors A, B and C to the set. As my actors are scurried off in a car, I am quickly bagging up each actor's make-up (they all have their own) to take with me to the set. The kit I take with me also contains small bottles of every make-up imaginable as the set is 20 minutes away from the make-up truck and I can't afford to find I have something missing once I'm there.

09.10

I arrive at the set shortly after Actors A, B and C. Rehearsals have now started.

10.00

Actors A, B and C each receive a touch-up before the first scene is shot.

10.30

With the first lot of shooting completed, I head back up to the mobile truck where I apply make-up to Actor D, a male.

11.00

Back down to the set. Now hanging around in the rain, waiting to touch up the actors' make-up in between filming, and sheltering them under an umbrella when they're not required on set. We were supposed to be stopping at 12.30 for lunch, but there's been a problem with the lighting so we've all been asked to keep working until the scene is finished.

13.15

The first scene is finally completed, so it's back to the make-up truck again for some lunch. In theory we have an hour for lunch but after 30 minutes or so, I'm checking my actors' make-up and hair and tidying my work area, etc.

14.15

Lunch break is over and the actors return to set but I stay in the truck.

14.30

Actor E arrives, a male, who needs make-up and a hair trim – it's been a couple of weeks since he was needed on set and I can see from photos in the Continuity File that his hair has grown since he was last filmed.

15.00

Back to the set where I spend the rest of the day re-touching make-up and keeping the actors dry between shoots. We have a hot snack at 6.00pm, which is much appreciated as I'm starting to feel quite cold now. The rain hasn't stopped all day!

19.00

'It's a wrap!' Back to the mobile truck where actors are de-rigged and faces cleansed, etc. Brushes are cleaned and my work area prepared for tomorrow morning. Photos that have been taken throughout the day are then sorted through and placed in the continuity file.

19.30

I leave the location and finally get home at just gone 8.00pm. I clean off my waterproofs, boots and make-up bag and stand, which are all caked in mud.

20.30

I have a bath, then it's time for a much-deserved glass of wine, a meal and some time with my loved ones. Then it's bed at 10 pm so that I have the energy to start all over again tomorrow!

Reality Check!

Many people who study beauty therapy hope to work eventually in film and television, and no doubt a small percentage will be lucky enough to do so after obtaining just their NVQ 2. However, most of today's successful make-up artists went on to take further qualifications in make-up, arming themselves with as much knowledge and hands-on experience as possible to get ahead in what is a highly competitive job market. If you do find work, contracts tend to be short, lasting between 8 – 10 weeks, so it is important to get noticed by all the relevant people if you do manage to get your foot in the door. It can also mean travelling up and down the country to find or follow work, and often the conditions are not as glamorous as many would think: filming could be entirely outdoors, or you may have to spend most of your 10-hour day working in cramped conditions surrounded by stressed actors and crew members. If you feel this is the career for you, you will need to be flexible but determined and prepared to work long and hard hours.

professional
BASICS

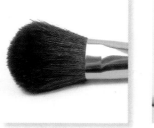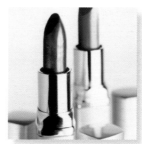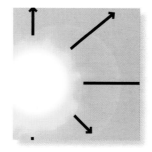

Professional basics

The professional basics is all about getting you started as a beauty therapist.

Before you can decide upon the most suitable treatment for your client, or prepare treatment plans, you need to have a clear understanding of the underlying principles of what you are doing.

This section covers the basic knowledge you will need before you start working through any practical unit. You will need to refer back to this section each time you start a new practical unit.

At the end of the **Professional basics** section you will be able to:

- list the importance of personal presentation when in the workplace
- name the various types of communication and their meaning
- describe the many salon services available and gather price lists of local salons for comparison
- compare assessment techniques and discover the right one for you
- distinguish between contra-indications and contra-actions and how this affects the client and the therapist
- relate the hygiene rules to a practical situation within the salon
- know your rights as an employee and how to protect yourself and your client within legislation
- record all treatment plans for the client and keep excellent client records
- be able to prepare in full for the treatment to be carried out.

There are three main topics in this section:

- You – the therapist
- You and your client
- You, your client and the law.

You – the therapist

In this element you will learn about:	
• professional presentation • effective communication • salon services	• treatment preparation • treatment planning • record keeping.

Professional presentation

As required by your awarding body, a professional appearance is expected not only to achieve your assessments but also to set the standards within your working life as a fully qualified therapist.

A professional appearance gives the client confidence in your ability as a therapist. This presentation should include:

Hair

Hair should be tied back and kept away from the face. The style should not interfere with the treatment. It is very distracting for the client if you have to keep flicking hair out of the eyes, and hygiene rules are broken if you keep touching your hair.

Nails

Nails should be clean, short and unvarnished (unless the employer states that, as a nail technician, you can have varnish on). Clients may develop an allergy to varnish, and chipped nail varnish is not a good advert for your trade! Unvarnished nails can also be seen to be clean. Long nails may scratch the client's skin when performing massage.

Jewellery

Most awarding bodies state that the only jewellery permitted is a plain wedding band and small unobtrusive earrings. Rings could scratch the client and carry germs. Remember that other body piercing may cause offence to some clients and does not reflect a professional image.

Uniforms

Most salons and training establishments require a professional uniform to be worn. This should be clean, pressed, and of a suitable length to work in. It is advisable to go up a size to allow free movement, or at least try it on with arm movements tested!

It is also wise to have several uniforms in order to allow one to be in the wash, and to prevent one uniform getting too soiled. Regular washing is essential to prevent body odour build-up as this can give off an unpleasant stale smell to the client.

Make-up

Subtle make-up may be worn, but heavy make-up or stale-make-up (e.g. left over from last night) is not professional. If the skin is clear and the eyebrows tidy the therapist may decide not to wear make-up at all – this is personal choice. The key should be how the therapist feels and looks on the day! Light make-up can hide minor blemishes and help tired eyes. If you need a 'pick me up', use it wisely.

Perfume

Remember that strong perfume may be as unpleasant to the client as body odour. Choose a light fragrance that does not over-power, and remember that stale perfume can be very unpleasant.

Also bear in mind that perfume cannot hide body odour, so the use of anti-perspirants and deodorants is recommended, as well as daily bathing to prevent an accumulation of smells. An anti-perspirant will prevent perspiration building up, and a deodorant will help prevent odour. Most of the products available do both jobs.

Shoes

Your shoes should be clean and comfortable for a full day's work. If your shoes do not fit securely, you could have or cause an accident.

Open shoes do not provide enough support for the feet, and high heels can damage your posture. Leather shoes allow the feet to breathe and are therefore more hygienic, preventing a build-up of bacteria, which may cause odour problems and lead to athletes' foot developing.

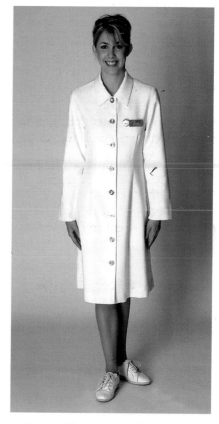

A clean uniform is part of your professional appearance

Oral hygiene

Regular dental care will prevent decay in the teeth, and so stop bad breath forming. Regular brushing, mouth sprays, mints and breath fresheners are also advisable to prevent stale breath being passed over the client. Remember that bad breath can be a sign of illness, so it may be worthwhile getting a dental or medical check-up if you think you may have a problem. It is only polite and courteous to your client to avoid strongly flavoured foods, such as curry, garlic and onions, especially at lunchtime. Smoking can also cling to the breath and the clothing – a good excuse to give up smoking, even if only at work.

Professional presentation: preparing to work

It is not only personal presentation that makes a professional beauty therapist but your attitude, too. Beauty therapy is a service industry. The general public are our clients and they pay for our service and our expertise. Therefore they should also be entitled to our full attention and care.

It is not just the décor of a salon that creates atmosphere, it is the ambience created by the people within it. How the therapist mentally prepares for work goes a long way to producing the calm, relaxed feeling of a salon which allows the client to gain maximum benefit from the treatment.

Put on a smiling, caring expression when you are working – you may have lots of your own personal problems, but passing them onto your client is not acceptable. Never gossip to your client about others: either staff or clients. Do not shout, swear or curse at work – you will develop the habit and not even realise when or to whom you are doing it.

It is said that you get out of life what you put in – and that is also true about a beauty therapy treatment. A quiet, relaxing facial should be as pleasurable to give as it is to receive – make sure that it is. A good therapist will gain satisfaction from a tranquil hour and you will find that giving a facial massage is very soothing to both of you.

As a quality check after a treatment a good therapist should ask herself:

- Would I like to be treated as I have just cared for that client?
- Would I pay for the treatment I have just given to that client?
- Could I have improved upon the quality of my service?
- Was it as restful and as peaceful as it could have been?
- Has the client re-booked?

Effective communication

Whatever your position at work you will need to communicate with others. If your business is to be successful you will need to communicate effectively with a variety of different people, as can be seen in the diagram. This communication can be verbal, non verbal or written.

Verbal communication

This is what you actually say and so it must be:

- clear
- to the point
- easily understood – using everyday language – technical terms should be put into easy terms, where possible
- spoken in a friendly manner.

Remember

A good appearance not only promotes confidence but leaves a lasting positive impression on the clients – regardless of how long they have been coming to your salon. Would you want to be treated by someone with less than perfect personal hygiene?

Reality Check!

Be totally attentive to your client and her needs. If you do not show interest in her, then she will lose interest in coming for any other treatments.

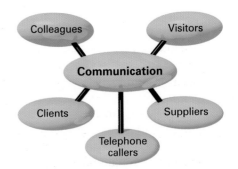

Communication at work will be with many different people

Remember those who may be hard of hearing – eye contact reinforces the message.

Non-verbal communication

This is another term for **body language**. Your body conveys messages through your:

- posture
- facial expressions
- gestures.

These unconscious gestures tell you a lot more about your client than verbal communication can. The therapist should be aware of body language and learn how to interpret it.

Watch for signs that understanding is not clear, or the client is not satisfied or following what you are saying.

- **Positive body language** – expressions and gestures such as smiling, nodding in agreement, lots of eye contact and open gestures, such as arms uncrossed.
- **Negative body language** – frowning, tension, no eye contact, and closed gestures, such as the arms crossed.

Communicating and working together

When you work in a salon you may have a manager who supervises what you do, or you may have junior staff whom you guide through the working day. Good communication means being understood: the message sent out is the message received.

Working under someone

This means that you:

- accept that someone is in charge
- should take instructions and act upon them
- communicate effectively
- take responsibility for your job role and do it to the very best of your ability.

Working together

Good teamwork means:

- supporting each other, not being in conflict with one another
- giving the salon a good atmosphere, which the client senses
- providing a reliable service
- giving effective results.

The ability to listen

Communication is a two-way process and having effective listening skills means:

- knowing when to stop talking and listen to what is being communicated
- listening with interest and understanding
- providing encouragement and confirming you have understood what has been said – nodding or agreeing with the point raised.

Written communication

Communication that is written down must be:

- **clear** and easy to understand
- **concise** – only information that is required should be given
- **legible** and easy to read
- **well presented** – handwritten or word processed
- **correct** – *all* the information should be included.

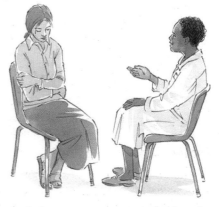

Body language can give you a lot of information – what can you tell from the body language of the client, on the left?

Check it out

Observe those around you, and analyse their communication skills. If you have part-time employment, quietly observe people in various skill areas, and in different positions, e.g. managers, and make some notes on this. How does your direct boss communicate with you?

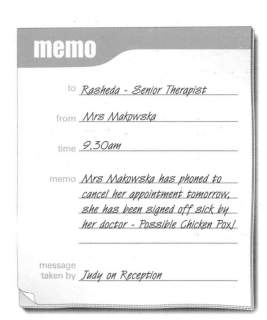

memo

to *Rasheda - Senior Therapist*

from *Mrs Makowska*

time *9.30am*

memo *Mrs Makowska has phoned to cancel her appointment tomorrow, she has been signed off sick by her doctor - Possible Chicken Pox!*

message taken by *Judy on Reception*

Written communication must be clear and concise

Clear written communication is important for many aspects of work within the busy salon environment, including health and safety, accident reports and record cards. For example, the client could be placed in danger if an allergic reaction warning on her record card is not readable.

Salon services

A good therapist is pleasant, patient, and helpful to everyone who comes into the salon. The needs of each person will vary and you must be able to give correct information. If you do not know, you must be professional enough to admit your knowledge is not sufficient, and get a salon manager to help – rather than making something up.

Treatments offered

Even if you personally cannot perform the entire treatment list, it is important to be aware of all the treatments and sell them. A professional therapist will have a thorough knowledge of the treatment process, the advantages or disadvantages of each, and each of the topics mentioned below. The salon will lose business if you just shrug and say you don't know.

Suitability of treatment

Not all treatments are suitable for all clients. Some treatments require a patch test, prior to the appointment, in order to assess the sensitivity of the skin or eyes. If a client has a treatment that was not entirely suitable for her, she will not be pleased. A dissatisfied customer will not return to the salon and may spread bad advertising instead.

Treatment timings

The timings of treatments should be accurately given. Do not mislead the client or underestimate how long a treatment may take or your credibility will be undermined. In addition to this, the smooth running of the salon will be disturbed if timings are not given correctly.

Reality Check!

Sales-related bonuses are common in the beauty therapy industry: a basic salary is boosted by commission on sales of products and of services – especially if you work on cruise liners. Linking treatments and products, and selling them to your client, should become second nature. With confidence and knowledge of products and services, selling is very straightforward. Remember that the client will want your products.

TIME	(1) SUSAN	(2) YASMIN	(3) LOUISE	(4) HAYLEIGH	(5)
9.00	MRS AUSTIN	MISS ALLEN	MISS BROWN	MR SIMONS	
	PHONE 823181	PHONE 631212	PHONE 761047	PHONE 471151	
	1/2 LEG WAX	ACRYLIC NAILS FULL	WEDDING	FULL BODY	
9.30	MRS WOOLFORD	SET	PAMPER	MASSAGE	
	PHONE 621148				
10.00	FULL BODY				
	MASSAGE			MRS SINGH	
				PHONE 821356	
10.30	MRS J.STREET			EYE LASH &	
	PHONE 521683			BROW TINT	
	EYELASH PERM				
11.00	MRS K GAROGHAN	MISS COLLINS			
	PHONE 356987	PHONE 712185			
	AROMATHERAPY	BRIDAL MAKE-UP			
	CANCELLED				
	BACK MASSAGE				

Accurate treatment timings are helpful for both the client and the therapist

Time is money and in order to be cost effective the timing of treatments must be accurate. Standard timings also help maintain the quality in the salon, so that all therapists offer the same time for each treatment. Clients are then all treated equally and get the same value for money.

The frequency of treatments given should also be negotiated with the client and will be dependent upon:

- the time available
- financial considerations of the client
- the condition or suitability of the area of the body to be treated.

Prices

Prices will vary from salon to salon, and area to area. Price lists should always be on display. This allows the client to view the costs for herself and is also additional advertising.

Costings given should be truthful, with no hidden extras – no one likes to be conned.

In the salon

Professional salons like to give an explanation of each treatment along with the price. This helps the client to understand the differences between the treatments and helps make the decision about which one to go for. Rona had been on placement for several weeks and thought she had just about got the hang of everything. But a client asked about a kind of waxing treatment which she didn't understand. She didn't want to seem silly – so she gave the client lots of information and most of it was wrong, including the timing and the price.

In your group discuss all the effects that might have had:

a on the salon
b on Rona's colleagues
c on Rona.

Special offers

If the salon has any offers to pass onto the client then you need to be aware of them. This helps to promote the offer and provides a chance to sell additional treatments that your client may not be aware of.

Most people like a bargain, or offer, and if they get to hear about it after the offer closes they will be very cross.

Remember that there is legislation in place regarding sale prices (refer to the Sale of Goods and Services Act, page 39, in the legislation section) so be careful when advertising a sale in your window.

Retail sales

As mentioned earlier, retail sales form an important part of any busy salon, and can help boost your wage packet at the end of the week.

Many salons offer a full retail sales service to complement the products used in the treatment. You need to be aware of what your salon sells, whether it is in stock, and what its benefits and selling points are.

Reality Check!

A manicure should have a time of about 45 minutes, but if the receptionist has only allowed half an hour, and it is the first appointment of the day, you will be at least a quarter of an hour behind all day. If you then over-run by ten minutes with every client, your last client of the day may be kept waiting for nearly an hour.

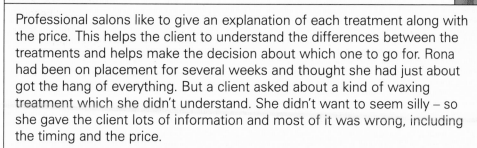

Body Treatments
We offer a comprehensive range of treatments designed to relax, invigorate and revitalise you.

Body Massage
In a relaxing atmosphere, tired muscles, aches and pains are revived reducing tension, easing away stress; skin, blood and lymph are improved, helping remove toxins and increasing metabolism.

Full body massage: £22.50
Back, neck and shoulder massage: £12.50

G5 Massage
The ultimate stress buster .... A mechanical massage designed to reduce tension, soften fatty deposits and detoxify problem areas. £18.00

Clients need to know what the different treatments involve and how much they cost

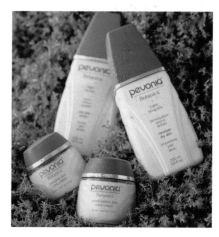

Retail sales can be an important part of a salon's business

Money will be lost if you ignore the customer who wants to buy the product that has just been used within the treatment. Most suppliers provide large sizes of product for use in the treatment room, with a smaller retail size for the client. In the course of conversation you will be asking about your client's homecare routine and which products she uses. Continuous care at home with the right products boosts the benefits of a salon treatment and good results can be seen.

Complaints

Realistically, a busy salon will encounter complaints sometimes. It is therefore important for salons to have a complaints procedure, which staff are aware of and have been trained to follow. This will mean that when a complaint does arise, however minor, the correct salon policy can be followed. An example of a complaints procedure follows.

- Deal with any complaints pleasantly in a professional manner.
- Calm the client and remove her from the reception desk to a more private area.
- Listen to her. Be objective and not defensive – the complaint may be valid.
- Be prepared to apologise if you are in the wrong and offer some form of compensation – a free treatment perhaps.
- Try to reach a mutually satisfactory outcome. This will minimise the damage that a complaint may have on other customers, and prevent further legal action being taken.
- Should the complaint be about another person, ask the staff member later in a calm manner. Do not blame the others in front of the customer.
- Record the complaint in the customer comments book.
- Be aware of the legal implications of further action – check out the insurance topic within legislation for public liability insurance, the client may decide to sue!

Treatment planning and preparation

Treatment planning is essential for the smooth organisation of a salon with more than one therapist working. Through good organisation, the relaxed, calm atmosphere that a salon should have will be in place, and that will be reflected in the mood of both customers and staff. Even if there is only one therapist employed, treatment planning will help with time management in order to ensure that money is not lost.

Remember the old saying:

Time = money

Treatment planning should be viewed as an investment. The more planning carried out 'behind the scenes' the more professional the treatment becomes. The key is to be organized.

The receptionist

A great deal of planning for the treatment starts with the receptionist and the initial booking in of treatments. The receptionist needs to be aware of:

- what treatments are being offered through the day and therefore which preparations can begin early, e.g. turning on the wax heaters
- what any treatment involves and therefore how much time should be booked out
- if this is a first treatment for the client or the middle of a course
- if a full consultation is needed, therefore needing more time
- the 'before and after' of the treatment – undressing / dressing / shoes etc.

A safety net of time should be included so that a client relationship can be built up.

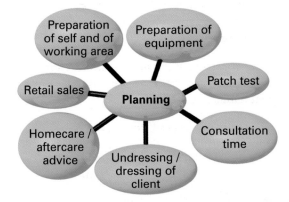

Treatment and planning should include these tasks

Unexpected occurrences

An organised therapist will make the receptionist aware of any alterations to the day, any time out of the salon, and any change of plans, well in advance of them happening.

Obviously the uncontrollable factor is **sickness**. If you have a full column of clients booked in and are unable to attend work because of illness there is very little that can be done. Therefore, the earlier you notify the salon, the better.

The receptionist should be able to rearrange some clients for another day, or at least notify them, as they may wish to cancel. The other therapists in the salon then have the task of covering all the clients that cannot be contacted. This is dependent upon the goodwill of the other staff members, and a good relationship is vital for the health, growth and atmosphere of the salon.

You should discuss at the initial job interview what the establishment policy is regarding illness and sick cover, as well as sick pay.

Good working relationships between staff should also be part of the planning for the salon manager or owner. **Teamwork** is very important and regular training and team building is essential.

If you as a therapist are continually unreliable and dependent upon the goodwill of others, then resentment will soon start to build up. The good atmosphere of the salon is lost, tensions will rise and arguments may occur – not very good public relations.

Develop and improve personal effectiveness within the job role

You must prepare for the working day ahead and contribute to the planning of the salon. Look back to the 'personal presentation' section and the 'preparing for work' section, which deals with your expected appearance and presentation.

Remember, however, that treatment planning is not just about appearance and personal presentation. It really is down to your approach or mind-set, as well. Most organisational skills develop from having the right attitude.

Being organised and planning ahead can actually become second nature and almost part of your personality at work. Being prepared, tidy and forward thinking are very good habits to cultivate!

You should ask yourself these questions:

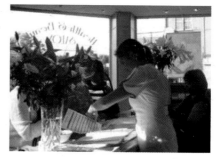
Treatment planning starts at the booking-in stage

Reality Check!

As part of your evidence for Units 2 and 3 you may be asked to be the salon manager for the practical workshop session, when practical assessments are taking place. This puts *you* in charge of your fellow trainees and you may face the problem of clients in reception, with no therapist to treat them because of sickness. You will see the other side of the coin.

Reality Check!

Treatment planning should actually begin right at the start of the day, as you get out of bed. As evidence for Unit 3 you will be expected to analyse your own performance within your job role and set your own targets for improvements. Self-evaluation really helps with the development of organising skills.

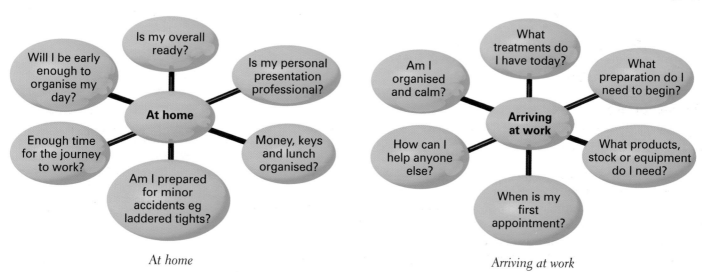
At home | *Arriving at work*

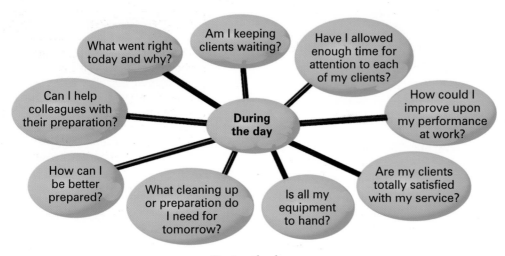

During the day

By continually evaluating these questions you can recognise and improve upon your working pattern towards planning and preparation time. If being disorganised is a habit that you have fallen into, with the attitude that 'it really doesn't matter, because someone else will do it', then bad habits need breaking.

How will disorganisation be recognised? By:

- clutter in the salon
- complaints from customers
- grumbles from other members of staff regarding extra workload
- continual poor time keeping
- confusion regarding treatments and equipment.

Effective teamwork and relationships

The salon manager plays a vital role and it is important that you understand how what he or she does affect how the salon operates.

The manager

The role of the salon manager is vital to the treatment planning and preparation of the working day. A good manager should:

- have a set salon system in place for morning and evening preparation and jobs to be done (these should be on a rota basis for all to do)
- have procedures and rules for everyone to follow – this will provide a consistent standard of service
- have clear guidelines on treatment times and expected preparation time
- provide realistic times for specific treatments
- hold regular training sessions for everyone so that all members of staff knows what is expected of them
- praise and reward those who perform well
- appraise and direct those who are not organised
- instruct clearly and without favour
- instruct clearly – with regard to being cost effective, not wasting products and being uneconomical
- lead by example and be professional at all times.

Reality Check!

Poor treatment preparation and planning ultimately leads to stress. This is the feeling of not coping and always being in a muddle.
If you feel stressed ask yourself why?

You – the therapist – should reflect upon the following.

Would I like to be a client of mine?

Did I offer the very best of service?

Would I pay for the treatment I have just given?

If the answers are No then a review of planning and preparation could make a big difference.

Record keeping

Good record keeping is absolutely essential to any beauty salon. You should create and use good systems in order to keep track of your work and your clients.

Record cards

The functions of a record card are:

- to record relevant details so as to be able to contact the client if necessary
- to provide full and accurate information which will ensure client safety
- to ensure consistency of treatment – regardless of who performs the treatment
- to record the number of treatments in a course and the date of each
- to note changes to the treatment programme or contra-actions if they occur
- to record the progress of the condition or treatment success
- to safeguard the salon and the therapists – to prevent clients taking legal action for damages or negligence.

The record card should be filled out in full for every treatment the client has. It should be written accurately, neatly and legibly.

In the salon

Siobhan and Kirsty work in a busy salon, giving a full range of treatments. Siobhan uses her record cards faithfully and even writes little notes to remind herself of the clients' particular needs / problems. For example, Mrs Barr's record card says – *Recently lost her husband. Went on holiday with her sister*. When Mrs Barr came in for her facial, Siobhan was able to ask, 'How was your holiday?' and knew to give a little extra kindness to this newly widowed lady. Kirsty hasn't bothered to fill her cards out, except for the most basic of information, and has been known to be tactless and even cause a reaction, as she hasn't noted the client's allergy to cotton wool.

Would you rather be treated by Siobhan or Kirsty?

Record systems

Most salons have a number system in place, or keep records on computer. This is both for safekeeping and for easy retrieval. Most software packages for computers have a database system for easy recovery of names and storage. A computer system is a large cost to start with, but can be very easy to use, with the correct training. It is ideal for use in a larger salon, with a wide client base. If this is the case, the **Data Protection Act** needs to be upheld. Please go to the section on legislation for more details.

The storage of record cards should be given consideration. They need to be accessible to the receptionist or therapist, but not so open that others can view them. A locked filing cabinet or drawer is most common, with limited access to the keys.

The two most common ways of filing names is to use:

- a number system i.e. client 1, client 2, etc.
- or an alphabetical system i.e. A, B, C, etc.

Alphabetical systems tend to use the first letter of the surname and if two names begin with the same letter then the second letter is used and so on.

Remember

Be safe – check for clients with nut or wheat allergies as these ingredients can be used in oils, creams and masks.

FACIAL TREATMENT	NAME			TEL	HOME			
					OFFICE			

ADDRESS							AGE	

DOCTOR Name:		TEL :		SMOKE		DRINK		MEDICATION:

MEDICAL HISTORY	ASTHMA		HEPATITUS		DIABETES		ALLERGIES:	

GENERAL HEALTH	GOOD		POOR		CONSTIPATION		BLOOD PRESSURE	NORMAL	HIGH	LOW

SKIN ASSESSMENT	A	B	C		A	B	C		A	B	C
SEBORRHOEA				DELICATE				SUNTAN			
OPEN PORES				DRY				PIGMENTATION			
BLOCKED PORES				DEHYDRATED				DILATED CAPILLARIES			
BLACKHEADS				MATURE				SKINTAGS			
ACNE				AGEING				MOLES			
SCARS				SLACK				SUPERFLUOUS HAIR			

	TREATMENT	MACHINE SETTINGS	PRODUCTS	AMPOULES	ADVISED FOR FOR HOME USE	THERAPIST	AMOUNT £	DATE
1								
2								
3								
4								
5								
6								

HOMECARE ROUTINE: ADVICE FOLLOWED   YES ☐   NO ☐   REGULAR HOME USE ☐   IRREGULAR HOME USE ☐

NOTES

INDEMNITY: I confirm that to the best of my knowledge the answers that I have given are correct and that I have not withheld any information that may be relevant to my treatment.

Signature ....   *Date* ....

A facial treatment record card

However it would be unrealistic to assume that there is only one Mrs Thomas in the area! This is how confusion can occur.

Be very careful about which client is which. Always take the client's full name and initial, along with address details. Repeat them back to the client as a double check that there is no confusion with clients of the same name.

Subject-specific record cards

Obviously each client will have a slightly different record card, depending upon the treatment needs. The more detailed the record card is, the better picture will be drawn of the client, so that each therapist who treats that client is aware of all possible details that may affect the treatment outcome.

Many manufacturers of beauty therapy products supply record cards to salons, and they can be purchased in bulk for ease of use. Many have an area for illustration for both face and body treatments. This is especially useful with make-up charts and skin diagnosis. These can be very useful and will save the therapist writing a lengthy description.

Both skin problems and make-up application can be recorded on a simple diagram. Most record cards will provide this facility.

Remember

The more detailed the card the easier the treatment will be, and the safer the salon will be.

You and your client

In this element you will learn about:

- assessment techniques
- questioning the client
- contra-indications
- contra-actions
- hygiene and avoiding cross-infection
- treatment and client expectations.

Assessment techniques and questioning the client

This is a vital part of your role as a successful therapist. All treatments are based upon what you discover within the initial consultation. The only way to make a correct diagnosis of the client's needs is through questioning and then tailoring your plan to the information you receive. All practical assessments are based upon successful client consultations and recognising your client's needs.

All successful salons earn their reputation by providing an excellent personal service. Care and attention to your client is the key to good business. Your consultation should be carried out in privacy, and the service should be free. It is standard practice to link a consultation with a treatment plan.

A good therapist will use all the skills mentioned and follow the client's body language to help obtain the information required for a good effective treatment plan. It must be agreed mutually that the time and money involved and the results suit both your client and yourself. If the plan is unrealistic your client will not stay with your salon. She will go elsewhere.

Questioning techniques

Asking questions is a skilled task. If you really want to find out what your client thinks and needs from you, you need to ask her. How you ask, what you ask and the type of question will dictate the reply you get. So, it is important that you give some care to your questioning technique. This information should be included on the record card, which you will be filling out as you discuss details in your consultation. Use your record card as your guide. As already stated, verbal questioning will determine all the personal details – refresh your memory by going back to the record card. There are two types of questions – open and closed.

Open questions

Open questions are much better for making the conversation flow, as they require a response. For example: 'How are you today?' The client cannot respond with just a 'yes' or a 'no' reply, a more detailed answer is needed and so these questions are good to break the ice.

Closed questions

Closed questions usually only need one word answers. For example: 'Have you ever had high blood pressure?' These questions confirm or eliminate information: 'Yes I have' or 'No, I have not'. Sometimes you have to use a closed question if you just require facts, but try to keep them to a minimum.

A professional therapist will use open or leading questions to help put her new client at ease. For example, the following open questions could be asked as she greets the client at the door.

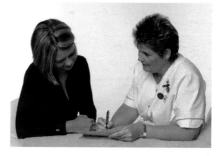

A successful consultation leads to a good treatment

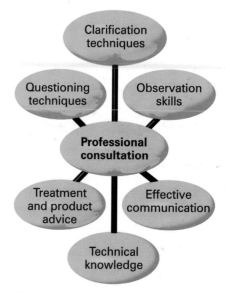

Your professional consultation will include all this

- What's the weather doing out there now?
- Where did you manage to park the car?
- How far have you come?
- How did you hear about us?

It is better to use open questions than closed questions, such as the following.

- Is it still raining?
- Did you get the bus?
- Have you been here before?
- Is this your lunch hour?

Can you spot the differences? Try making up some of your own open and closed questions and try them out within your group.

Listening skills

Communication is a two-way process and the ability to be effective in listening skills means:

- knowing when to stop talking and *listen* to what is being communicated
- listening with interest and understanding
- providing encouragement and confirm you have taken in the conversation: nodding or agreeing with point raised.

Listening is a good skill to develop and is different from hearing. It is so easy to talk and not really listen. So:

- always maintain eye contact with the person who is speaking, and let them finish their sentence – never interrupt
- remember that really understanding what the client is trying to say may mean you also pick up on what she is *not* telling you
- do not formulate your reply whilst you are being spoken to – you will not have all the facts until the client has finished.

Observation skills

Diagnosis of the client's well-being is not only discovered by the consultation questions but also through observation. It can reveal as much as, and sometimes more than, questioning alone. The unconscious body language of the client can speak volumes about her general attitude and state of mind.

A dropped pair of shoulders and dragging feet will indicate that she is nervous, a bit low in self esteem or worried or anxious about something. A confident client will have a more direct body language, more eye contact, with a spring in the step and an upright deportment. So, when your client arrives it is important to observe:

- how she walks
- how she stands
- how she sits
- your client's body language generally
- whether there is a mobility or handicap problem to be aware of.

In addition to this, you may be able to view the area to be treated, if on the face, the condition of the client's skin, the amount of care and attention previously given to the area as well as, of course, your client's body language and her reactions to you.

Clarification techniques

Clarification means checking the details given by the client to ensure the information that she gives you is correct. You need to do this whenever information is being passed on to you. It will happen at all stages of client contact. The following are examples.

1 When the client makes a **telephone booking**, all information regarding date, time, the nature of treatment, and the client's name and number should be repeated back as confirmation. Avoid saying what the treatment is too loudly, as it

Check it out

Listen to someone talk for a full five minutes, without interrupting or formulating an answer before he or she has finished speaking. Do you find this difficult? List your comments and discuss within your group.

Remember

In the early stages it is quite a compliment if the client wants to talk freely to you; but it may be some time before you fully gain the client's trust and confidence.

could be of a sensitive nature e.g. if the client is booked in to have a bikini wax she may not appreciate everyone in reception knowing about it!

2   When the client arrives at reception for the appointment, the time of the booking and the name of the therapist can be repeated to the client.

3   When the client is having the consultation.

Repetition of details will enable the correct treatment plan to be prescribed and reinforces what the therapist may already know. For instance: 'So, Mrs Gupta, your skin has been dry for most of the winter months, what products are you using?' This also gives the client lots of opportunities to respond to your open questioning techniques and therefore rapport builds up between you.

Technical knowledge

It is very important that you fully understand the treatments you are talking about. Do not make anything up – this is very unprofessional. Always refer to the manufacturer's instructions and product information if you are unsure.

You should always have a copy of your salon's price list at hand to refer to. A good price list should have the treatment description, time of the treatment and the cost.

Be straightforward and use words that your client will recognise. For example, she may not know what a comedone is – but she is sure to understand blackhead!

Product knowledge

Products, like treatments, require some time and effort so that you fully understand what they can do and how to use them properly. Be sure the information, benefits and effects you are claiming are true. It is also professional to ensure that the product you wish to sell to your client is appropriate and in stock. Selling an unsuitable product just to close the sale is very bad practice.

Regular training and visits from manufacturers will ensure that your information is up to date and accurate. Many companies are happy to visit training establishments to introduce their product knowledge.

Treatment and product advice

The client has come to you (and is paying) for your skill and expertise. Some of her issues may be of a personal or sensitive nature. Be gentle with her and treat her kindly.

When giving advice remember never to patronise or talk down to your client. All clients should be treated with the same respect and courtesy, regardless of how trivial their problems or questions may seem. Be both honest and realistic with aims and objectives in the treatment plan, especially with courses of treatment.

Make sure your client realises that results may take some time and are often not instant. Perhaps some small treatments that do have instantly visible results could be used as a morale booster, such as a pretty nail varnish with a manicure, or an eyebrow tidy.

⚠ Contra-indications

A contra-indication is the presence of a condition which makes the client unsuitable for treatment. A contra-indication means that treatment should not take place at all or that the treatment needs adapting. A treatment is normally unsuitable because the client has a medical condition which may be external and /or visible, or it may be 'hidden' and discovered during the consultation.

> ### Remember
>
> Clarification of information gives you the chance to help the client examine their lifestyle, health and homecare routine. It is also extremely flattering for the client when you take such an interest taken in them. After all, we all like to talk about ourselves. Having a loyal therapist who takes notice, with genuine concern, is very good for the ego and helps to boost the feel-good factor in the salon.

> ### Reality Check!
>
> Be careful of talking to your client, using technical terms that could cause confusion. It may be thought that you are showing off!

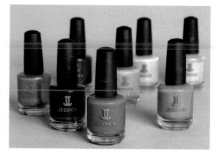

Accurate knowledge of your products is essential

> ### Reality Check!
>
> Under the Trades Description Act 1968 and 1972 it is a crime to describe goods falsely and to sell, or offer for sale, goods which have false claims about them. So, you cannot claim that a cream will make your client look twenty years younger, or that a treatment will make all her facial lines disappear. It is much better to say that the product will help replace lost moisture within the skin.

It is important that you do not treat the client because:

- the disease could be contagious and therefore there is a risk of cross-infection to both therapist and other clients
- the condition may be made worse by a treatment
- there may be a reaction later, which puts the client's health at risk.

This is why it is essential to complete a thorough consultation, prior to any treatment being given.

If the contra-indication is small and localised in one area, treatment **may** take place with some adaptation. For example, a minor cut would be covered with a plaster.

But a larger problem, such as a leg with open, weeping eczema, would be a total contra-indication and further advice should be sought from the client's GP.

Be warned that some doctors' surgeries do demand a small fee for administration costs. However, this is preferable to risking a reaction to drugs taken, and a possible court case for negligence.

The GP permission slip could then be placed in the client's record card so that all therapists are aware of medical problems for that client and therefore all therapists are protected.

General contra-indications

To help you remember different contra-indications, try to visualise looking from the outside of the body and work inwards. So, what you may see on the skin comes first, then muscles, bone, blood and so on.

Reality Check!

A therapist should not name specific contra-indications when referring a client to a GP. This is because, as a therapist, you do not have medical qualifications with which to make a diagnosis, and it is unacceptable to cause the client any concern, which may be unfounded.

Reality Check!

It is important that the contra-indications are discovered prior to the treatment taking place, rather than half-way thorough the treatment. This is fundamental to both your clients' safety and to your professionalism.

Skin	Muscles	Bones	Body systems
Skin infections, diseases and disorders	Dysfunctional muscular conditions (such as Parkinson's disease or multiple sclerosis)	Broken bones	High or low blood pressure
Cuts, bruises and abrasions			Heart conditions
Thin papery skin			Diabetes
Raised and hairy moles	Loss of sensation in the area		Epilepsy
Unknown swellings	Dysfunction of the nervous system (such as motor neurone disease)		Severe asthma
Recent scar tissue			High fever, colds and flu
Varicose veins and phlebitis			

Contra-indications

Specific contra-indications are listed at the beginning of each unit. Please refer to them prior to commencing your treatment.

 Contra-actions

A contra-action is the unfavourable reaction of a client to a treatment. Some treatments do cause some slight reaction, which is normal and to be expected, e.g. a waxing treatment will cause the skin to go red, there may be some blood spotting. It is a normal reaction to the slight trauma that the skin has undergone. However, an abnormal reaction to a treatment would be a severe response, as shown in the diagram.

Remember

Some of these contra-indications will not prevent treatment from taking place if the treatment is adapted or a doctor gives written permission. It may be that the condition is slight and not serious. Some clients find that treatments do help them, but it is not a therapist's job role to decide that. A GP must recommend it.

It is up to the therapist to respond quickly to any adverse reaction that happens within the salon, in order to minimise the problem and not make it worse. The client must also be informed of what to look for *after* the treatment has finished and what action to take at home.

Contra-actions can occur with the application of any product – even one your client has used for years can suddenly produce a reaction not seen before.

For specific contra-actions please refer to the individual units.

Hygiene and avoiding cross-infection

A dictionary definition of hygiene is: 'The science concerned with the maintenance of health / clean or healthy practices or thinking.' So for you, as a professional therapist, hygiene could be described as good practice to maintain:

* your own health
* your clients' health
* your colleagues' health.

However, there is no such thing as a completely sterile environment; perhaps the closest to it would be an operating theatre within a hospital. Germs are all around us and, while some are beneficial to humans, many of them are not. Beauty therapy treatments demand close human contact, so care must be taken to provide the maximum protection against cross-infection of germs.

Expert advice on hygiene can be confusing. Conflicting reports have been seen in the media with regard to AIDS and hepatitis. The most valuable information can be gained from the professional body's code of ethics or practice. (Refer to your own awarding body for more details.) These guidelines have been established after a great deal of research on behalf of the beauty industry, and are most likely to be current.

It is important to understand the responsibilities we each have under the Health and Safety at Work Act, and under COSHH, so please also refer closely to the legislation section for extra guidelines (see page 34).

Micro-organisms

In order to understand how to maintain the highest hygiene standards it is important to know how infection can occur. Micro-organisms are organisms that are too small to be seen by the naked eye. These micro-organisms are ever-present in the environment and can cause different types of infection.

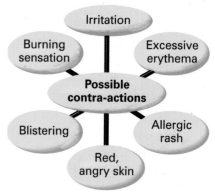

An abnormal reaction to a treatment can lead to unpleasant contra-actions

Type of micro-organism and the diseases they can cause

Micro-organism	Disease
Bacteria	Boils, impetigo, sore throats, meningitis and pneumonia, diphtheria, tuberculosis, and typhoid fever, tetanus (or lockjaw), whooping cough
Viruses	The common cold, flu', cold sores (herpes simplex), warts, measles, rubella (German measles), mumps, chickenpox, hepatitis A, B and C and HIV
Fungi / yeast	Ringworm of the foot, body, head and nail, thrush, infection to the heart and lungs, which may prove fatal
Protozoa	Diarrhoea, malaria and amoebic dysentery

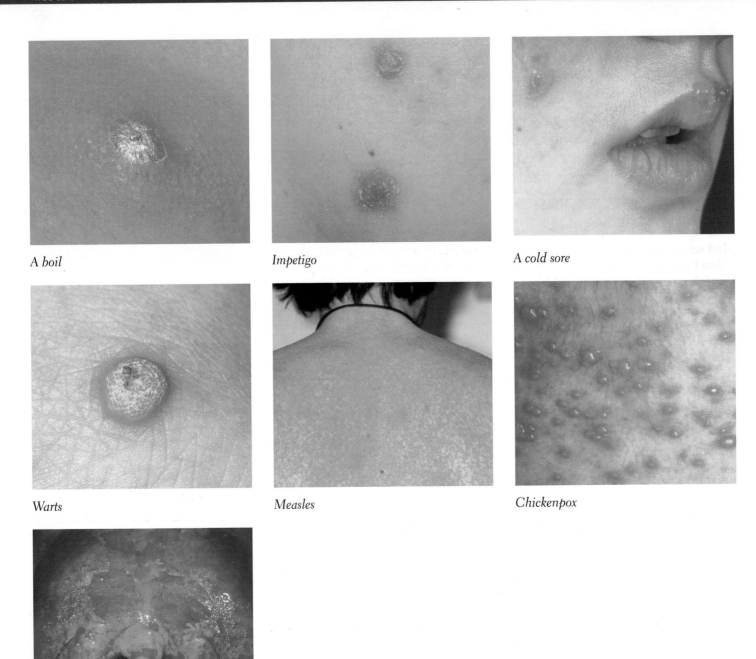

A *boil*

Impetigo

A *cold sore*

Warts

Measles

Chickenpox

Oral thrush

Micro-organisms enter the body through any route they can:

- through damaged, broken skin
- through the ears, nose, mouth and genitals
- into hair follicles
- into the blood stream via a bite from blood-sucking insects (e.g. malaria).

The symptoms and severity of the infection or disease will depend on the type of invasion, the person's immunity system being able to defend the body and general health. If a person is run-down then the micro-organisms have more chance of multiplying rapidly. They also thrive in poor hygiene. The best methods of avoiding these are prevention – through good hygiene practices.

Obviously some of these diseases are life threatening, but many are not and can be prevented by good hygiene. For example, protozoa can be transmitted from contaminated food and water, which grow and infect the bowel, causing ill health with diarrhoea.

Many of these diseases are also radically reduced by vaccination. Precautions can be taken against both Hepatitis B and tetanus – recommended for beauty therapists. Most school children are given immunisation against measles, mumps and rubella, unless there are medical complications against having the injections. Whooping cough has been dramatically reduced by the same method of immunisation.

Please refer to the contra-indication section for recognition of the common diseases that may prevent the treatment from taking place.

Good hygiene practices

How do you maintain good hygiene practices in a beauty salon?

A guide to controlling micro-organisms

Ammonia

Ammonia is commonly used as a base for trade liquids used to kill bacteria, e.g. barbicide that is used to soak suitable instruments in salons.

Antibiotics

An antibiotic is a chemical substance that destroys or inhibits the growth of micro-organisms. They are usually used to treat infections that will respond well to them, such as fungal or bacterial infections, and are given to humans and some animals for treatment.

Antiseptic

An antiseptic is a chemical agent which destroys or inhibits the growth of micro-organisms on living tissues, thus helping infection when placed onto open cuts and wounds.

Autoclave

An autoclave is a piece of equipment rather like a pressure cooker, used to sterilise equipment. It works by heating water under pressure to a higher temperature than 100°C, therefore creating an environment where germs cannot survive. It is most suitable for small metal equipment, such as eyebrow tweezers and manicure items.

Refer to individual manufacturer's instructions for use.

Bactericide

A bactericide is a chemical that will kill bacteria but not necessarily the spores, so reproduction may still take place. It can also be called biocide, fungicide, virucide or sporicide.

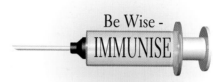

Be wise – immunise

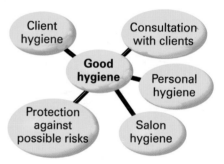

Good hygiene practices must include these aspects

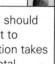
Remember

All good hygiene practices should be continuously carried out to ensure that no cross-infection takes place, that the client has total confidence in the salon and to ensure the best results are gained from each treatment carried out.

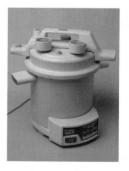 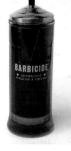

An autoclave   *A bactericide jar*

Chlorhexidine

Trade names for chlorhexidine include Savlon and Hibitane. Chlorhexidine is widely used for skin and surface cleaning and some sunbed canopies. Check individual manufacturer's instructions for cleaning.

Detergent

A detergent is a synthetic cleaning agent that removes all impurities from a surface by reacting with grease and suspended particles, including bacteria and other micro-organisms. Detergents need to be used with water, but are ideal for cleansing large surface areas.

Disinfectant

This is a chemical that kills micro-organisms but not spores – most commonly used to wash surfaces and to clean drains.

Phenol compounds

Phenol compounds are ideal for large areas that need cleaning but phenol does have a chlorine base and should not be used on the skin. It is used in industrial cleaning preparations and the old-fashioned carbolic soap.

Sanitation

This is the term used to describe conditions that are favourable to good health and preventing the spread of disease.

Sterilisation

Sterilisation is the complete destruction of all living micro-organisms and their spores.

Surgical spirit

Surgical spirit is widely used and easy to purchase from chemists. It can be used for skin cleansing, and the removal of grease on the skin. Surgical spirit comes in varying strengths of dilution. A 70% alcohol base concentration is acceptable for cleansing.

There are a great many commercial products on the market for cleaning and sterilisation – with lots of different trade names. This is merely a general guide. Please consult with the manufacturer's instructions for each individual piece of equipment. Most companies have their own particular favourites that they recommend. Also investigate the recommendations from beauty wholesalers and suppliers.

Your personal hygiene

- Always wash your hands – ideally with bactericidal gel – before and after every treatment.
- Wear disposable gloves for treatments if there is a possibility of an exchange of body fluids, e.g. waxing.
- Wear protective clothing for protection and to sustain a professional appearance, i.e. an apron for waxing.
- Cover cuts or broken skin with a waterproof plaster.
- Keep nails short and scrub under them with a nail brush.
- Do not come into work if you know you have an infection or disease likely to put anyone else at risk, e.g. impetigo.
- Wash hands thoroughly after every visit to the toilet.
- Follow the guidelines given in the personal presentation section for clean overalls etc.

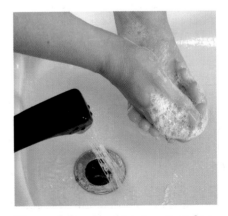

Thorough handwashing is essential to good hygiene

- Attend training programmes about hygiene and the use of sterilising equipment.
- Do not use equipment that is cracked or broken, as germs will be present. This includes chipped cups, plates or glasses.

Salon hygiene

- Sanitise used equipment, as fully as possible. This means following the manufacturer's instructions for individual equipment, such as using the recommended cleaner for make-up brushes so that the bristles do not fall out. Some cleaners will dissolve the glue that holds them in place.
- Invest time and correct training in the use of sterilisation equipment, such as an autoclave or sanitising unit.
- Clean the treatment area or room thoroughly. Clean daily and also wipe generally after each treatment has taken place. There are many preparations on the market for use on walls, floors and work surfaces, trolleys and couch and stool.
- All work surfaces should be cleaned regularly with hot water and detergent.
- Couch roll and towels can be used as a barrier between blankets and the clients – these can then be disposed of, and fresh ones put on for each client.
- Tissues tucked into the headband or turban can be disposed of after use, so keeping the headband / turban looking fresh.
- Towels should be washed after use – so your training salon needs to invest in plenty of towels to ensure you do not run out.
- The same applies to towelling robes for clients. Big fluffy robes are very luxurious, but the image would soon be spoilt if dirty ones were given to clients.
- Disposable brushes for applying make-up will prevent cross-infection from lips and eyes.
- Make-up pencils should be wiped clean with spirit and resharpened to get rid of any contamination.
- Powder eye shadows and blushers need to be scraped onto a palette and then applied to the client, to avoid contamination.
- Creams and oils need to be decanted into a smaller bowl, using a spatula, and any excess should be thrown away. Never pour back into the original container any product that has been in contact with your hands or the client. In order to be cost-effective, be careful not to pour out too much, as it may be wasted.
- Disposable spatulas should be used for waxing, i.e. one use from pot to client, to avoid contamination.

Client hygiene

- It is a good idea to have some form of notice in the reception area asking clients to state that they are not knowingly suffering from any contagious diseases.
- Always carry out a full consultation to discover any contra-indications.
- Always perform a physical check of the area to be treated for infection etc.
- Do not treat if any unrecognised problems are present.
- Ask the client to sign the declaration on the record card stating that all medical and other information is correct to date, to avoid possible repercussions later.
- Before you start, always wipe the area to be treated with the appropriate lotion e.g. surgical spirit, Hibitane or the recommended choice of your training establishment.
- Provide all possible protection for the client and insist that clients use the recommended procedure, for example: treading on the couch roll with bare feet to avoid touching the floor surface.
- Discourage the client from having a treatment if she has the beginnings of an illness – she may really want the treatment but spreading a cold or 'flu to you and to other clients is not fair.

In the salon

Fiona was about to start a pedicure, when she noticed that her client's feet had an unpleasant odour. Fiona asked her client whether she had noticed this smell, and when she had first noticed it. She also asked the client whether she wore leather shoes, to help the feet breathe.

On discovering that the client's hygiene was good, and that the problem had only just started, Fiona examined the feet in close detail. She found between the toes the beginnings of an infection called athlete's foot.

Fiona is not a doctor, and is not qualified to suggest what might have caused this problem, but she was able to suggest tactfully that her client seek advice from her doctor.

The treatment had to stop, as athletes' foot is highly contagious, and could be spread to both clients and therapists. Fiona's tact and diplomacy stopped an infection from spreading, safeguarded herself and her salon, and helped her client, who was very grateful and returned for further treatments.

Treatment and client expectations

It is important to explain the treatment thoroughly to the client, and it is important that the client understands what the treatment involves.

This will help to:

- ensure client satisfaction
- avoid misunderstandings
- dispel any unrealistic expectations
- give the client confidence in the salon and the therapist.

Honesty between therapist and client is part of the ethical conduct expected to maintain the high professional standards for all beauty therapists. The table opposite gives some examples of unrealistic and realistic expectations.

The client must also be aware of:

- the time involved in a treatment
- the total cost of the treatment or course of treatments
- the position to be in – on the couch, sitting etc.
- the expected outcomes
- the length of time the treatment should last
- the possible contra-actions to the treatment
- the aftercare and homecare for the treatment
- the cost of items they may wish to purchase
- the cost of maintenance, e.g. for artificial nail structures
- how often the treatment should be given for maximum effect
- the reasons for a patch test, consultation and record-cards.

The entire list above has a part to play in creating the complete picture for the client, so that the therapist gains the client's full trust and confidence.

Remember

Ensure your client is fully aware of homecare routines and how to treat a possible contra-action to avoid infection. If the skin is broken or there is blood spotting, such as after waxing, this is especially important.

Remember

A satisfied customer is more likely to return and to recommend the salon to others.

Reality Check!

The Advertising Standards Authority states that adverts should be 'Legal, decent, honest, and truthful' so salon owners and therapists should be very careful about exactly what they advertise and what they guarantee a treatment does. For example, an anti-ageing cream must state that it can temporarily help to reduce fine lines; it cannot state that it permanently makes the skin look twenty years younger – that cannot be proven!

Remember

The client needs to know about every aspect of the treatment in order to feel comfortable and relaxed – that way, maximum enjoyment and benefit can be gained from the treatment. The customer feels she has got value for money, the salon has some excellent advertising and everyone is happy!

Treatment aim	True	False
Waxing is permanent hair removal		✓
Waxing makes the hair growth weaken		✓
All the hairs grow back at the same time		✓
Waxing lightens the hair colour		✓
The hairs grow back with a sharp spiky feel to them		✓
Waxing does not hurt		✓
Waxing lasts for 3–6 weeks depending on hair growth	✓	
As the blood supply to the hairs are increased with waxing the hairs may grow back slightly more thick and coarse	✓	
The hairs grow back spasmodically as the hair growth cycle for each follicle is different	✓	
Waxing does not change the hair colour	✓	
Shaving and cutting blunts the end of the hair, making it feel spiky; after waxing the hair grows back with its natural tapered end, feeling smooth to the touch	✓	
Waxing feels like a plaster being taken from the skin. Pain thresholds will vary and some clients will feel more than others	✓	
Tinting the eyelashes makes them thicker		✓
Tinting darkens the existing lashes but does not 'build them up' to look thicker in the same way mascara does	✓	
Tinting is permanent colour on the eyelashes		✓
The tint lasts as long as the life cycle of each eyelash and will vary	✓	
All the eyelashes grow back at the same time		✓
The eyelashes grow back spasmodically as the hair growth cycle for each follicle is different	✓	
Eyebrow shaping changes the shape of the face		✓
Eyebrow shaping creates space for make-up application and can open up the eye area but will not change a person's basic face shape	✓	
The hairs grow back with a sharp, spiky feel to them		✓
After plucking the hairs grow back with their natural tapered ends, feeling smooth to the touch	✓	
Eyelash perming makes the eyelashes look thick and full		✓
Eyelash perming will curl the existing lashes but will not bulk up the lashes like mascara does	✓	
Make-up application can transform a client into looking like a supermodel		✓
Make-up can enhance facial features and bring out the best features of the face ~ it cannot transform that face into someone else's!	✓	

Unrealistic and realistic aims of a treatment

You, your client and the law

There are many regulations and lots of legislation covering you and your work in the salon. Any person dealing with members of the public and working with other people has to be aware of the law, and how to use it to be safe. You do not need to know all the regulations in detail, but you do need to know what your responsibilities are.

You will learn about:	
• legislation	• industry codes of practice
• local by-laws	• salon guidelines.
• insurance	

Reality Check!

Each of us must take responsibility for our deeds and actions, and we are liable for the consequences if we do not. Insurance cover will be null and void if it is proven that legislation or establishment rules have been broken, and an accident or damage has occurred as a result.

Legislation

All businesses are covered by laws as set down by the government in Acts of Parliament. These Acts of Parliament are continually being updated to fit into modern society, so you will find that Acts have dates after their title stating when they were updated, such as Trades Descriptions Act 1968 (amended 1987).

These Acts are the law of the land. Breaking or ignoring them is therefore an offence, and can lead to punishment. You could be fined, your business could be closed or you could go to prison.

As well as the UK law decided in London, i.e. the Houses of Parliament, there is European law to follow, too. The European Union (EU) is made up of 15 countries. Britain joined in 1993 so we all follow the same legislation. (These laws were signed at the Treaty of Rome in 1993.) The EU laws are decided in Brussels, where the European courts are based.

Specific legislation that you need to know

In order to be fully competent in employment it is essential that you have a sound knowledge of the basis of consumer protection and health and safety legislation. You need to understand how these laws protect you, your colleagues and your clients.

Health and Safety at Work Act 1974

This requires all employers to provide systems of work that are, as is reasonably practicable, safe and without risk to health.

The employer's duty is to provide:

- premises – a safe place to work
- systems and equipment
- storage and transport of substances and material
- access to the workplace exits
- good practices in the workplace.

Employers' responsibilities	Shared responsibilities	Employees' responsibilities
Planning safety and security	Safety of the working environment	Correct use of the systems and procedures
Providing information about safety and security	Employees have responsibilities to take reasonable care of themselves and other	Reporting flaws or gaps within the system or procedure when in use
Updating systems and procedures, with five or more employees	people affected by their work and to co-operate	
Safety of individuals being cared for	with their employers in the discharge of their obligations	

Health and safety responsibilities

The employer's duty to other persons not in employment includes: not exposing them to health and safety risks – this includes contractors, employees, and self-employed people.

The **employee** has a responsibility to:

- take care during time at work to avoid personal injury.
- assist the employer in meeting requirements under the Health and Safety at Work Act
- not misuse or change anything that has been provided for safety.

The employee has a duty to herself / himself, to other employees, and to the public.

The Act allows various regulations to be made, which control the workplace. The Act also covers self-employed persons who work alone, away from the employer's premises.

In 1992 EU directives updated legislation on health and safety management and widened the existing Acts. These came into being in 1993. There are six main areas:

- provision and use of work equipment
- manual handling operations
- workplace health, safety and welfare
- personal protective equipment at work
- health and safety (display screen equipment)
- management of health and safety at work.

Some provisions of the EU directives are:

- the protection of non-smokers from tobacco smoke
- the provision of rest facilities for pregnant and nursing mothers
- safe cleaning of windows.

Manual Handling Operations Regulations 1992

The Health and Safety Executive (HSE) has drawn attention to skeletal and muscular disorders caused by manual handling and lifting, repetitive strain disorders and unsuitable posture causing low back pain. The regulations require certain measures be taken to avoid these types of injuries occurring.

1 Think about the lift. Where is the load to be placed? Do you need help? Are handling aids available?

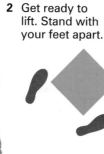

2 Get ready to lift. Stand with your feet apart.

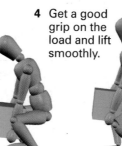

3 Bend the knees. Keep the back straight. Tuck in your chin. Lean slightly forward over the load to get a good grip.

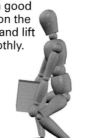

4 Get a good grip on the load and lift smoothly.

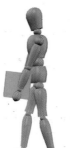 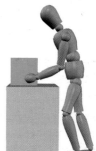

Safe lifting procedures must be observed

Think of all the situations that may apply in the salon:

- stock unpacking and storage – lifting heavy objects
- couch height is adjustable for individual therapists
- chairs or stools used in the treatment rooms
- trolley height
- reception desk and chair

> **Remember**
>
> Follow the golden rule: always lift with the back straight and the knees bent. If in doubt – don't lift at all!

- rotation of job roles so that the therapist is not in the same position for every treatment
- height and size of nail art desk.

It is worth considering all of these factors when purchasing your equipment, as you then have to work with the consequences!

When purchasing a couch for home or mobile use, it is well worth actually pretending to carry out a body massage, complete with client lying on the couch, for the right height. Working at a couch at the wrong height is very bad for the back in the long term, and may cause considerable discomfort.

Heat stress

The Health and Safety Executive draws attention to heat stress at work. The best working temperature in beauty therapy is between 15.5 and 20 °C.

Humidity (the amount of moisture in the air) should be within the range of 30 to 70 per cent, although this will vary if your salon has a sauna and steam area. They should be in a well-ventilated area away from the main workrooms, whilst still being accessible to clients. There should also be sufficient air exchange and air movement, which must be increased in special circumstances, such as chemical usage. Treatment rooms used for nail art, aromatherapy, bleaching or eyelash perming will need specialist ventilation methods.

Mechanical ventilation: extractor fans, which can be adjusted at various speeds.

Natural ventilation: open windows are fine, but be careful of a draught on the client.

Air-conditioned ventilation: passing air over filters and coolers brings about the desired condition, but of course this is the most expensive method!

A build-up of fumes, or of strong smells (for example, from manicure preparations), will cause both physical and psychological problems, which affect not only clients but staff, too!

Physical effects	Psychological effects
Headaches	Irritability
Sweating	Aggressive behaviour
Palpitations	Nervous fatigue, which may result in mistakes being made
Dizziness	
Nausea or fainting	Lethargy

The effects of heat stress

Remember

It is very good practice to investigate what your professional body states about protective clothing. It may null and void your insurance if you do not follow their directives.

Protective clothing

This covers both equipment and protective clothing provisions to ensure safety for all those in the workplace. The regulations also provide that workplace personnel must have appropriate training in equipment use. Protective clothing, such as white overalls for work wear, ensures cleanliness, freshness, and professionalism. For certain treatments it may be advisable to wear extra disposable coverings. The client's clothing must also be protected.

Protection against infectious diseases

Caution: It is important to protect against all diseases, which are carried in the blood or tissue fluids. Protective gloves should be worn whenever there is a possibility of blood or tissue fluid being passed from one person to another i.e. through an open cut or broken skin. Two specific infectious diseases to mention are:

• AIDS

Acquired Immune Deficiency Syndrome (AIDS) is a disease caused by the Human Immuno-deficiency Virus (HIV). The virus is transmitted through body tissue. Most people are aware of AIDS because of media coverage. The virus attacks the natural immune system, and therefore carries a strong risk of secondary infection, such as pneumonia, which could be life threatening. As there is no known cure, prevention through protection is vital.

• Hepatitis variants (A, B and C)

Hepatitis is an inflammation of the liver. It is caused by a very strong virus also transmitted through blood and tissue fluids. This can survive outside the body, and can make a person very ill indeed; it can even be fatal. The most serious form is Hepatitis B and you can be immunised against this disease by a GP. If a person can prove they need this protection for their employment there is no cost involved. Most training establishments will recommend this.

Control of Substances Hazardous to Health Regulations 1999 (COSHH)

This law requires employers to control exposure to hazardous substances in the workplace.

Most of the products used in the salon are perfectly safe, but some products could become hazardous under certain conditions or if used inappropriately. All salons should be aware of how to use and store these products.

Employers are responsible for assessing the risks from hazardous substances and must decide upon an action to reduce those risks. Proper training should be given and employees should always follow safety guidelines and take the precautions identified by the employer.

The COSHH regulations require that the containers of hazardous substances are labelled with warning symbols. These symbols are shown on the right.

Here are some examples of potential hazards:

- **highly flammable substances**, such as solvents, nail varnish remover or alcohol steriliser are hazardous because their fumes will ignite if exposed to a naked flame
- **explosive materials**, such as hairspray, air freshener or other pressurised cans, are also highly flammable and will explode with force if placed in heat, such as an open fire, or even on top of a hot radiator
- **chemicals** can cause severe reactions and skin damage – vomiting, respiratory problems and burning could be the result if chemicals are misused.

COSHH precautions

Employers must, by law, identify, list and assess in writing any substance in the workplace. This applies not only to products used for treatments in the salon, but also to products that are used in cleaning e.g. bleach or polish. Potentially hazardous substances must be given a hazard rating, or risk assessment, even if it is zero.

Remember

Always cover cuts with a plaster.

DUST   Dust   Toxic   Flammable

Irritant   Corrosive   Oxidising Agent

Symbols showing types of hazardous substances

TIPS

Manufacturers **have** to supply COSHH data sheets for all their products. Get one for each product.

Remember that a reaction can happen if the client is using products at home that may not mix well with salon preparations, eg home hair colorants.

Clients may be more susceptible to reactions if they are taking long-term medication, such as HRT or the contraceptive pill. This must be included on the client record card.

Invest in all the leaflets and latest information regarding COSHH from your local Health and Safety Executive office. **Keep up to date and keep safe.**

Remember these COSHH tips

Finally, you should read all of the COSHH sheets used in the salon, and be safe: follow what they say, never abuse manufacturer's instructions and attend regular staff training for product use. You never know when you might need it!

Gas Safety (Installation and Use) Regulations 1994

These relate to the use and maintenance of gas appliances. You may think that this does not apply to you as a therapist, but read on! The **Rights to Entry Regulations** 1996 give gas and HSE inspectors the right to enter premises and order the disconnection of any dangerous appliances. The inspectors themselves are not normally trained gas fitters, so they will instruct you to contact your local service engineer. Gas fumes are silent, with no smell, and very, very deadly.

Electricity at Work Regulations 1989

These regulations affect the use of electrical equipment in every salon, clinic or health club. Regulation 4 of the act states:

'All electrical equipment must be regularly checked for electrical safety. In a busy salon this may be every **six months**. The check must be carried out by a "competent person", preferably a qualified electrician. All checks must be recorded in a book kept for this purpose only.'

A 'competent person' need not be a qualified electrician, but must be capable of attending to basic safety checks. Manufacturers often supply their own technical staff to attend to safety checks.

If electrical apparatus is found to be faulty, the equipment must be withdrawn from service and repaired. An electrical safety record book should be used to record dates and the nature of the repair and by whom. It should also contain a list of tests carried out on the equipment under inspection, the results of those tests, and be signed by the competent person who carried them out.

This is essential for public liability insurance purposes and in case of legal action being taken for accidents due to negligence.

> ## Remember
>
>
> Around 1000 electric shock accidents at work are reported to the HSE each year.

Reporting of Injuries, Diseases and Dangerous Occurrences Regulations 1995 (RIDDOR)

These regulations cover the recording and reporting of any serious accidents and conditions to the local environmental health officer, whose remit covers beauty therapy and hairdressing salons. This officer will investigate the accident and make sure that the salon prevents the accident from happening again in the future. The officer can also assess the risk factors in each instance.

An accident or death at work must be reported within ten days of it happening. If the accident does not require a hospital visit, but the person is absent from work for more than three days, a report needs to be given.

If an employee reports a work-related disease a report must be sent; a work-related disease could include occupational dermatitis, asthma caused through work or even hepatitis. Accidents as a result of violence or an attack by another person must be reported. A car accident when on company business is reportable in the same way as an accident at work.

A dangerous occurrence in which no one was actually injured must also be reported, for example if the ceiling of the salon collapses overnight.

If you are a mobile therapist working in someone's home and you have an accident yourself or you injure the client you must report it.

Employer's Liability (Compulsory Insurance) Act 1969

Employers and self-employed persons must by law hold employer's liability insurance. This will reimburse them against any legal liability to pay compensation to employees for bodily injury, illness or disease caused during the course of their employment.

Employers must insure for at least £2 million per claim, but check with your own insurance company. Also follow the recommendations of your professional association.

It is worth remembering the following points.

- A legal claim made against your salon could result in very large financial losses and possibly the sale of the owner's business or even private home.
- Public prosecution results in a heavy fine for those not having this essential insurance cover.
- Damage to the salon could be so great that the business might never recover.
- Some cases can take up to ten years to come to court and with inflation the claim against you could be very much more than your original cover, if you only go for the minimum requirements.

The Consumer Protection Act 1987

This Act follows European laws to safeguard the consumer in three main areas:

- product liability
- general safety requirements
- misleading prices.

Before 1987 an injured person had to prove that a manufacturer was negligent before suing for damages. This Act removes the need to prove negligence.

An injured person can take action against:

- producers
- importers
- own brand manufacturers
- suppliers such as: wholesalers or retailers.

In the salon this means that only *reputable* products should be used and sold. Care should be taken in handling, maintaining and storing products so that they remain in top condition.

It is important that all staff are aware of consumer protection laws when selling products and when using products in a treatment.

Cosmetic Products (Safety) Regulations 1996

These regulations are all part of consumer protection legislation. The EU has laid down strict regulations about the composition of products, labelling of ingredients, how the product is described and how it is marketed. American cosmetic companies have had to list all ingredients on their labels for years, and Europe is now following suit. This is ideal for the easy identification of products that some clients may be allergic to, such as lanolin.

Trades Descriptions Act 1968 and 1987

This Act is concerned with the false description of goods. It is important to realise the relevance of this Act.

It is illegal to mislead the general public. This also applies to verbal descriptions given by a third party and repeated. So, if a manufacturer's false description of a product is repeated you are still liable to prosecution. The law states that the retailer must not:

- supply information that is in any way misleading
- falsely describe or make false statements about either a product or a service on offer.

The retailer may not:

- make false contrast between present and previous prices
- offer products at half price unless they have already been offered at the actual price for at least 28 days prior to the sale.

Be mindful of using statements saying something is 'our price'. Comparison of prices can be misleading and can be illegal – be sure that the product is identical in every way. You should also check that products are labelled with their country of origin.

Sale of Goods Act 1979 and Sale and Supply of Goods Act 1994

This Act has several others under its umbrella of protection:

- the Supply of Goods and Services Act 1982
- the Unfair Contract Terms Act 1977
- the Supply of Goods (Implied Terms) Act 1973.

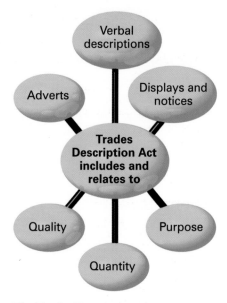

The Trades Descriptions Act covers several different areas

The Sale of Goods Act recognises the contract of a sale between the retailer and the consumer when purchasing a product, which applies when the salon sells a product to a client. Of course, it can also apply to us all as consumers when we purchase any goods (this Act is a good one to quote when returning something to a shop!).

The Act states that the retailer:

- has a responsibility to sell goods of the very best quality, which are not defective in any way
- must refund the money for the purchase if it is found to be defective (some retailers will only offer an exchange of goods, if there is no receipt)
- must then make a complaint to the supplier.

The Supply of Goods and Services Act 1982

This Act also deals with rights for the consumer and the trader's obligations towards the consumer. It has two branches: goods and services.

- **Goods** This allows the consumer to claim back some or all of the money paid for goods. When we buy something, in good faith we expect it to be:

    – of merchantable quality
    – fit for the purpose for which it was sold
    – as described in the advertising.

    This applies to all goods, regardless of whether they are on hire, in part exchange, or as part of a service.

- **Services** This means that the person or trader providing a service (such as a beauty therapist) must:

    – charge a reasonable price
    – provide the service within a reasonable time
    – give the service with reasonable care and skill.

    This means no two-hour manicures, no charging over the top prices, and no slap dash treatments! Your customer can complain and contact the trading Standards Office, if they feel they have a case against you. Be careful!

The Unfair Contract Terms Act 1977

This Act was prior to the Sale of Goods Act 1979 and defined the term 'of merchantable quality' for the first time.

The Supply of Goods (Implied Terms) Act 1973

This Act attempts to exclude or restrict statutory terms related to title, description, and fitness of the goods.

Both of these Acts covered consumer rights before The Sale of Goods Act 1979, when definitions became tighter and the law was better defined regarding consumer rights.

Performing Rights – within Copyright, Design and Patents Act 1988

This Act is designed to protect the people who write music but then do not get the royalty payments they should when the music is played! Any use of music in the treatment room, reception or in exercise groups is classed as a public performance.

The Phonograph Performance Ltd (PPL) collects licence payments from people wishing to use music on behalf of artists and record companies. Under the **Copyright Designs and Patent Act 1988** the PPL can take legal action against persons who do not pay a licence to use music – and they do! This can mean a considerable fine for those who try to avoid paying. So, legally, all salons and exercise / aerobic instructors need to purchase music that has a built-in licence. Although more expensive to purchase in the first place (a CD can cost about £30) it does save all the worry of a heavy fine, if caught!

Most good specialist music shops have a section of licensed music – just ask.

Data Protection Act 1998

Businesses that use computers or paper-based filing systems to hold personal details about their staff and clients may be required to register with the Data Protection Registrar.

The Data Protection Registrar will place your business on a public register of data users and issue you with a code of practice which you must comply with, stating:

* you must keep information secure
* you must ensure information is accurate and relevant to your needs
* you must comply with individuals' requests for information that you are holding on them and failure to do so means you are contravening the Act.

Contact: Data Protection Registrar, Springfield House, Water Lane, Wilmslow, Cheshire. SK9 5AX. (tel. 01625 545745).

The information held by an organisation about any one of us can be revealed if requested within 40 days for a fee not greater than £10.00. It is possible to gain compensation through a civil court action if you feel there has been any infringement of rights, in which information that was given for a specific purpose has been abused.

Local Government (Miscellaneous Provisions) Act 1982

This relates back to the local authorities in your particular area. Section 8 of this Act is concerned with the registration of any practitioners who pierce the skin. This applies to:

* acupuncture
* ear and body piercing
* tattooing
* epilation.

This applies to both salons and mobile therapists.

The concern of most local authorities is that through registration they will be able to keep some control of hygiene regulations and ensure that people have recognised qualifications. The amount of enforcement of these regulations will depend upon the individual authority, as does the amount of inspection that takes place, and the scale of fees for registration.

This does not include people working in hospitals.

Local by-laws

Local government by-laws are laws decided by the local authority or borough council of an area, and they can differ from region to region. Therefore, London has different local by-laws from Birmingham. However, both these authorities have a register of salons offering body massage as a treatment. This is to maintain a professional qualified salon base and to eliminate the 'massage parlour' image.

You need to investigate the by-laws in your own area from your borough council – these by-laws relate to hygiene, and the registration of ear piercing, and epilation salons, as well as tattoo parlours.

Insurance

Professional indemnity insurance

Every single professional beauty therapist should have this insurance protection, regardless of how few or how many treatments they carry out.

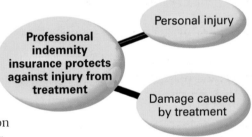

The best deal for these kinds of insurance policies can usually be found via your professional body – professional bodies are often able to offer the best rates because they negotiate on behalf of members and get a considerable discount.

As an employee you need to check with your employer whether you are covered on its business insurance, or if you need to organise your own cover. A salon owner or employer should include this liability in the public liability policy, so that *all* employees are protected against claims made by clients.

Indemnity insurance could save you a lot of money

Public liability insurance

This insurance is not compulsory, but it is certainly advisable. It will protect the employer should a member of the public be injured on the premises. This could be something as simple as a roof tile hitting the client on her way into the salon. If this results in the client being unable to work for a long period of time, the client can seek legal advice and the salon owner could be sued for compensation.

Insurance is important – so protect yourselves and your clients.

Industry codes of practice

Industry codes of practice or ethics are a guide to **correct procedures** and etiquette as dictated by professional therapists associations, of which there are several. Which professional body you join is a matter of personal choice, and may depend upon the one favoured by your training establishment.

The cost involved in joining depends on your level of entry – a student membership is normally available and with your joining pack you will be given a code of ethics or a code of practice.

This code is a book of rules that the therapist agrees to abide by, as part of the contract of membership. If these rules are broken or ignored, membership can be withdrawn.

Being a member of a professional body brings benefits, which can include:

- a good insurance deal negotiated on the members' behalf
- support and advice upon leaving college
- a monthly magazine, with useful articles and adverts for jobs and equipment
- regular legal updates
- free legal help lines, for all aspects of your business
- discount cards for suppliers
- a business guide for setting up on your own.

> **Remember**
>
> When you are in a training establishment there are lots of people to seek help and advice from – but when you are out in the working world you are on your own. It can be very reassuring to have the support of a professional association behind you.

Salon guidelines

All the legislation mentioned above should be considered within the normal working life of the beauty therapist. Working safely and following the correct legal procedure is very important.

It is also very important to follow the salon guidelines for the particular establishment you are in – be it a training establishment, salon or health farm, ocean liner or renting a room in a health suite.

It is vital that you are aware of the policies on health and safety, safety training and what *exactly* is expected within the job role. Normally salon rules are very similar, regardless of where the salon is located, but the safety procedures to follow if your salon happens to be floating in the Caribbean Sea will be very different.

> **Remember**
>
> Regular training is the key to following salon guidelines.

It is very important that the salon expectations and the required behaviour for therapists is set out at the beginning. This could be at your induction training, or even at the initial interview.

Regular reviews of policies and regular training for updates is essential, as is your attendance. If a member of staff continually ignores safety requirements, whether through negligence or through ignorance (if they have not attended training), this could form the basis for dismissal. Worse still, should an accident happen through negligence, injury may occur, and the person responsible may be found liable.

Health and safety rules

These will encompass all aspects of the Health and Safety at Work Act, plus COSHH guidelines and the Electricity at Work Act.

You should be in no doubt about:

- therapists' responsibilities
- salon procedures
- treatment safety
- equipment safety
- protection against cross-infection.

Client safety	Storage procedures	Stock regulations
Positioning of client	Electrical equipment	COSHH regulations are followed
Minimum risk of hazard for bed height – getting on and off	Chemicals	First aid procedures in place
Correct use of equipment and products	Valuables	Stock rotation
Correct diagnosis of treatments needed	Stock	Spillage management
Correct evacuation procedures	Money	Correct storage and containers

Salon procedures for health and safety

Your employer or head of the training establishment should have all these standard procedures in place. If you are not instructed within your first few weeks of beginning your new post – then ask.

Test your knowledge

1   List five points that you think contribute towards a professional consultation.

2   a   Give three examples of open questions.
    b   Give three examples of closed questions.

3   As a student, what would your responsibilities be regarding the following pieces of legislation?
    a   The Health & Safety At Work Act
    b   The Consumer Protection Act
    c   COSHH

4   a   How do the Electricity at Work Regulations affect the use of electrical equipment in the salon, clinic or health club?
    b   If electrical apparatus is found to be faulty, what action must be taken?

5   Why should you be insured?

6   When would you need to wear protective clothing? Why?

7   What are your salon guidelines regarding client safety?

8   If a face cream states on its label that it can guarantee loss of wrinkles, under which Act would you be liable to prosecution?

9   Which body provides a code of practice or ethics that you have to follow as a beauty therapist?

the workplace
ENVIRONMENT

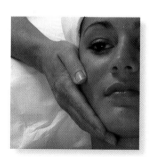

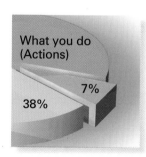

What you do
(Actions)

7%

38%

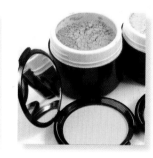

Support the health, safety, and security of the salon environment

Unit 1

Health and safety is an important part of your working day and this chapter will help guide you through the things you need to know, in order to ensure your safety, that of your client, and the people working with you.

We all need to help make the workplace a safe, secure and healthy place for everyone. It is a consideration that should be part of every treatment that you carry out and every unit for which you are assessed. If you don't follow health and safety guidelines during the treatment or assessment, then at best the assessment cannot be competent, at worst, the action could result in injury or damage – and you may be legally responsible.

Within this unit you will cover the following elements.

Element 1.1   **Follow emergency procedures**
Element 1.2   **Support health, safety and security at work**

In addition to this unit, you need to read the information in the **Professional basics** section on legislation, local by-laws and the industry codes of practice.

Follow emergency procedures

1.1

This element requires a practical demonstration that you have met the emergency guidelines for your establishment regarding fire evacuation. Obviously, setting fire to the building is not very practical, so a simulation will be acceptable. You must be able to find the emergency personnel required for firefighting and first aid and be able to find the firefighting equipment for electrical and non-electrical fires. First aid and accident report procedures, and understanding exactly what is required of you, is also essential knowledge.

In this element you will learn about
• fire and evacuation procedures   • first aid
• emergency procedures and personnel   • accident reporting procedures.
• firefighting equipment

Fire and evacuation procedures

Fire Precaution Work Place Regulations 1997

The law requires all premises to undertake a fire risk assessment. If five or more people work together as employees, the fire risk assessment must be in writing. Employers must also take into account *all other persons* on the premises, not just employees. This will include clients and visitors to the salon.

In every period of one year there must be at least one fire drill, which involves everyone. All staff must be fully informed, instructed and trained in what is expected from them and some people have special duties to perform. All employees, trainees, temporary workers and others who work in any undertaking, must – by law – agree to co-operate with the employer so far as is necessary to enable them to fulfil the duties placed upon them, by law. This means everyone has to co-operate fully in training courses and fire drills, even when everyone knows it is only a practice.

Most large training establishments will have their own policy on fire and evacuation procedures and may carry out a fire drill once a term, i.e. three times per year. This is especially important with large groups of people or students, and any people with disabilities who will need special consideration.

Many fire-training exercises are organised with a fire safety officer from the local fire station. Often the fire engines will take part in the exercise so that the firefighters can test their own attendance time from the station to the premises. Everyone should be made aware of his or her own particular rules for evacuation.

When first joining any business or establishment new employees should be briefed regarding all health and safety issues, and especially in fire evacuation procedures. It is standard practice to include the information in a staff handbook containing all the establishment policies.

Below is an example of an evacuation procedure.

Check it out

Find out where your own staff handbook is and what your fire evacuation procedure is. Do you know your assembly point?

Building evacuation procedures in the event of fire or bomb alert

The following procedure has been agreed and must be followed. Any staff member who does not comply is committing an infringement of the college disciplinary code. Whenever a fire occurs, the main consideration is to get everybody out of the building safely. Protection of personal or college property is incidental.

Raising the alarm

Anyone discovering a fire must immediately raise the alarm by operating the nearest fire alarm and report to the controller the fire location.

On hearing the alarm the receptionist will immediately contact the emergency services and then evacuate the building.

In the event of a fire being discovered when the reception is unmanned – the premises officer on duty will contact the emergency services and assume control.

On hearing the alarm

All those in senior positions proceed to the control point, normally at a main entrance to the building – where one person must take control of the proceedings.

All other staff: close windows; switch off machinery and lights, and close doors on leaving the room.

Assist less able colleagues, leave the building by the nearest marked route and proceed quickly to the appropriate assembly point. Staff must supervise their class.

Staff evacuating the building must check their locality is clear.

Assembly points

Everyone must remain at assembly points well away from buildings and clear of access roads.

Report to control in person or via two-way radios where allocated.

Everyone must remain at assembly points until further instructions.

DO NOT re-enter the building until you are told it is safe to do so.

An evacuation procedure

Emergency procedures and personnel

Fire drill relevant to the working area

- All electrical equipment to be switched off.
- Shut windows.
- Clients should be led by the therapist to a safe area. Wrap client up warmly if necessary using blankets and towels – this is especially important where the client has been having a body treatment.
- If possible, take the client's valuable possessions with her, such as a handbag and jewellery, but not if they are safely locked away, or if it puts the client or therapist in any danger.(Usually, clients' belongings are kept under the trolley and therefore are within easy reach.)
- Be aware of the treatment being performed before the evacuation – if the client has chemicals on the skin, it may be better to remove these immediately. (This would need to be at the judgement of the lecturer in charge of the workshop – certainly a client having a eyelash tint will need to have it removed before being able to proceed to the assembly point.)
- Take appropriate remover and damp cotton wool or tissues to remove products on the skin such as facemasks. Whilst not dangerous to the skin if left on, the client will probably be more comfortable if it can be removed.
- Be aware of the client's footwear and, if possible, encourage her to wear shoes, to prevent an accident occurring during the evacuation.
- Report to the named emergency person at the specified assembly point.

Bomb alert

Follow the procedures for fire drill. Do not look inside a suspicious package but act quickly if an abandoned parcel or bag arouses concern.

Gas leak

Open all windows.

Evacuate the building following the fire drill instructions.

Do not turn off or on any electrical equipment – it may cause a spark, which may ignite the gas.

Sensible fire precautions

- Be informed – know what to do and where to go when the evacuation begins.
- Be sensible and do not panic – this will only make the client feel panicky, too.
- Make sure that the location of the fire bell, fire extinguishers and fire exit are familiar.
- Never ignore smoke or the smell of burning – it is always safer to have a false alarm. Better safe than sorry!
- Do not misuse or mistreat electrical appliances that are a potential hazard – a healthy respect is needed.
- Do not ignore manufacturer's instructions for the storage and use of highly flammable products, which are very common within the salon.
- Do be sensible with naked flames and matches or disposal of cigarette ends – a smouldering tip can burst into flames that will destroy the salon in minutes.
- Be accountable to clients – the appointment book can be taken outside, as a master check against which clients should be present.
- Do not use a lift for the evacuation – it may be that the fire affects the electric mechanism and that then becomes another emergency.

Remember that you must report to your specified assembly point after leaving the building, otherwise you may not be accounted for. This could mean that firefighters risk their lives to go back into a burning building to check – when all the time you are around the corner!

Firefighting equipment

Fire extinguishers

There are different types of fire extinguishers, and not every fire extinguisher is suitable to fight every fire – using the wrong one can make the situation worse. Only a person who has been specially trained in the use of a fire extinguisher should attempt to use one. Never put yourself at risk: personal safety is more important than saving material items that can be replaced – a human life cannot be replaced.

Extinguisher	Type	Colour	Uses	NOT to be used
Electrical fires	Dry powder	Blue marking	For burning liquid, electrical fires and flammable liquids	On flammable metal fires
	Carbon dioxide	Black marking	Safe on all voltages, used on burning liquid and electrical fires and flammable liquids	On flammable metal fires
	Vaporising liquid	Green marking	Safe on all voltages, used on burning liquid and electrical fires and flammable liquids	On flammable metal fires
Non-electrical fires	Water	Red marking	For wood, paper, textiles, fabric and similar materials	On burning liquid, electrical or flammable metal fires
	Foam	Cream / yellow markings	On burning liquid fires	On electrical or flammable metal fires

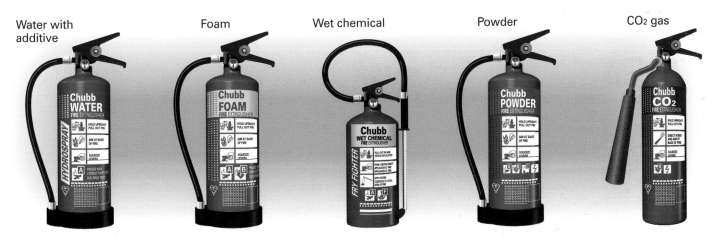

Water with additive　　Foam　　Wet chemical　　Powder　　CO₂ gas

Different types of fire extinguishers

Fire blankets

Fire blankets are made of fire resistant material. They are particularly useful for smothering fat pan fires or for wrapping around a person whose clothing is on fire. A fire blanket must be used calmly and with a firm grip. If the blanket is flapped about it may fan the fire and make it flare up, rather than put it out. The hands should be protected by the edge of the cloth and the blanket should be placed, rather than thrown, into the desired position.

Never lean over the fire and remember – if you cannot control the fire, leave the room, close the door and phone the fire brigade.

Fire blankets conforming to British Standard BS6575 are suitable for use in the home. These will be marked to show whether they should be thrown away after use or can be used again after cleaning in accordance with the manufacturer's instructions. Fire blankets are best kept in the kitchen.

Sand

A bucket of sand can be used to soak up liquids, which are the source of a small fire. However, it is impractical to have large quantities of sand available to try to stop a large fire. Therefore the instructions would be the same as for fire blankets – **if in doubt never risk injury, get out and phone the fire brigade**. Fire safety officers always advise that you leave the firefighting to the experts, i.e. the fire brigade.

Even small fires can spread very quickly, producing smoke and fumes, which can kill in seconds. If there is any doubt do not tackle the fire, no matter how small.

Remember

Every year hundreds of people die and thousands of people are injured in fires, which are caused by lack of concentration or carelessness. Your responsibility is to prevent a fire starting in the first place.

First aid

The Health and Safety (First Aid) Regulations 1981 set out the essential aspects of first aid that employers must address, because people at work can suffer injuries or fall ill. It does not matter whether the injury or illness is caused by the work they do. It is important that they receive immediate attention and that an ambulance is called in serious cases.

First aid can save lives and prevent minor injuries becoming major ones. First aid in the workplace is the initial management of any injury or illness suffered at work. It does not include giving tablets or medicines to treat illness.

This means that sufficient first-aid personnel and facilities should be available to:

- give immediate assistance to casualties with both common injuries and illness and those likely to arise from specific hazards at work
- summon an ambulance or other professional help.

This will depend upon the size of the workforce, the type of workplace hazards and risks, and the history of accidents in the workplace.

Two aspects of first aid need further consideration: trainees and the public.

- **Trainees** – students undertaking work experience on certain training schemes are given the same status as employees and therefore are the responsibility of the employer.
- **The public** – when dealing with the public these regulations do not oblige employers to provide first aid for anyone other than their own employees. This means the compulsory element of public liability insurance *does not cover* litigation resulting from first aid to non-employees. Employers should make extra provision for this themselves. Education establishments must also include the general public in their assessment of first aid requirements.

First aid kits

The minimum level of first aid equipment is a suitably stocked and properly identified first aid container.

First aid containers should be easily accessible and placed, where possible, near to handwashing facilities. The number of containers will depend upon the size of the establishment, and the total number of employees in that area. The container should protect the items inside from dust and damp and must only be stocked with useful items. Tablets and medications should not be kept in there.

There is no compulsory list of what a first aid kit should contain but the following would be useful:

- a leaflet giving general guidance on first aid (such as the HSE leaflet *Basic advice on first aid at work*)
- 20 individually wrapped sterile adhesive dressings (assorted sizes) appropriate to the type of work
- two sterile eye pads
- four individually wrapped triangular bandages (preferably sterile)
- six safety pins
- six medium-sized individually wrapped wound dressings
- two large sterile individually wrapped unmedicated wound dressings
- one pair of disposable gloves
- antiseptic cream or liquid
- eye bath
- gauze
- medical wipes
- a pair of tweezers
- cotton wool.

Do not forget that if in doubt, do not treat – phone for an ambulance immediately.

First aid training

First aid certificates are only valid for a certain period of time, which is currently three years. Employers need to arrange refresher training with re-testing of competence before certificates expire. If a certificate expires, the individual will have to undertake a full course of training to be re-established as a first-aider. Specialist training can also be undertaken if necessary.

Records

It is good practice for employers to provide first aiders with a book in which to record incidents, which require their attendance. If there are several first aiders in one establishment then a central book will be used.

The information should include:

- date, time and place of incident
- name and job of the injured or ill person
- details of the injury or illness and what first aid was given
- what action was taken immediately afterward (e.g. did the person go home, go to hospital, get sent in an ambulance)
- name and signature of the first aider or person dealing with the incident.

This record book is not the same as the statutory accident book, although the two might be combined. The information kept can help the employer identify accident trends or

Reality Check!

A first aid kit must be in a proper first aid container.

An old biscuit tin just will not do.

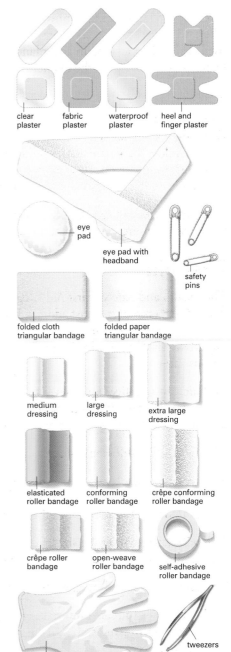

clear plaster — fabric plaster — waterproof plaster — heel and finger plaster

eye pad

eye pad with headband

safety pins

folded cloth triangular bandage — folded paper triangular bandage

medium dressing — large dressing — extra large dressing

elasticated roller bandage — conforming roller bandage — crêpe conforming roller bandage

crêpe roller bandage — open-weave roller bandage — self-adhesive roller bandage

disposable gloves

tweezers

cotton wool

gauze pads

wound cleansing wipes

ANTISEPTIC WIPE
Moist tissue to clean and sooth cuts and grazes

Items a first aid box should contain

patterns and so improve on safety risks. It can also be used to judge first aid needs and assessments. This record book is also very useful for insurance and investigative purposes.

ACCIDENT / ILLNESS REPORT FORM

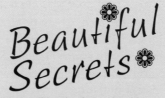

This form is to be completed by the injured party. If this is not possible, the form should be completed by the person making the report. If more than one person was injured, please complete **a separate form for each person.**

Completing and signing this form does not constitute an admission of liability of any kind, either by the person making the report or any other person.

This form should be completed immediately and forwarded to the Health and Safety Officer and Salon Manager.

If it is possible that an accident has been caused by a defect in machinery, equipment or a process, isolate / fence off the area and contact the Health and Safety Officer or Manager immediately.

SECTION 1 PERSONAL DETAILS

Surname: _Lung_   (Mr/Mrs/Ms/Miss) Forename(s): _Jenny_

Date of birth: _29/01/57_   Address: _89 New Street, Glasgow_

STAFF ☐   CONTRACTOR ☐   VISITOR ☐   GENERAL PUBLIC ✓

SECTION 2 ACCIDENT / INCIDENT / ILLNESS DETAILS

Accident (Injury) ✓   Illness ☐   Date: _19/04/02_   Time: _13.07_   (24-hour clock)

Location: _Salon room 3_

Nature of injury or condition and the part of the body affected:

Slipped on floor, twisted ankle

Account

Describe what happened and how. In the case of an accident state clearly what the injured person was doing. _Small patch of water on the floor – client got off couch and slipped on it._

Name and address of adult witness(es): _Jo Benfield, Beautiful Secrets_

Details of action taken

Ambulance summoned ☐   Taken to hospital ☐   Sent to hospital ✓

First aid given ☐   Taken home ☐   Sent home ☐   Returned to work ☐

SECTION 3 PREVENTATIVE ACTION

Recommended: _to ensure that all spillages are mopped up straight away_

Implemented: Yes / No   Date: _19/04/02_

Report raised by

Name: _Catrina Waldron_

Position: _Therapist_

Signature: _C Waldron_   Date: _19/04/02_

FOR OFFICE USE ONLY	
Copy sent to: Salon Manager	☐
Health and Safety Officer	☐

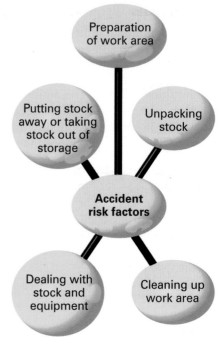

There are potential accidents in many areas of your work

An accident report form

Accident reporting procedures

Accidents can happen even to the most careful of people. However, it is important to react in a correct manner – to stay calm and follow the proper accident procedures.

Therapists should be aware of all of the possible risks in all aspects of salon life.

In the salon

In Poona's salon there are two small steps leading from the reception area down to the changing room. Mrs Lions had an early appointment for a leg wax, and was running a little late. Being in a hurry, Mrs Lions tripped down the steps and landed on her knees. Offering sympathy, Poona helped her client stand up, and after checking that Mrs Lions was fine, Poona got on with the treatment. Nothing more was said, and the incident was forgotten.

However, two months later the salon received a letter from a solicitor, which claimed that Mrs Lions had, in fact, hurt her knee so badly that she was unable to work, and was therefore suing for damages and compensation for loss of earnings. The letter asked the salon to inform its own solicitor and to forward details of its insurance cover and a copy of the accident report form.

What are the consequences for the salon of Poona not taking any notice of the salon policy of always filling out an accident report form?

Who is liable?

Discuss this situation in class, and research the end result of who pays!

Remember

All of the above should be continuously reviewed for accident potential. If equipment is continually being broken because of lack of storage space or because a trolley is too near to a windowsill then a review should take place. If accidents keep happening then the question must be why?

Check it out

All establishments should have a set procedure to follow in the event of an accident. What is yours?

Support health, safety and security at work

1.2

In this element you will learn about:

- salon guidelines for health and safety
- personal health and safety
- security
- hazards.

Salon guidelines for health and safety

All professional salons should have a set of rules and procedures for everyone to follow regarding health, safety and security. This is not to be kept a big secret – it should be common knowledge for the safety and protection of all within the salon. Regular staff training and updates are vital to keep new information circulating *and* remembered.

Why?

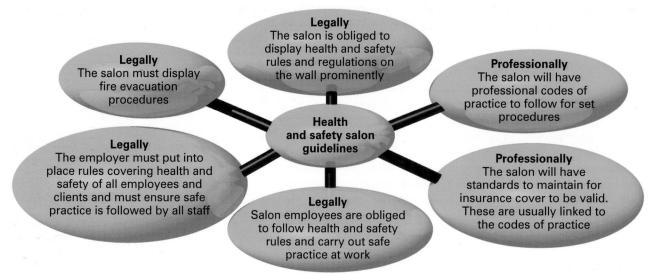

Legally
The salon must display fire evacuation procedures

Legally
The salon is obliged to display health and safety rules and regulations on the wall prominently

Professionally
The salon will have professional codes of practice to follow for set procedures

Legally
The employer must put into place rules covering health and safety of all employees and clients and must ensure safe practice is followed by all staff

Health and safety salon guidelines

Professionally
The salon will have standards to maintain for insurance cover to be valid. These are usually linked to the codes of practice

Legally
Salon employees are obliged to follow health and safety rules and carry out safe practice at work

How?

✓ **Regular training** with staff meetings to update on safety issues.
✓ Clear outline given at the initial interview as to what is expected.
✓ **Maintaining records** of injuries or first aid treatment given.
✓ **Monitoring and evaluating** health and safety arrangements regularly.
✓ Providing a written **Health and Safety booklet**.

Remember that it is important to ask the experts and improve your knowledge on health and safety issues. Ignorance is not an excuse in the eyes of the law and could lead to a court appearance for negligence. Please consult the **Professional basics** section for a full breakdown of legal obligations of the employer and employee.

Personal health and safety

It is not only the employer's responsibility to provide health and safety management; it is the responsibility of each employee to follow the rules.

All beauty therapists work very hard, long hours, and are often on the go all day. They are in a busy salon environment, with other people present all the time – their own clients, other clients, other staff, outside representatives, management and receptionists, cleaners and so on. A therapist must have a sense of personal safety and respect for the safety of others in order to prevent accidents occurring. This will involve:

- personal appearance
- high standards of cleanliness
- good personal conduct.

Personal appearance

A therapist's personal appearance should always combine safety with professionalism – starting with the feet. High-heeled shoes are not only uncomfortable but are also not very safe or stable to walk on. Open-toe sandals will not protect the toes from damage from either spillage or impact injury. Therefore, shoes should be smart but essentially comfortable and safe.

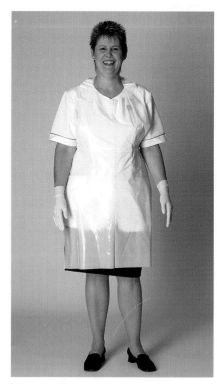

Personal appearance should be a combination of safety and professionalism

It is important to avoid stooping and slouching to prevent back problems from occurring. A therapist should have good posture and evenly distribute the body weight by standing correctly with both feet slightly apart. This will prevent accidents and damage to the therapist.

Always wear the correct protective clothing provided to shield a uniform. Always wear gloves when using chemicals or if there is a possibility of coming into contact with body fluids. Remember also that it is necessary to follow the correct disposal regulations for gloves and waste materials. If an establishment provides a uniform as part of a corporate image then it must be worn.

Hair should be neat and tidy and if it is long it must be tied or pinned back – otherwise it may fall in your eyes and cause eye problems.

High standards of cleanliness

This will ensure that no cross-infection can occur.

Good personal conduct

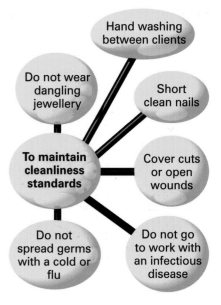

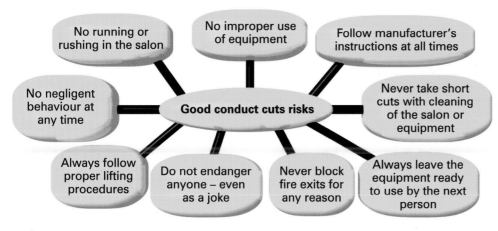

Remember

You should take responsibility for yourself, the machinery you use and problems such as spillage that may occur – do not expect someone else to clean up behind you!

Reality Check!

The old saying 'Do as you would be done by' applies here. Always leave the salon and its equipment as you would wish to find it – it is dangerous to do otherwise.

Security

It would be a foolish salon owner who ignores the subject of security. There are many areas to keep secure in a business and possible risk areas are shown in the diagram below.

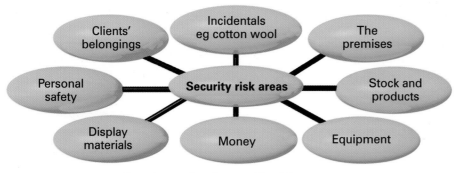

Security needs to be considered in many areas

The premises

The salon owner must have adequate security measures in place for the salon in order to get insurance and a mortgage. It is worth consulting the local police station for guidance. The Crime Prevention Officer will come to survey the premises and give advice regarding the most vulnerable areas and the most common forms of entry by a burglar.

Externally

It is important to deadlock all doors and windows. Double glazing is expensive but makes a property more difficult to break into – the older the window and frame, the easier the entry. Fit a burglar alarm, if possible, or even fit a dummy box on the wall, which may deter a burglar. These false alarm boxes are quite popular with householders.

Closed circuit television (CCTV) may be available if the premises are in a shopping area with other well-known named stores. Metal shop front shutters are very popular with jewellery stores and shops that sell expensive electrical items. If the premises have a shutter system, use it, as this is probably the most effective deterrent to a burglar.

Internally

Internal doors can be locked to prevent an intruder moving from room to room. Fire doors and emergency exits should be locked at night, and re-opened by the first person in at the start of business every morning.

A light left on in reception may also deter the would-be burglar who may feel that well-lit premises makes them more obvious.

Stock and money should be locked away or kept in the bank, so that nothing is visible to entice a burglar to break in. Lock expensive equipment away in treatment rooms or in the stock cupboard, to avoid tempting fate!

Very large businesses employ night watchmen to patrol their premises, but, along with alarmed infrared beams, these are not affordable for the average small salon owner. If, however, the salon is situated within a shopping centre or business park, night patrols may be included in the lease or purchase agreement, or offered for a set fee per year. Costs would need to be considered, but it may be an investment and save money in the long term.

The local police station can be contacted and the police patrol vans will regularly check the building as part of their normal evening beat.

Stock and products

Beauty products and stock that is on display and in use in the treatment rooms can be vulnerable to theft. Of all the temptations to the thief these smaller items may prove irresistible – they are small enough to fit in a pocket, and are very accessible. Unfortunately this form of shoplifting costs many businesses a great deal of money, as stock can be expensive to replace and can be a large part of the capital outlay for a salon.

A sad fact is that the average 'thief' may be rather closer to home than is comfortable. Staff may 'borrow' an item of stock for home use, and think that their behaviour is acceptable. Also, clients may like the look of a lipstick and 'forget' to pay for it! Small items that are stolen are referred to as 'pilfering', which is a polite word for stealing, and larger items stolen are referred to as 'shoplifting'.

Precautions

Tight precautions are called for to prevent stealing and loss of stock. These can include the following.

- Have one person in control of the stock and limit keys and access to stock. This person is usually a senior therapist or senior receptionist.
- Do a regular stock check – daily for loss of stock and weekly for stock ordering and rotation.

Reality Check!

Goods which may have been pilfered or stolen can cause problems. It means the salon has bought an item of stock from the wholesaler that is not paid for by the customer, so the salon has to absorb that financial loss. It could eventually bankrupt the business.

- Use empty containers for displays, or ask the suppliers if they provide dummy stock – this will also save the product deteriorating whilst on display.
- Keep displays in locked glass cabinets that can be seen but not touched.
- Encourage handbags for staff and customers to be kept away from the stock area (usually in reception) to stop products 'dropping' into open bags.
- Have just one member of staff responsible for topping up the treatment products from the wholesale sized tubs.
- Hold regular staff training on security and let the staff know what the losses are and how it may affect them. Some companies offer bonus schemes for reaching targets for sales and to minimise pilfering. Staff need to know that heavy losses may affect potential salary increases.
- Carry out banking of money in the till at differing times of the day and do not keep too much money in there at any one time.

Personal security for staff

The salon should provide lockable storage cabinets or cupboards for staff so that personal belongings can be locked away. Handbags and purses are always vulnerable to the opportunist thief, who may look just like a client but will come in off the street and be gone with someone's valuables before anyone realises what has happened.

Staff should be discouraged from bringing large amounts of cash into work. They should also be encouraged not to wear expensive jewellery to work, which has to be removed during treatments and is therefore vulnerable to loss or theft.

If a daily job is to take large amounts of takings from the salon into a bank or night deposit safe, it is best to avoid taking the same route to the bank at the same time each day. Someone may be watching.

Therapists should always be very aware of their clients' jewellery. Let clients see that their rings etc. are placed in a bowl on the trolley, do not forget to return them when finishing the treatment and do not compromise yourself by slipping them, for safety, into your overall pocket.

It is important to be aware of any suspicious packages which are left unattended: inform a supervisor, and, if necessary, call the emergency services.

The salon should have a list of emergency numbers by the telephone, such as, for example, for the security guard room or the local police station. This will help save time in an emergency.

Never leave yourself unprotected: do not leave outside doors open when working in a treatment room; do not leave the till drawer open; do not be naïve enough to think that it could not happen to you. If you are at all unsure it is always helpful to seek professional advice from the local crime prevention officer or local police station, both for building security advice and also for personal safety hints – for staff and clients.

As a professional therapist do not allow yourself to become a victim – follow your professional guidelines.

- Do not treat a male client alone in the salon late in the evenings.
- Always work in pairs at least, in the winter evenings.
- Always lock up the premises in the company of other staff.
- Be aware of car parking places at work. In daylight that alley might look fine, but it might not be so pleasant in the dark after work.
- Do not travel home after work alone in the dark – phone a taxi or friend.
- Do not put yourself at risk in any way.

Reality Check!

Think ahead and be safe.

Know what to do and be safe.

Be responsible and be safe.

Hazards

A therapist needs to be able to recognise when a hazard can be dealt with immediately, or when help may be required, and the hazard must be reported to someone else, such as a supervisor or manager.

Hazard	Way to avoid	When referral may be necessary
Breaches of security	Shut windows, lock cupboards and doors	When something is found open or something is believed to be missing, complete full stock checks
Faulty / damaged products, tools, equipment, fixtures and fittings	Correct handling, correct storage, treat with care, follow manufacturer's instructions	When something is found to be broken
Spillage	Take care when mixing, pouring and filling etc.	When spillage material is corrosive or an irritant
Slippery floors	Make others aware by blocking the area with a chair to prevent an accident. Sweep up powder spills, mop up spills of liquid, refer to COSHH sheets for correct method	When acid is spilt, or grease or polish is spilt
Obstruction to access and exit	Move large equipment away from doorways if able to do so, put bags and coats on a rack or shelving	When object is too heavy to be moved

Dealing with hazards

In the salon

In the Ocean Blue Beauty Salon, all products are bought in bulk, and transferred into smaller bottles, for use at individual work stations. These small bottles are the same size and shape, with labels on them for easy identification. It is the junior staff's job to make sure that each work station does not run out of any product. Unfortunately, because someone had oily hands, one of the bottles lost its label. When Sara, the therapist, took off her client's eye make-up, she used cuticle remover instead of the correct product, as the bottle had no label. Cuticle remover is alkaline and caustic and makes the nail dry and sore if left on for too long. Imagine what it did for the client's eye area. Sara was quick to remove the product and to give suitable first aid.

Although the client needed hospital treatment, she was fine, and there was no long-term damage – the point is knowing how to recognise the potential hazard in putting all products, regardless of how harmless or dangerous they are, in the same type of bottle. Being alert to all sort of hazards, and the prevention of accidents is so much better than the cure.

Fulfil salon reception duties

Unit 2

In this unit you will explore the different areas necessary to learn about to become a successful beauty therapy receptionist. The reception area and receptionist are what a client sees first as she enters the salon, so it is essential to have a warm and inviting entrance, with a confident and effective receptionist.

First impressions really *do* count – and they become lasting impressions – so it is vital that they are positive. You will need to learn your own salon's guidelines for dealing with both general enquiries and more specific problems as they occur. You will also have to gain knowledge regarding each treatment, how long the treatments take, and linked services offered, as well as appointment bookings. This information will enable you to offer a professional service, guarantee client satisfaction and allow maximum cost effectiveness to your employer.

Within this unit you will cover the following elements:

2.1 Attend to clients and enquiries
2.2 Make appointments for salon services
2.3 Handle payments from clients for the purchase of services and retail products.

You should also read the **Professional basics** section in conjunction with this unit.

Before looking in detail at the requirements of this important unit, it is a good idea to explore two essential parts of a working salon environment: the receptionist's role and the way the salon's atmosphere can affect the work you do.

The receptionist's role

In order for a receptionist to be professional and confident with clients she needs to know and understand in detail everything her job role demands. It is also important that the receptionist recognises the limits of her authority and when to refer a problem to the manager or the salon owner.

A receptionist is often employed for her office and managerial skills – she may not be a therapist at all. Some receptionists do take small qualifications, such as a manicure certificate, so as to be able to help out in the salon when busy, but often they will have no formal training as a therapist. In this case a good receptionist must have a thorough knowledge of all the treatments, their contents and duration, so they can advise clients and plan the working day correctly.

The best way to achieve this is through good staff training. All staff members should have a working knowledge of the treatments available, so demonstrations and regular staff meetings are essential, with the therapists giving treatments to other members of staff. The receptionist can then talk with confidence about a treatment, for example, 'Well madam, I can tell you that a leg wax feels a little like a plaster being pulled off – and the girls here are very quick, so you will be finished within half an hour'.

Good training should be seen as an investment for the future healthy growth of the business. If the receptionist is not a beauty therapist she should have all the treatments – as a client – to understand fully what is involved, and so she can offer information to clients from experience.

Check it out

Think about the qualities of the receptionist in the salon where you work. Alternatively, you may want to look at another salon where you have some experience as a client. Note these qualities. You will need to refer to them for evidence collection for this unit.

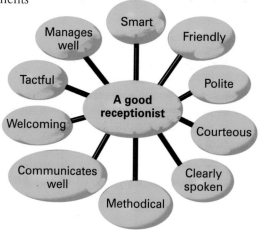

The qualities of a good receptionist

Why is a receptionist important?

- The receptionist is the first person the client sees, or hears, on the telephone.
- The receptionist represents the business – and first impressions do count!
- The receptionist sets the atmosphere for the salon: her duties and the correct methods of using them will determine just how smoothly the business will run.
- The reception area is the central pivot around which the business revolves, and its success will largely depend upon the skills of the person in charge of reception.

What happens in reception?

- Appointments are made – remember, appointments mean money! The appointment book should have a simple, easy-to-follow format and be kept at reception at all times. Appointments will be made in person or by telephone.
- Clients are greeted and welcomed into the salon.
- All enquiries are dealt with.
- Retail products are displayed and sold in reception.
- Payments are taken for services given or products purchased.
- Complaints may begin here.
- Business enquiries may begin here, from wholesale representatives, staff applicants, or even the bank manager.
- Price lists are given, and further bookings made.

The atmosphere of reception

Because it is so important to have the right atmosphere, time and planning should go into making the reception area as welcoming and friendly as possible. The décor should be light and gentle on the eye and be a positive reflection upon the rest of the salon. It needs to be very clean, warm, and tidy.

Client comfort needs to be considered so the reception should be enticing and encourage the customer to want to stay, and to see more .

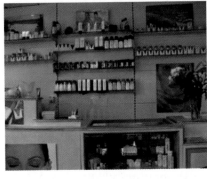

The reception area should encourage clients to stay in the salon

Check it out

Have a closer look at other places that may employ a receptionist. For example, how are you treated at the dentist, the doctor's surgery or opticians? What is the atmosphere like? Is the receptionist calm and in control? Make notes that you can refer to later.

Attend to clients and enquiries   2.1

The client or visitor's first impression of the salon is often formed by the way she is greeted by the receptionist rather than just by the décor. Receiving clients into the salon is a little like greeting a guest into your home, and there should be similar levels of hospitality and friendliness from the receptionist. It may be the client's first or twenty-first visit but the polite and welcoming greeting from the receptionist should be the same.

All visitors should be made welcome and treated with equal courtesy and importance. This is achieved through effective verbal and non-verbal communication, good listening skills and questioning techniques. These topics are fully covered within the **Professional basics** section. In this element you will look at good practice in handling a wide range of clients and their enquiries: vital requirements for a successful business.

In this element you will learn about:

- handling enquiries
- taking messages
- confidential information.

Handling enquiries

The approach to clients, customers and visitors can be summed up in a simple word – **PLEASE**.

- Posture
- Listen
- Expression
- Appearance and attitude
- Speech
- Eagerness to help others.

Posture should be good – both to give a create a good impression (slouching gives the impression of boredom or not caring), and to protect the spine.

Listen with your whole body, not just your ears. Look as if you are listening, as eye contact encourages the talker to continue, and facing the client shows you are giving the visitor your full attention. You are saying to your visitor, 'You are important to me and to the salon and I give you my full attention'.

Expression should be welcoming, open and positive – you are not there to challenge the visitor or make her feel threatened. Smile and show that you are pleased to see her.

Appearance and attitude should reflect total professionalism and mirror the high standards of the salon.

Speech should be clear, not patronising in any way, and free of any technical terms a client may not understand.

Eagerness to help is a charming quality and very flattering to the client – use it wisely to give attention without appearing insincere.

What to do

What should the receptionist do when the visitor or client first comes in? Remember that eye contact and a pleasant initial greeting are important. The receptionist should not keep a visitor or client waiting but should ask for the person's name and the purpose of the visit e.g. an appointment, or to see the manager.

Visitors should be dealt with as soon as possible, and the right action taken or the appropriate staff member informed of their arrival.

DO NOT:

- ignore clients
- hide under the counter and pretend they are not in view
- huff and puff as though serving a client is the last thing you want to do
- patronise a client by talking down to them.

The receptionist's role

For the receptionist to be professional and capable, she needs to know about everything that her job role can demand. As with all life skills, knowledge leads to confidence. However, it is equally important that the receptionist knows the limitations of her authority and when she should refer a matter to the manager or salon owner.

Reality Check!

Making a client cross is a sure way to lose them.

Check it out

After your first couple of days as duty receptionist at your training establishment, pause for thought – how good were you at putting people at their ease? Did you remember the PLEASE approach? What would you change about your behaviour?

In the salon

In Beauty Secrets salon, the manageress, Carmine, had several dealings with a client who continually bought products back for an exchange, even though they were nearly finished with. Carmine got a little suspicious and phoned a few of her friendly competitors in the area. Yes, they had heard of this client, and several salons had actually blacklisted her, as she was definitely 'on the fiddle' and trying to get something for nothing. Carmine gave strict instructions that refunds were to be given only with her permission, and staff had to know the limit of their authority. Unfortunately, when Carmine was at lunch, the client appeared at reception with a half empty cream, with no receipt or box. She cleverly picked on the youngest of the staff and started to make a scene, and aggressively demanded a refund.

The young receptionist was embarrassed, unused to being shouted at. Feeling intimidated, the receptionist gave a large cash refund to the woman, without a thought – really to stop her making such a scene.

When Carmine returned, she was very cross. The receptionist had gone over the limits of her own authority and had cost the salon a lot of money.

What should the receptionist have said to the client?

What would you have done?

As mentioned above, the receptionist may be employed for her managerial and office skills and so she may not be a beauty therapist. However, in order to be able to book in a client and talk knowledgeably about treatments, she must be fully aware of everything contained within her salon price list. She should have a clear understanding of:

- each treatment on the price list
- what it involves
- how long it takes
- how much it costs
- what the benefits and effects are
- what the aftercare and homecare is
- what products can be sold in conjunction with the treatment.

This knowledge will mean the receptionist can speak with confidence about each treatment, and will also allow her to book appointments correctly, schedule the working day into logical sequence and advise clients correctly.

First responses

The receptionist should be asking herself these questions about her visitor.

- Why has the client come?
- What is she / he here for?
- Where has the client come from?
- What action do I take to help them?

After the receptionist has worked out what she has to do for her visitor, one of the following responses might be appropriate.

- Please take a seat; the manager won't keep you a moment.
- Would you like a drink or magazine while you wait?
- I will just inform your therapist that you have arrived for your appointment, Mrs Smith.

Remember

Many different clients with different needs can walk through the salon door – so it's best to be prepared.

Customers with special needs

People with physical disabilities may require some help negotiating doorways and getting into the treatment area. Always offer to help, but do not assume that they cannot manage – and **never** patronise or 'talk down' to the client. It may only be their legs that don't work properly.

People who are hard of hearing are usually good lip readers, so the receptionist should face the client and speak clearly; this allows the client to see the words forming. Depending upon the severity of the disability, a notepad could be provided to jot down a message. A price list can be a good visual aid to help clarify what the client wants.

Visitors from overseas may have slight problems being understood, although some cultures have a better command of English if they have been taught it in school. Again, speak clearly, use visual materials to help clarify what is required, and seek help if available.

Older clients may have problems with their mobility or hearing. However, never assume this to be the case – never judge. Be on hand to offer assistance and, if the client is very frail, then it should be explained that some treatment adaptation might be needed.

Taking messages

During the course of your reception duties you will often be asked to take messages: for other staff members, the manager or even a client having a treatment. This valuable service also provides evidence for your portfolio, so make sure you get your message signed and dated by the person it should go to (and include an assessor number, where appropriate). It can then go into your evidence portfolio.

It is very important to write down the exact and whole message given to you. You may think it odd, or a bit difficult to understand, but if that is the message sent, it should be the one given to the person.

You will need to include:

- date and time of the call
- a brief description of the nature of the message
- whether the caller needs a reply – a return telephone number is then essential and is often useful
- how important the message is – if necessary, write urgent on it in large letters.

It is important to listen carefully and ask the caller to repeat any part of the message that you did not understand, or hear properly. Always repeat the whole message back to the caller to make sure you have all the details correctly written down – especially the return telephone number.

Confidential information

You should always be sensitive to any confidential information you come across in the course of your work. Confidential information includes details of your clients' address, telephone numbers, health status / problems, medication and other personal details. You are allowed to give these details to authorised people only, such as your salon owner, manager or fellow workers. No one outside the salon should have access to your clients' personal details, and you should never gossip about your clients or mention anything about them to your friends or family.

MESSAGE

FOR	*Deepak*
FROM	*Mrs Alessi*
TEL. NO.	*0208 321 145*

TELEPHONED	✔	PLEASE RING	✔
CALLED TO SEE YOU	☐	WILL CALL AGAIN	☐
WANTS TO SEE YOU	☐	URGENT	☐

MESSAGE: *Needs to speak to you asap - you can call her on the tel. no. above up to 5.30pm*

DATE: *10.05.02*　　TIME: *9.03am*

RECEIVED BY: *Amber*

Reality Check!

If a client's health status or other sensitive or personal details are not kept confidential, you are breaking rules of confidentiality. If you use a computer to store clients' personal details, you need to be aware of, and abide by, the Data Protection Act. Please refer to the Professional basics section (page 41) for further information.

Make appointments
for salon services

2.2

In this element you will learn about:

- appointment systems
- confirming appointments.

Appointment systems

It is usual for the appointments for each therapist to be kept in a large book, with either a column for each therapist or a page for each. This allows the therapist to see at a glance what treatments are booked in for the day, in order to make the appropriate preparation.

The golden rule is to have a system and to use it properly.

Pages should be set out for several weeks in advance so that clients booking ahead or clients wanting special days (for example, for pre-wedding make-up etc.) can book in confidence. It is also useful when planning a course of treatments for a client, such as twice a week for six weeks. This also allows the therapist the opportunity for advanced planning, should she need time off for her personal needs or holidays.

Booking

When booking the appointment the receptionist requires the following details:

- name
- telephone contact number
- treatment.

She also needs to know how long to book the appointment for. Time must be allowed for:

- greeting the client and consultation
- client undressing
- client preparation during the treatment
- client getting dressed, homecare and aftercare advice given.

Reality Check!

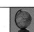

If sufficient time is not allowed for all aspects of the appointment, the first treatment will overrun, making the next appointment late. This can continue all day and the knock-on effect may be that the last client is kept waiting for far too long. The therapist will become stressed under pressure, the client may feel rushed, and the benefits of the treatment will be lost.

In the salon

Mrs Ahmed phoned in, a day before her appointment, to see if Sofia, her therapist, could squeeze in a leg wax and lip wax with her facial. Mrs Ahmed had been given a surprise – a weekend break in the sunshine – and wanted to look her best. Anita, the receptionist, had a look at the page, and told Mrs Ahmed that yes, it would be possible to add these extra treatments, as there was a gap in Sofia's column. Anita had a busy day, with lots of pressure, and not only forgot to add in the extra appointment time, but also forgot to leave a message for Sofia, to remind her to put on a wax pot, prior to Mrs Ahmed's appointment.

When the client arrived for her appointment, she was furious that her needs could not be met. Sofia's column had, by that time, filled up, so there was no gap to squeeze the extra treatment into.

Sofia was left feeling embarrassed, as she knew nothing about it, and she lost a valued customer, because Mrs Ahmed felt that the salon had poor communication and took her business elsewhere. What could Anita have done to avoid this situation?

Date: **Tuesday 13th October 2000**

	Lucy	Hellena	Anetta	Siobhan	
AM 9.00	Mrs Khan	Mrs Hughes			9.00 AM
9.15	full	full			9.15
9.30	Body wax	B/Massage			9.30
9.45	01234 45678	223335			9.45
10.00					10.00
10.15					10.15
10.30		Mrs Inder			10.30
10.45	Miss Jones	Pedicure			10.45
11.00	Aroma	+ ½ leg wax	Miss Westerby		11.00
11.15	Back massage	01235 771540	French		11.15
11.30	357928		Manicure		11.30
11.45			+ facial		11.45
12.00			01329 815242	Mr. Vallete	12.00
12.15		Mrs Green		Back massage	12.15
12.30	LUNCH	Eye tint		+ pedicure	12.30
12.45		444321		02271 881570	12.45
PM 1.00	Mr. Walsh				1.00 PM
1.15	Manicure		Miss Rudman		1.15
1.30	+back wax	LUNCH	Miss Allen	Miss Binder	1.30
1.45	02392 815815		x2 eyebows	waxing	1.45
2.00	Mrs Suling		335215	e/b + lip & chin	2.00
2.15	Eyebrow tidy	Miss Murphy	LUNCH	07807 577211	2.15
2.30	413927	Arm wax			2.30
2.45		+ u/arm wax			2.45
3.00		223792	Miss Nair	Mrs Pattel	3.00
3.15			Bridal	Sugaring	3.15
3.30		Miss Woolford	Top to toe	to x2 leg	3.30
3.45		Basic facial +	447 812	221 335	3.45
4.00	Mrs Wang	eye lash tint			4.00
4.15	Non-surg.	445 877			4.15
4.30	facial lift				4.30
4.45	08729 815 111				4.45
5.00		Mrs Townsend			5.00
5.15		M/up			5.15
5.30		lesson			5.30
5.45		315579 ext. 222			5.45
6.00					6.00
6.15					6.15
6.30					6.30
6.45					6.45
7.00					7.00

(Siobhan column note: lunchtime cover only)

A page from an appointment book

Remember that if the salon has a system of coding then you should use it – it will make life easier. For example: C – cancellation, L – late arrival, A – client has arrived and so on.

Some salons do not have columns for each therapist, they allot a work station number or couch position and then fit the staff around the treatments that need to be completed. The advantage of this system is that the workload can be easily distributed between staff and the manager can allot the jobs as fairly as possible. The disadvantage is that regular customers do not always get the same therapist.

When booking an appointment, it is important to do the following.

- Fill out the details in pencil. This allows any alterations or cancellations to be changed without making the page too messy.
- Have an easy code to identify any potential problems.
- Make sure that everyone can easily understand start and finish times.
- Make sure that all names and numbers are clear and legible.
- Allow the hardworking therapist a break for lunch. Do not be pressured by a persistent client into giving a lunchtime appointment to a therapist who has had no break during the day. It is better practice to stagger the lunch breaks, so that there is always a therapist covering a busy lunchtime session.
- Do give an appointment card to the client with all the details recorded on it – she then has a record of when she has to come in and this cuts down the possibility of a missed appointment.

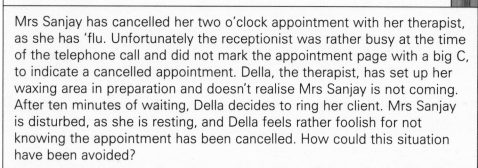

In the salon

Mrs Sanjay has cancelled her two o'clock appointment with her therapist, as she has 'flu. Unfortunately the receptionist was rather busy at the time of the telephone call and did not mark the appointment page with a big C, to indicate a cancelled appointment. Della, the therapist, has set up her waxing area in preparation and doesn't realise Mrs Sanjay is not coming. After ten minutes of waiting, Della decides to ring her client. Mrs Sanjay is disturbed, as she is resting, and Della feels rather foolish for not knowing the appointment has been cancelled. How could this situation have been avoided?

Missed appointments

There should be a clear salon policy on missed appointments.

Some salons have a small cancellation charge if the appointment is missed – rather like the dentist or physiotherapist. There is usually no cancellation fee if the appointment is cancelled with twenty-four hours notice. Both staff and clients need to be clear on this policy and it could be displayed on a notice in the reception area.

Receptionists need to be flexible and should be prepared to fit in the client who arrives without an appointment. The receptionist should always check first and where possible fit the client into a suitable slot – and then inform the therapist who might not otherwise be aware that another client is waiting.

In the salon

Mrs Smith turns up for her appointment for an eyelash and brow tint, in readiness for her holiday tomorrow. She has never had a patch test, and has not been informed that she needs one. How is she going to react, and what can Aiysha, the therapist, do? Whose fault is it?

Remember

Be aware of the new client and have a code to alert the therapist. This allows patch testing (if required) to be carried out and a full consultation, if needed.

Dealing with telephone enquires

Using the telephone is now second nature to us all – very few homes do not have one, and mobile phones are now commonplace. However, not everyone uses the telephone effectively. Good telephone communication skills are very useful for business, and it is worthwhile learning how to use the telephone well.

How to use the phone

There are some definite key steps to acquiring a good telephone manner, ensuring that the person on the end of the phone is treated courteously, efficiently and accurately. These include the following.

- Always have a pen and paper handy as a jotting pad, so you are prepared to take messages.
- Answer the phone promptly, even if you are busy.
- If you do feel harassed, pause and take a deep breath before lifting the receiver. Smile and sound friendly – it is very easy to sound abrupt on the telephone.
- Identify the salon quickly, after making sure you are connected properly and the caller can hear you.
- Be cheery – no matter how pressurised you may feel, it should not be obvious from the tone of your voice, and no one wants to be greeted with a miserable-sounding receptionist. Redirect the call quickly, if going through to another extension. If the call cannot be put through, ask if the caller wishes to leave a message.

Remember the dos and don'ts

- **Don't** sigh into the phone– it gives the impression that the caller is a nuisance, and that you are doing a huge favour by answering.
- **Do** answer with a smile on your face – just as if you can see the person's face.
- **Don't** be curt, rude or irritated when you first pick up the phone – you never know who is on the other end, and no one deserves rudeness.
- **Do** write a message down clearly, so that anyone can read it, not so that it is incomplete, or missing a valuable piece of information – such as who called.
- **Don't** make up an answer – if you don't know something or where someone is, then honesty is the best policy. Unless you tell the truth you will only get caught out and lose credibility.
- **Do** be honest with all callers.
- **Don't** ever slam down the phone in temper, cut someone off, or talk about the caller in a rude manner – the person will almost certainly hear and be offended.
- **Do** remember that all calls are from existing or prospective clients.
- **Don't** use the telephone for private calls. Itemised phone bills now show who made a call, for how long and to whom. No employer would mind the odd essential local call, or emergency message, but do not abuse an employer's goodwill.
- **Do** ask to use the phone if it is a quick personal call.
- **Don't** forget that there might be telephone calls outside office hours, or when everyone is genuinely busy. An answer machine is a simple solution, and most people are comfortable about leaving a message. Revenue may be lost if there is no one to answer that important phone call; but remember you have to follow up on the messages.

Confirming appointments

Appointment details always need to be confirmed in order to be sure that what the client said was what you heard. Names, times, and services can sound similar, and confirming the details just means a bit of double checking – which may save confusion later on.

Reality Check!

It can be just as easy to give a bad impression over the phone as it is in person – perhaps more so, because the caller only judges what is heard, and may not know the background leading to an irritable telephone manner. So: smile when you dial!

Check it out

Make a list of all the enquiries you answer throughout a working day. How many were telephone enquiries? How many were there in person? Keep a note of these by writing down a brief account of the nature of the enquiry, the client's name, date and time, and include this as evidence for your portfolio of evidence.

You will need to make sure that you confirm with the client all the details: 'So, Mrs Patel, just to confirm your appointment for Wednesday, the 10th, at 4 pm for a facial – can I give you an appointment card with that on?'. Look to the client and she will usually agree with you, 'Yes, that is correct, and yes, you had better put it on a card for me, thank you'.

If the client's treatment is a little more personal in nature, then you should not repeat it too loudly. Remember the importance of confidentiality.

Handling payments   2.3

In this element you will learn about:	
• methods of payment • discrepancies • security measures.	

The client should be treated as courteously at the end of her treatment as at the beginning, so politeness is still of prime importance when she is paying for her treatment. The way in which the financial side of any business is approached is as vital as the treatment side.

Methods of payment

The client's method of payment is very much her choice, and the receptionist must be prepared and able to cope with any payment method. The client should feel that her treatment was so special that she is delighted to pay for a service she has thoroughly enjoyed and which was worth every penny!

Several methods of payment are possible, and most common in the salon are:

- cash
- cheque
- credit or debit card
- gift voucher.

All of these are equally acceptable and should be handled with care.

Cash

When a customer is paying with cash (a rarity these days), there are several things to be aware of. The most important is to check that bank notes for large amounts, e.g. twenty or fifty pounds, are genuine and not counterfeit. You need to check for the following.

- Look for the watermark – every note has a watermark, which can be seen when the note is held up to the light.
- Look for the metallic strip which is woven into the paper – it should be unbroken.
- Compare the feel of bank note paper – often a forged note is not printed on the same quality of paper, and may have a thin papery feel.

The police often circulate a list of forged notes to look out for. The bank note numbers are on a stop list, which should be kept near the till, so that numbers can be compared.

If any irregularity occurs, it will usually be because the client has been given this money from another source, and the authorities should be notified. Quietly ask the client to step

Remember
It is important not to feel embarrassed about checking money; it will save the salon and protect the customer.

into the office, out of reception, to avoid embarrassment. Ask a supervisor or the manager or owner to deal with the situation. You can then return to your duties at the front desk.

The client will have taken a forged note in all good faith, so it is not up to the receptionist/therapist to accuse her or him. However, it is important that the note is removed from circulation, and the police are informed.

Even when accepting money from very regular customers, remember that it should still be checked thoroughly.

Procedure for handling cash payments

Dealing with cash involves a lot of responsibility, so care must be taken when handling it to avoid errors.

- Place a client's money on the till ledge, to ensure you remember what amount has been given to you – do not put the money straight into the till drawer. This may lead to confusion – was it a ten pound note or a twenty?
- Count the change required from the note, and then re-count it into the client's hand.
- Place the client's money in the till drawer, and close it.
- Give the client the receipt to confirm the cost of the treatment, how much was given to you, and the change to be given back.

Cheques

A cheque is essentially no more than a letter to the bank telling them to pay a certain sum to a specified person. Most banks and building societies offer a cheque service, although a switch service (see below) is also available. A cheque payment is very acceptable, providing certain checks and precautions are carried out.

You should always check that:

- the date is correct – day, month and year – this is especially important in January
- the name of the salon is spelt correctly – the client could be offered a stamp with the full name pre-printed on it
- the amount of money is right, and is in words and numbers
- the signature is completed correctly and matches the signature on the cheque guarantee card.

Reality Check!

Payments for all treatments should be acknowledged by a receipt, either hand written or from the till, regardless of which type of payment it is.

Reality Check!

If a cheque is faulty in any way, the bank the salon uses will reject it, and it will be returned to the salon. It is then up to the salon to contact the customer, and inform her, the client will then have to call into the salon and alter and initial any necessary changes. It may be wise to re-write the cheque altogether. It is much easier to get it right first time.

In the salon

A large department store in London contained a busy beauty salon, with twenty therapists, with full bookings every day. The salon needed to employ receptionists to cope with the demands on booking in clients. All the receptionists had to undergo thorough till training for the store, and had a personal till number that they keyed in, every time they put a payment through.

One client paid a very large bill by cheque, and Lesley, a new receptionist, talked to the client while keying in all the treatments. The client asked for an extra hand cream and moisturiser to be added to the bill, as a present for her mother. Lesley keyed in all the till details and told the client how much the total was. The client left quite

happily, with her parcel of goodies. It was only when Lesley looked again at the cheque that she saw that the date was wrong. Lesley decided that it didn't matter, and she just got out her pen and altered it.

The next day Lesley's supervisor and the store's floor manager came to reception, and asked Lesley about the altered cheque. Yes, she said, I couldn't find the client, so I changed the date myself. Lesley was asked to get her things and was escorted off the premises, with instant dismissal. Tampering with cheques is considered to be fraud, and it was against the store's policy. What should Lesley have done when she noticed that the cheque had been dated wrongly?

Cheque cards

A cheque guarantee card should always support a cheque to the bank, and it has two functions.

- It acts as proof of identity.
- It guarantees that the bank will honour the cheque up to the limit of the card. The limit on most bankcards is now one hundred pounds.

Always check the expiry date on the card, which is written as, for example 03\04 – this is the month and year when the card will need to be re-issued. You also need to check that the signatures match, and that the card type is the same as the cheque i.e. both are from HSBC, Barclays etc.

The cheque is then treated exactly like cash, put into the till, a receipt given, and the till closed.

Credit cards

Credit cards are often referred to as plastic money or a flexible friend. All leading banks offer credit cards to those customers they consider credit worthy.

If your salon has a contract with a credit company, it will usually display a sign stating that credit cards are accepted. The card is simply taken onto an imprinting machine, which takes all the details down on a special carbonated triplicate voucher provided by the credit card company. The customer then signs the voucher and if the amount is a large one, it is standard practice to phone the credit company to see whether the credit limit will support the payment. Some salons use the computerised till unit for this service (see below).

The salon submits the details of the bottom two pieces of the voucher to the credit card company, which then pays for the goods or services the customer has bought in the salon. There is usually a small handling fee of 1.5 or 2%.

Debit cards

Most banks now also offer the convenience of a debit card, often known as a Switch or Connect card. This is when the payment is made electronically, transferring money straight from the customer's bank account to the salon's own bank account. This saves having to write a cheque.

Debit cards are usually also the same as the cheque guarantee card.

The card is swiped through the computerised till unit, using a sliding action so that the information stored on the metallic strip on the back of the card can be read. The details are then printed onto a duplicated slip, which the customer is asked to sign, the slip is torn off the till, and the customer can be handed back both the card and the top copy of the slip, which acts as a receipt.

Discrepancies

Unfortunately, there may be times when payment discrepancies and disputes arise. They should be dealt with calmly, without causing too much embarrassment to the client.

Possible problems could include the following.

- Invalid currency is presented – perhaps a foreign note or even a forged note.
- An invalid card is presented – it may be out of date, or if it is a cheque guarantee card, it may not match the cheque details.

Remember

Remember to check credit cards just as you would cash, or a cheque.

- Is the card within its expiry date?
- Is the name or title clear, and is it the same name by which you know the client?
- Does the signature match the name on the front of the card?
- Is the card on a stop list issued by the local police?
- Is the hologram on the front clear and definite?

If the card passes all these security checks, carry on with the procedure.

Reality Check!

Be careful with debit cards.

All information is stored on a metallic strip. If this strip comes into contact with a magnet the information is destroyed. Even the magnetic clasp on a purse or handbag is enough to disable all information. Some retail stores that use a magnet to remove security tags can also interfere with your debit card.

- A cheque is filled out incorrectly, or does not have a current cheque guarantee card.
- Fraudulent use of a payment card is suspected – perhaps it has been put onto the stop list.

Security procedures

At the end of the day's business the till must be totalled and the takings should match the recorded amount taken, either through the till roll or a docket system. If a float has been used to provide a base of change at the beginning of the day, then it needs to be deducted. This can then be used for the next day's trading and the balance of the takings should be paid into the salon bank account.

Most large banks offer a night safe facility, in which the takings can be deposited. It is not a good idea to keep large amounts of money on the premises overnight – there is always the risk of a burglary.

Reality Check!

If depositing money avoid using a big bank bag, which advertises exactly what it is you are carrying! Never take the same route to the bank at exactly the same time every day: someone may be watching. Being a victim of a snatch robbery would be a dreadful experience so do not be a willing victim – be safe!

Develop and maintain effective teamwork and relationships

Unit 3

This unit is all about you: how you relate to your job role, your colleagues and how to analyse your performance for personal improvement and career growth. If you can be objective about your own performance, i.e. learning to stand back and view your behaviour from the outside, it will help in all sorts of ways. Your personal attitude and emotional growth will develop; your relationships with the people you have to work with will improve, and the resulting relaxed atmosphere within your salon will be beneficial for your clients. That has to be good for everyone.

Therefore, in this section you will need to demonstrate in your everyday work that you have met the standards for developing and maintaining good working relationships with your colleagues.

Within this unit you will cover the following elements:

3.1 Develop and maintain effective teamwork and relationships with colleagues
3.2 Develop and improve personal effectiveness within the job role.

The Professional basics section also needs to be read in conjunction with this unit, to refresh your memory about the importance of good communication skills.

Develop and maintain effective teamwork and relationships with colleagues

3.1

In this element you will learn about:

* working with others
* communicating effectively
* working arrangements
* good teamwork

Reality Check!

It is a fact of life that no one gets to choose who they work with – unless they own the salon. It isn't like a college or training environment where you are very close to your best friends and can stick together in little groups. You may enter an established salon with a variety of employees, with differing backgrounds, skill areas and ages.

Working with others

When you leave college with a good beauty therapy qualification, you will have worked as a student with others in a salon environment, but usually under the close eye of an assessor or salon manager. In a busy salon that then employs you as a beauty therapist the supervision is not as close, and you are expected to work sensibly, effectively and responsibly at all times. This is part of the employment agreement.

Working with others is a hard lesson to learn, and is part of growing up. In order to work well with others we must first analyse ourselves. The pie chart shows a breakdown of how we see one another, and what we are judged upon.

So the old saying 'Actions speak louder than words' is true.

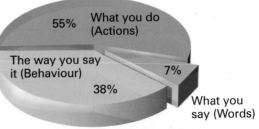

The way in which others see us

Communicating effectively

When you work in a salon you may have a manager who supervises what you do, or you may have junior staff who you guide through the working day. Good communication skills enable you to get on with all your co-workers.

Working under someone

- You accept that someone is in charge.
- You should take instructions and act upon them.
- You communicate effectively if you need to check or ask something.
- You take responsibility for your job role and do it to the best of your ability.

Working together

- Good teamwork means supporting each other – not being in conflict with one another.
- It gives the salon a pleasant atmosphere, which is obvious to the client.
- Provides a good and reliable service.
- Gives effective results.

Listening skills

Communication is a two-way process. You can develop the ability to be effective in listening skills. It means:

- knowing when to stop talking and listen to what is being communicated
- listening with interest and understanding
- providing encouragement for the other person to continue
- confirming that you have understood the conversation so far – nodding or agreeing with the point raised.

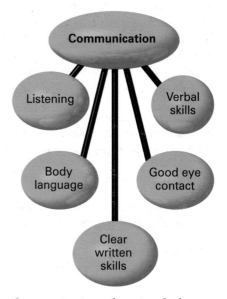

Communication = listening, body language, clear written skills, good eye contact, and verbal skills.

Working arrangements

Professional staff hold the key to an effective, friendly and efficient salon. Effective working arrangements and good relationships among staff lead to an efficient and harmonious salon. Professional staff can achieve this through:

- ✓ good communication
- ✓ knowledge of requirements
- ✓ competence
- ✓ initiative
- ✓ responsibility
- ✓ identification of strengths and weaknesses
- ✓ up-to-date skills and knowledge
- ✓ flexibility
- ✓ teamwork.

- **Good communication** between colleagues will build rapport, and that will be reflected in the smooth running of the business. It will also mean that there is less chance of any misunderstanding among staff.
- **Knowledge** is very comforting and prevents confusion or worry. Make sure you know what is asked of you, if given an area of responsibility. A clear understanding of issues and requirements leads to a good treatment and a happy client.
- **Competence** – do the job as well as you have been trained to. Do not attempt to bluff your way through a job, and put a client or colleague at risk in doing so. This comes back to knowledge. Never attempt a job you have not been taught to do. If you do not know something, do not guess – ask.
- **Initiative** means taking the first step or action – without being prompted to do so. If a job needs doing, do it without being asked. This will prove to your employer that you can be relied upon to work effectively without having to be prompted all the time.

- **Be responsible** for all your actions. Also take responsibility for mistakes and take appropriate action to minimise damage, rather than trying to cover up mistakes and so making matters worse.
- **Identification** of strengths and weaknesses allows for professional growth and development of skills. Working out your weaknesses should not be seen as a personal attack, but a chance to receive some constructive guidance and evaluation of performance. A supervisor, manager and colleagues can carry this out in staff review sessions.
- **Up-to-date skills and knowledge** can be gained through regular training, reading trade journals, attending the organised beauty trade shows or exhibitions and through the media. Be enthusiastic to learn new skills and regard it as a challenge rather than a chore. The more skills a therapist has to offer, the more employable she is, and will be seen as a valuable asset to any salon.
- **Flexibility** is a skill worth cultivating. Therefore, try to accommodate the client who arrives without an appointment, with help from your colleagues. Do not make her feel that it is just too inconvenient or stupid of her to even ask. You could book another appointment if you cannot help at that particular time. If a client is late for her appointment or there is an over-booking, then do the same. Re-scheduling of appointments can work both ways – it could be that, owing to staff sickness, clients have to be juggled into other time slots.
  If this is done in an open and genuinely apologetic manner, most clients will be just as flexible. If a client changes her treatment booking, again be flexible. If time permits, and the client's needs can be accommodated, then do so. The receptionist may need to be made aware of this, so as not to double book the time slot, but flexibility is the way to keep encouraging new business.
- **Teamwork** is essential for any group of people working together. To be part of a team takes patience, a willingness to help each other, and respect for the others in the team. Respect cannot be bought – it has to be earned through hard work and commitment. Whilst a little competitiveness may be healthy in the salon (e.g. the person with the most retail sales in a month wins a prize), a person determined to undermine her colleagues at every available opportunity could not be considered a team player. The consequences can be a build-up of bad feelings between staff, resentment and ill-will – all of which are very bad for business.

Good teamwork

As a vital part of the team you need to know:

- who is who within the salon
- who is responsible for what
- who you should go to if you need information or support.

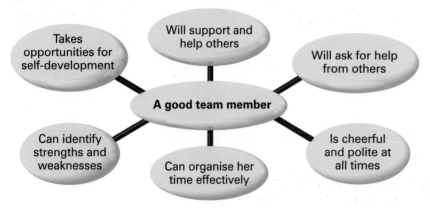

How to be a good team member

> **Remember**
>
> Being a team player involves offering lots of support, getting a good balance of assistance and never letting the other team member down. Could you consider yourself a team player?

A good team needs:

- an appropriate leader who is fair but decisive
- enthusiastic, committed team members
- good listening skills and an exchange of ideas
- clear objectives and a sense of direction
- good balance of planning and action
- good communication between members
- clear job roles – so you know what you are supposed to do
- flexibility and tolerance from all members of the team
- right mix of skills
- a safe environment to try things, make mistakes and learn from them
- a sense of humour.

Team problems

If problems arise that might affect the services offered by the salon, these must be reported accurately to the relevant person.

Team spirit can be lost if:

- one group member seems to be favoured more than another
- one member of the group works on her own and won't join in the team
- there is a breakdown in communications
- people are unwilling to be flexible and tolerant of others' mistakes
- there is too much work for too few people
- job roles become blurred and people encroach upon areas they shouldn't and for which they may not be qualified.

Develop and improve personal effectiveness within the job role

3.2

Self-development

Self-development is essential for the growth and maturity of the therapist within a salon environment. If a therapist keeps making the same mistakes, over and over, and clients complain or stop coming into the salon altogether this is a strong indication that something is wrong. Sometimes, with experience, it is easier to be reflective and spot our own mistakes and then change the action, or reaction, to break the cycle of behaviour. However, sometimes it is not so easy to be inward looking, and this is where a good manager can help. Regular work-related reviews, called appraisals, will also help to identify strengths and weaknesses, and so aid personal development.

Many large companies provide both self-assessment sheets for the employee to fill in, throughout a set period, and then a joint review sheet with the manager, to help improve performance.

Self-assessment

A self-assessment appraisal is not just about achievement within the job role, and how many sales have been completed – although that is important.

An appraisal should highlight how well the individual is coping within her job role and whether the salon is asking too much of an employee. It provides an opportunity

> **Remember**
>
> Appraisals should be viewed in a positive light so you can learn, and make progress in personal growth and development. They are also important for the maintenance of good working relationships. It is important to react in an optimistic way to any feedback or review. Nobody likes criticism, but it is essential to listen carefully to what is said and to learn from it.

for the therapist to offer her opinions on the development and improvement of treatments and services. An appraisal should also be viewed very much as a two-way discussion – not a 'telling off' for a bad performance at work.

An appraisal or team review should happen on a regular basis, perhaps every three months. It should:

- be at a mutually agreeable time, not an inconvenience to either party
- be constructive and open, not conducted in fear or concern about job loss
- be objective and as non-personal as possible
- be a review for both parties, not just a performance judgement
- be constructive and positive
- leave the employee feeling enthused and not depressed.

A self-assessment form can contain whatever the employer or manager feels is most relevant to the job role. Below is an example of a common format.

Reality Check!

Self-assessment is also about short-term plans and development of the individual and it opens up many areas for discussion for future plans between a manager and an employee.

Self-assessment form for appraisal

beauty SECRETS

Salon: Beauty Secrets **Date:** July 2002

Position held: Beauty therapist **Therapist:** Joanne Smith

Please add comments on how you feel you are progressing in each area listed.

Appearance: Good, I do try to look professional every day.

Absences: Could be better, as I have had a week off with flu this month. I haven't had any more time off.

Time keeping: Could be better. I have been late 5 times this month.

Job performance: Good, I feel my regular clients always ask for me, and I have worked hard this month.

Sales: Good, as above. My sales are from my regulars.

Strengths: I am confident with my treatments and I especially enjoy doing facial massage.

Weaknesses: Time keeping. I have missed my bus quite a lot in the mornings.

Any areas of change: I have been in the wet area, putting clients in the sauna this month, as Jane seems to have the flu bug that I had and is still off sick.

Staff development request: I would like to go on an eyelash perming training day if possible, as we have been asked for the treatment by our regular clients.

Action plan for next review: To improve on time keeping and do my course.

An example of a self-assessment form for appraisal

In the salon

Beenal and Fleur have been working together in a salon for two years. They started at the same time and have the same number of responsibilities. They catch the bus together in the mornings, and sometimes have a little moan about wanting to be given extra training and therefore able to give more advanced treatments. They each have their appraisal on the same day. Beenal says on the bus, 'I got the notice of my appraisal through, but nothing good ever happens to me, and I don't think the manageress likes me, so I don't think I'm even going to bother'. Fleur replies, 'I spent last night writing out some questions I want to ask, and I want to be put forward for extra training, even in my own time – it might lead to more money and experience in the long term'.

Who do you think got the best out of their appraisal?

Check it out

Copy out the self-assessment form (or ask your tutor for one) and use it to analyse your own performance.

Target setting

Linked into the appraisal system is the setting of targets for the action plan to improve performance at work. Targets should always be SMART, i.e. **S**pecific, **M**easurable, **A**chievable, **R**ealistic and **T**imed.

The SMART rule

Specific

Have particular aims in mind rather than too grand an idea. Set a goal specific to you, e.g. I want to complete two assessments each week.

Measurable

Make sure you can measure the aims with a start and a finish. Assessments can be measured against the NVQ performance criteria and ranges. You must know where you are now, and where you want to be. For example, product sales might be on average £50 per day now, and a 10% increase would take that up to £55 per day.

Achievable

Do not give yourself an aim that cannot be realised e.g. saving the world. A short-term target may be to complete an NVQ unit by a set date – that should be achievable.

Realistic

Can you save the world? No! Doing ten treatments per hour is not realistic – be sensible with your aims. For example, how long will it really take you to cover all the performance criteria ranges in one unit?

Timed

In order for the target to be achieved there should be a timescale for you to aim towards, for example: by next month I will improve my timekeeping by 50%; by Christmas I am going to have my portfolio for Unit 8 ready to be signed off by my assessor.

Joint review

The self-assessment form is a *personally set* identification of your own strengths and weaknesses, and your own personal targets can be set. A joint review with a relevant person, such as a manager or assessor / tutor can then identify whether your personal targets are realistic and achievable using the SMART formula. These targets can be short term or long term.

Short-term goals

Short-term goals are easier to measure and judge than long-term goals. They can bring a very positive glow to the therapist who achieves them and that will encourage her to go on and improve further.

A short-term goal for the therapist Joanne, in the example self-assessment form on page 76, is to complete an eyelash perming course and gain her certificate, and so offer her clients another service. This is rewarding and achievable.

Long-term goals

Long-term goals are not so easy to measure and may be harder to keep in view. They require much more dedication to achieve.

A long-term goal for Joanne might be to gain two years' salon experience and then apply for a job as a therapist on an ocean liner. This is still achievable but will take two years at least.

Joanne's joint review

Using the SMART theory for Joanne's joint review will help both her and her manager / assessor decide how best to help Joanne achieve her target. The main problem seems to be her late arrival in the salon on some mornings. This is not very professional so it is good that Joanne has identified this as a weakness – especially if she is relying on the goodwill of her team-mates to prepare her working area.

Specific

Is her target specific? Yes it is, but not enough. She wants to improve her time keeping but by how much?

Measurable

This will make her target specific – her time-keeping needs to improve by 100%. No lateness at all would be ideal.

Achievable

Do not put an aim that cannot be realised. A good short-term target would be to be punctual for a week.

Realistic

Is 100% improvement realistic? What are the problems? Joanne lives some distance away from the salon in a rural country area. The buses run only once an hour so if she misses the 8 o'clock bus she has to wait an hour for the 9 o'clock bus – by when she should already be in the salon preparing for her busy day. Can Joanne realistically get up half an hour earlier to get to the bus stop? Yes she can.

Remember

Short-term goals are like the proverbial carrot dangling on the stick. They provide incentive and reward. Lots of short-term goals can help to achieve a long-term goal, which is also very satisfying, and help you get where you want to go.

Timed

Agree a time limit of improved time keeping for the month of August, so at the end of the month her self-assessment and review will be ready to be done again.

Now Joanne has analysed the problem of her time-keeping, what are the solutions? She could apply any of the following:

- buy an alarm clock and set it at an earlier time to get up
- find out if another member of the staff could give her a lift, perhaps sharing petrol costs
- put an advert in the local shop for someone from her village who is working in the town who would be able to offer a car-share on a permanent basis
- learn to drive and save up for a car – so becoming independent regarding transport
- change the appointment booking in system at the salon, so that Joanne starts at 9.30 – when she can realistically get to work – and then either finish half an hour later or have only a short break for lunch
- try cycling to work and get fit at the same time.

Any number of these possible solutions would help Joanne achieve her goal, although some – such as learning to drive – would take longer than others.

Check it out

Now fill out your own self-assessment plan, and see if you can offer your own solutions to your problems.

Develop and maintain positive working relationships with customers

Unit 4

This section covers:

- methods of communication
- body language
- customer needs
- customer reactions and how to handle them
- when to ask for help.

All of these topics are found elsewhere in the book, so to avoid repetition, please refer to the cross-mapping table which will show you where to look.

The **Professional basics** section needs to be read in conjunction with this unit, along with units 1, 2 and 3.

Cross mapping of evidence for Unit 4

Element	Professional basics	Unit 1	Unit 2	Unit 3
Where information can be found				
4.1				
PC 1–5	●		●	
Ranges:				
Literature	●		●	
Stationery	●		●	
Forms	●		●	
Mechanical			●	
Electronic			●	
Consumables	●		●	
K1–4	●			
4.2				
PC 1–5	●			●
Ranges:				
Involve managers	●	●	●	●
Involve others	●	●	●	●
Cost	●	●	●	●
Time	●	●	●	●
Resources	●	●	●	●
Pro-active	●	●	●	●
On request	●	●	●	●
4.3				
PC 1–4	●	●	●	●
Ranges:				
Anxiety	●		●	
Anger	●		●	
Confusion	●		●	
4.4				
PC 1–5				
Ranges:	●		●	
Face-to-face	●		●	
Written	●		●	
Telephone	●		●	
Body language	●		●	
Physical disabilities	●		●	
Leaning difficulties	●		●	
Language differences (accents and dialects)	●		●	

related anatomy and
PHYSIOLOGY

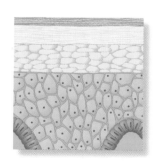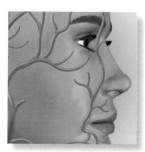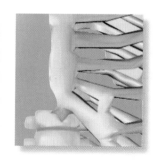

Related anatomy and physiology

As a beauty therapist you should have an understanding of the body and its basic functions so that you can give the most effective treatments to your client. When you can look at the body with knowledge and understanding you will be able to identify any problems and treat them with suitable products, and make recommendations to help your client.

The information in this section is compatible with the new standards for NVQ level 2 Beauty Therapy. It can also be used in conjunction with all non NVQ qualifications and follows the Vocational Awards International framework for anatomy and physiology.

The depth of knowledge for NVQ level 2 is very defined; the requirements for this section have been taken directly from the standards. Therefore no other anatomy or physiology is required to complete these qualifications. The related knowledge, to support anatomy links to a specific treatment given, is contained within the book. The areas where the anatomy links into the individual units is shown in the cross mapping which follows on page 85.

What you will learn

In this section you will learn about:

- Bones of the head, face, neck and shoulder girdle
- Structure of the skin
- Structure of the nail
- Muscles of the face, neck and shoulder area
- Hair
- Blood
- Lymph

A check it out activity is included at the end of each topic that you may like to undertake either with your study group or independently.

Cross-mapping: anatomy and physiology

Level 2 Your guide to the anatomy required in each unit/element

	5·1	5·2	5·3	6·1	6·2	6·3	7·1	7·2	7·3	7·4	8·1	8·2	8·3	8·4	9·1	9·2	9·3	9·4
The bones The position of the head, face, neck and shoulder girdle bones.				●		●												
The skin Structure and function of epidermis, dermis and subcutaneous layer, nerve endings and appendages.	●			●		●									●		●	●
The nails The structure of the nail unit (i.e. nail plate, nail bed, matrix, cuticle, lunula, hyponychium, eponychium, nail wall, free edge).															●		●	●
The process of nail growth (i.e. nail formation, growth rate, factors affecting growth, the effects of damage on growth).															●		●	●
The muscles The position and actions of the facial, neck and shoulder muscles (i.e. Frontalis, Corrugator, Temporalis, Orbicularis Oculi, Procerus, Nasalis, Quadratus Labii Superioris, Orbicularis Oris, Buccinator, Risorius, Mentalis, Zygomaticus, Masseter, Triangularis, Sternocleidomastoid, Platysma, Trapezius, Pectoralis, Deltoid, Occipitalis).				●		●												
The hair Basic principles of hair growth (i.e. Anagen, Catogen and Telogen).								●										
Types of hair growth and how to recognise its direction of growth (i.e. Terminal, Vellus).									●									
The blood The composition of blood and its role in improving skin and muscle condition.				●		●												
How to identify erythema and its causes.									●				●					●
The lymph The composition of the lymph and its role in improving skin and muscle condition.				●		●												

The bones of the head, neck and shoulder girdle

This section will teach you about the position of the bones of the head, face, neck and shoulders.

The arrangement of bones that are joined together is known as a skeleton. The skeleton gives the body shape, it provides attachment for muscles and protects delicate organs. For good facial work the therapist needs to identify the bones of the head, neck, face and shoulders.

Bones that form the skull

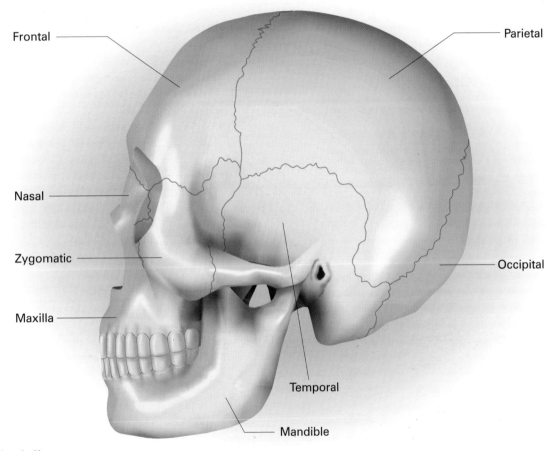

Bones of the skull

Bone	Position
1 Occipital bone (×1)	At the back of the skull
2 Parietal (×2)	Positioned at the back of the head and forms the roof of the skull
3 Frontal (×1)	Forms the front of the skull, forehead, and upper eye sockets
4 Temporal (×2)	At the side, around the ears
	These bones are fused together to form the shape of the skull, and their joins are known as sutures.

The skull is attached to the body via the vertebral column. The vertebral column enables the head to turn and tilt. The weight of the head is supported by the neck, the shoulder girdle bones and muscles.

The bones of the face

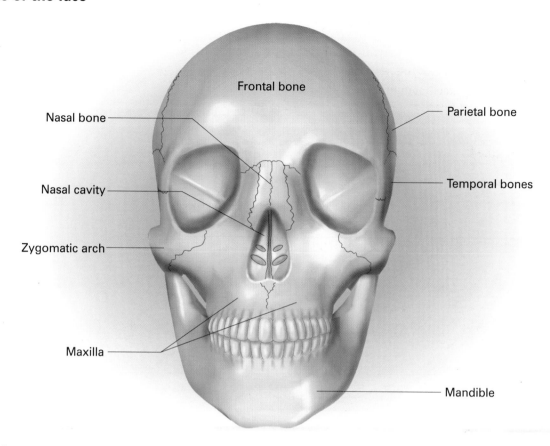

Bones of the face

Bone	Position
1 Zygomatic bones (×2)	These form the cheek bones
2 Maxilla (×2)	These form the upper jaw, most of the side wall of the nose and the front part of the soft palate
3 Mandible (×1)	This is the lower jaw and is the only moving bone in the face, allowing movement of the mouth for chewing and talking
4 Nasal (×2)	These form the bridge of the nose

The openings in the base of the skull provide spaces for the entrance and exit of many blood vessels, nerves and other structures. Projections and slightly elevated portions of the bones provide for the attachment of muscles. Some portions contain delicate structures, such as the part of the temporal bone that encloses the middle and internal sections of the ear. The air sinuses provide lightness and serve as vibrating chambers for the voice.

Bones of the shoulder girdle

The bones of the shoulder girdle allow the arms to move freely. The clavicle is more commonly known as the collar bone, and you can feel it in the area where the collar of a shirt or blouse would sit. The scapula is commonly referred to as the shoulder blade. The scapula is only secured to the skeleton by muscle, so it is fairly free to move about.

Check it out

Draw your arms back, and look in the mirror. Can you see your scapula? It may be easier to identify this on a partner.

Bones of the shoulder girdle

Bones	Girdle
1 Clavicle (x2)	Across the front of the chest, going from each shoulder to the breast bone
2 Scapula (x2)	At the back of the shoulder girdle, sitting on top of the rib cage

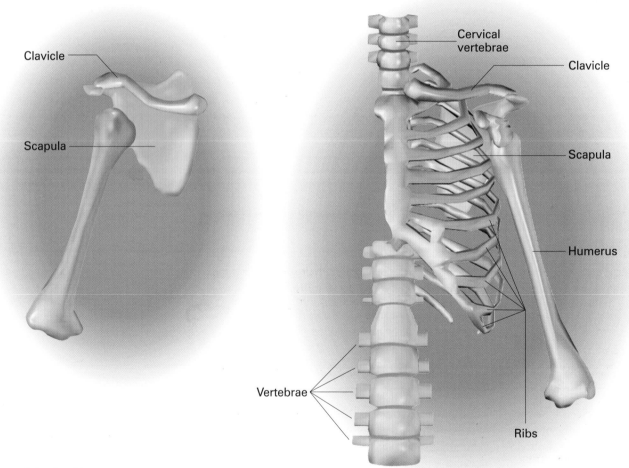

The bones of the shoulder

Skin

Skin is a remarkable organ that is able to adapt and perform various functions. It can mould to different shapes, stretch and harden, but can also respond to delicate touch, feel pain, pressure, hot and cold, so it is regarded as an effective communicator.

Skin makes up about 12% of an adult's body weight and consists of three layers: the epidermis, dermis and the subcutaneous layers. You can think of these layers like clothing.

The epidermis is the outer skin, like a breathable waterproof jacket – this is the skin we *see*. Our skin, or dermis, is under this and could be thought of as a blouse or shirt with lots of pockets containing many different items. Underneath this is a cushioned soft layer for protection, like a soft thermal vest. This bottom layer contains fat which helps to insulate and keep in warmth. The layers vary in thickness over different areas of the body. The thickest layers are over friction and gripping areas and the thinnest are over the eyelids, which must be light and flexible.

You can help yourself to remember the functions of the skin by the word **Shapes.**

S = Sensation
There are five types of nerve ending within the skin to help identify pain, touch, heat, cold and light pressure.

H = Heat regulation
The skin helps regulate the body's temperature by sweating to cool the body down when it overheats and shivering when it is cold. Shivering closes the pores. The tiny hairs that cover the body stand on end to trap warm air next to the skin and therefore prevent heat loss, when cold.

A = Absorption
Absorption of ultraviolet rays, from the sun, help with formation of vitamin D, which the body needs for the formation of strong bones and good eyesight. Some creams, essential oils, and some medication can also be absorbed through the skin.

P = Protection
Too much ultraviolet light may harm the skin, so the skin protects itself by producing a pigment, seen as a tan, called *melanin*. Bacteria and germs are prevented from entering the skin by a protective barrier called *the acid mantle*. This barrier also helps protect against moisture loss.

E = Excretion
Waste products and toxins are eliminated from the body through the *sweat glands*.

S = Secretion
Sebum and *sweat* are secreted onto the skin's surface. The sebum keeps the skin lubricated and soft, and the sweat combines with the sebum to form *the acid mantle*.

Structure of the skin
The skin is made up of three layers:

1   Epidermis
2   Dermis
3   Subcutaneous layer.

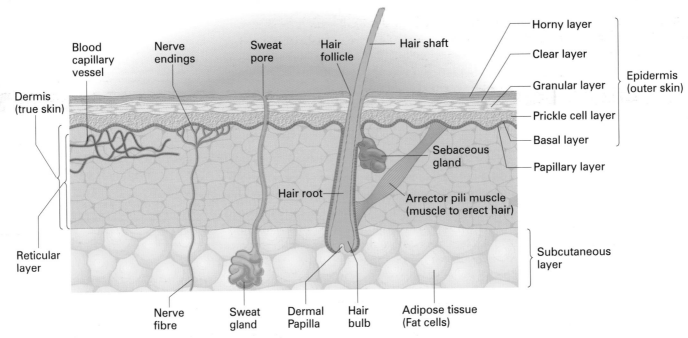

The structure of the skin

The epidermis

The epidermis is the outermost layer of the skin. It is made up of five layers:

1 Horny layer (*Stratum corneum*)
2 Clear layer (*Stratum lucidium*)
3 Granular layer (*Stratum granulosum*)
4 Prickle cell layer (*Stratum spinosum*)
5 Basal cell layer (*Stratum germativum*).

Layers 1 to 3 – the horny, clear and granular layers – are dead and are constantly being shed. But the prickle cell and basal cell layers – layers 4 and 5 – are still living because the cells contain a nucleus and can therefore reproduce. Skin renews itself every 28 days.

For assessment purposes you are only required to learn the English names for the epidermis. In some books you will find Latin names for the layers.

The layers of the epidermis need to be looked at in order of formation.

The five layers of the epidermis, or our outer skin, begin at the **basal** or bottom layer (5). This skin is constantly being reproduced, as the cells contain a nucleus or seed. As the cells reproduce the layers get constantly pushed up into the next layer. Each of the layers has its own specific function.

The **prickle** layer (4) is called this because the cells have spines, which prevent bacteria entering the cells and moisture being lost. These cells also have a nucleus and so reproduce.

The next layer is the **granular** layer (3). The prickle cells lose their spines and become flatter. The nucleus dies and a protein is formed called **keratin**. This protein prevents moisture loss and is found in skin, nails and hair.

The next layer is the **clear** layer (2). This layer is for cushioning and protection and is found only on the palms of the hands and soles of the feet.

The final layer is the **horny** layer (1), where the cells are dead and ready to be shed.
If you look at flakes of skin under a microscope they would resemble flakes of almond.
The name for the shedding of the skin is **desquemation.** This process speeds up as we age.

Layer	Function
1 Horny layer	Made up of many flattened dead skin cells which contain the tough keratin This is the final top layer of skin These cells are shed continuously to allow the new cells through.
2 Clear layer	3 to 4 rows thick of dead flattened cells Only found on the palms of the hands and the soles of the feet, above the granular layer. These cells act as protectors in areas of friction
3 Granular layer	2 to 4 layers thick, the cells begin to die and flatten The middle layer of the epidermis Waste and other substances from the cell get squashed together and harden.
4 Prickle layer	10 to 20 cells thick, with spines that connect with other cells Sits on top of the basal layer This layer of cells starts to harden and produce *keratin. Melanin* is also produced here which determines our colouring and helps protect against ultraviolet light.
5 Basal layer	A single layer of column-shaped cells The deepest layer of epidermis Continuously produces new cells

Functions of the epidermis

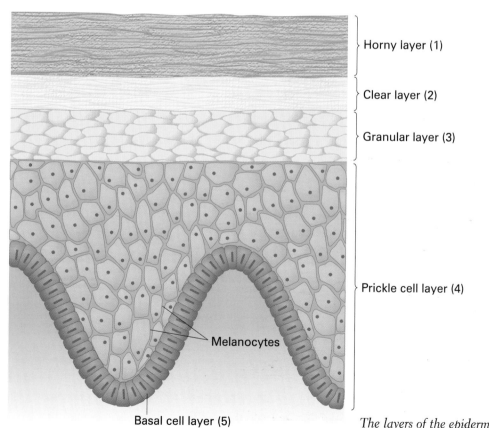

Horny layer (1)

Clear layer (2)

Granular layer (3)

Prickle cell layer (4)

Melanocytes

Basal cell layer (5)

The layers of the epidermis

Definition of terms

Carotene A pigment found in the granular layer.

Keratin A fibrous protein that forms in the body. It is found in the skin, hair and nails.

Keratinisation The process of cells hardening.

Melanin A pigment in the skin or hair that protects us from the sun. It determines our colouring and is determined largely by hereditary influences and location in the world.

Melanocytes Cells formed between the basal layer and prickle layer, which form the pigment melanin.

You may be required to label this diagram for a written skin assessment.

The dermis

The dermis or true skin contains many structures. It can be subdivided into two parts:

1 Papillary layer
2 Reticular layer

The dermis contains the main components of the skin such as nerve endings (for pain, pressure, hot and cold), the blood supply and the lymph vessels, hair follicles and our sweat glands for temperature regulation.

Papillary layer

- Undulating wavy tissue, rich in blood and lymph vessels and nerve endings.
- Joins the dermis to the epidermis
- Area of cell reproduction provides lots of nourishment and aids waste removal via lymph system.

Reticular layer

- Dense and fibrous, contains main components of dermis
- Found beneath the papillary layer
- Protects and repairs injured tissue, contains collagen, elastin, reticulin tissue.

The subcutaneous tissue

This is the fatty layer of the skin, underneath the dermis. Cells called *lipocytes* produce lipids, which are the fat cells from which we form subcutaneous tissue.

The job of the subcutaneous tissue is to:

- protect the muscles, bones and internal organs from being damaged
- provide insulation against the cold and to provide a source of energy if the body should need it.

Definition of terms

Lymphatic system A separate system of vessels that comes from the blood stream to filter toxins and waste by passing lymph fluid through a series of glands.

Collagen A protein found in white fibrous connective tissue. In the skin it provides strength and resilience.

Elastin Allows the skin to stretch easily, and then regain its original shape.

Reticulin Keeps all other parts of dermis in place.

Please refer to the diagram of the cross-section of the skin.

Structure	Location	Function
Sudoriferous glands There are two types:		
1 Eccrine glands (sweat glands)	Eccrine glands are found all over the body but dense on the palms of the hands and soles of the feet.	Eccrine glands produce sweat, water and urea, so help to regulate body temperature, remove toxin accumulations and help with the acid mantle.
2 Apocrine glands (post-puberty sweat glands)	Apocrine glands are fewer in number and larger tham eccrine. Only found in hairy parts of the body, i.e. armpits, nipples, anal and genital areas.	Apocrine glands are under the control of the nervous sysyem and respond to sexual attraction, emotional demands and psychological factors.
Hair follicle A threadlike outgrowth of the epidermis	Found in the dermis but not present on the soles of the feet or the palms of the hands or lips.	Produces and contains the hair during its life cycle
Hair Not present on the soles of the feet and the palms of the hand or on the lips	Grows in the follicles in the dermis and is then seen growing out through the epidermis	Believed to be connected to the production of body warmth. It is also a sexual characteristic.
Sebaceous glands Not found where there are no hair follicles present – see follicles	In the dermis, adjacent to hair follicles	Produces sebum to lubricate the hair and the skin. Combines with sweat to form the acid mantle. Helps to waterproof the skin
Erector pili muscle Muscle tissue	Attached to the hair follicle to the base of the epidermis	Raises the hair follicle to close the pore and so trap warmth in the body. Gives that goose pimple look to the skin
Nerves Sensory nerve endings	Found on the dermis and subcutaneous tissue	Responds to pain, pressure, heat, cold and touch. The nerves carry impulses to the brain for response by the body for protection.
Blood vessels These consist of arteries, veins and capillaries	Found in the dermis and subcutaneous layer	Arteries carry nutrients and oxygen to the skin via the capillaries. Veins remove waste products. Capillaries also help with heat regulation

Structures found in the dermis and subcutaneous layer

Check it out

1 Look in the mirror and see if you have any pigmentation marks, for example freckles. Do they appear more in the summer?
2 What causes your skin to change colour?
3 Feel the texture of your skin with the side of your little finger, is it smooth, oily, dry, or uneven, does it change on different areas?
4 Pull the skin up on the back of your hand – does it spring back quickly, or does the skin take a while to return to its place?

The nails

The nails are the hardened growth on the ends of the fingers and toes. Their cell formation is similar to that of the skin and hair follicle based on the protein keratin.

Structure	Location	Function
Matrix	Situated in the dermis in an area of dense fibrous tissue called the mantle	The reproductive part of the nail, where new cells are formed. It contains nerves, blood and lymph vessels
Mantle	An area of tissue that contains the matrix	Helps protect the matrix cells from damage
Nail bed	Underneath the nail plate	Continuation of the matrix, similar to ordinary skin, with a good nerve supply and blood vessels
Lunula (half moon)	At the base of the nail, linked to the nail plate. Sometimes hidden by the cuticle	Visible part of the matrix. It is crescent-shaped with translucent appearance
Nail plate	Lies on top of the nail bed	The compressed keratinised cells produced by the matrix from the nail. They lie in three layers
Nail wall	Around the three sides of the visible nail plate	The framework of skin to support the nail plate
Cuticle	The barrier that protects the matrix to prevent bacteria entering the nail	The horny layer of epidermis around the nail. It is constantly discarding old cells and producing new ones
Eponychium (Pronounced ep-on-nik-ee-um)	The extension of the cuticle around the nail	To prevent bacteria entering
Perionychium (Pronounced peri-on-nik-ee-um)	Surrounds the entire nail border	A framework of skin to support the nail plate
Hyponichium (Pronounced hy-po-nik-ee-um)	Underneath the nail plate where the free edge is formed	A horny layer of the epidermis for protection
Free edge	Extension of the nail plate which grows over and beyond the finger tip. Does not adhere to the nail bed.	For protection of the nerves at the fingertip. This is what we shape during a manicure. It is the hardest part of the nail

Structure of the nail

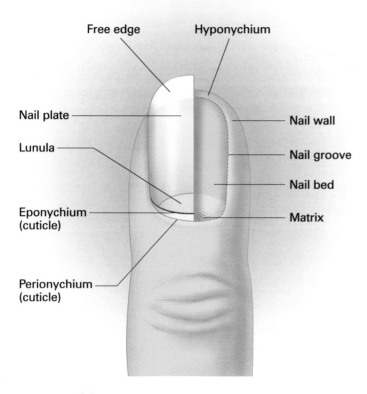
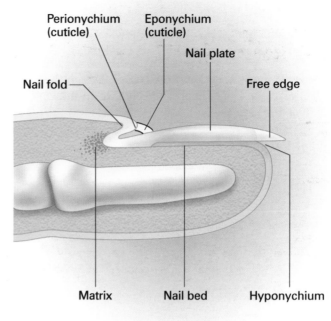

Structure of the nail unit

Nail growth

The cells in the matrix reproduce to form the nail plate. As the cells multiply they are gradually pushed up, before they die and harden. This process is called **keratinisation**.

For cells to reproduce, the matrix needs a good supply of oxygen and nutrients.

The growth of the nail can be influenced by:

- poor diet
- illness
- medication
- age
- time of year (more growth in summer)
- injury to the matrix or nail bed
- neglect.

If the cells in the matrix are damaged by illness or injury, the thickness of the nail plate can vary, showing itself as a furrow ridge or overgrowth of the nail plate.

A healthy nail grows at an average of 1 mm per week for finger nails, and 0.5 mm for toe nails, so it takes approximately six months for the nail to grow from matrix to free edge.

A healthy nail should have:

- supple unbroken cuticle
- no inflammation
- a natural sheen
- a pink glow from beneath the nail bed
- no ridges or spots
- an unbroken free edge.

> **Check it out**
>
> 1 Look at your hands and finger nails. Can you identify your lunula? Do your cuticles overgrow your nail plate and is your free edge growing over your finger tip?
> 2 How much does a healthy nail grow each month and what should your nails look like?
> 3 Are your nails healthy?

The muscles of the face, neck and shoulder area

Muscles

The body is made up of more than 600 voluntary muscles (i.e. muscles we can control). They make up 40% of a person's body weight. The contraction of these muscles causes body movement: it can be a large movement, for bending or running, or a small movement which brings about a change in facial expression.

The muscles of the face, neck and upper body (or trunk) are important when carrying out facial work, as in Unit 5 Application of make-up and Unit 6 Facials. An understanding of the position and the action of these muscles is vital for beauty therapists.

Forehead muscles

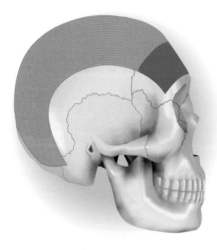 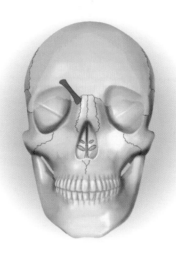 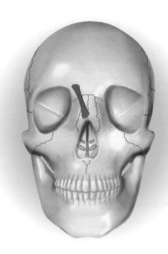

1 **Frontalis**
   - Upper part of the cranium
   - Scalp moves forward, raises eyebrow

2 **Corrugator**
   - Inner corners of the eyebrows
   - Draws eyebrows together – as in frowning

3 **Procerus**
   - Top of nose between eyebrows
   - Depresses the eyebrows, forming wrinkles over the bridge of the nose

Eye and nose muscles

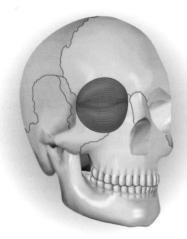 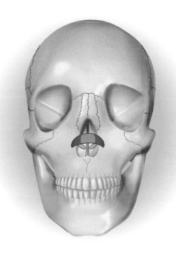

4 **Orbicularis Oculi**
   - Surround the eye
   - Closes eyes, blinking

5 **Nasalis**
   - Over the front of the nose
   - Compresses nose, causing wrinkles

Side of face muscles

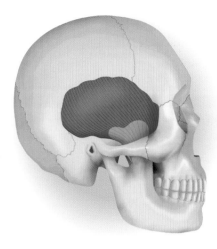

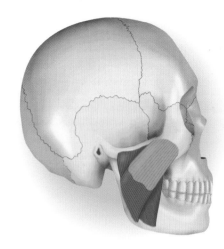

6 **Temporalis**
- Runs down side of face towards upper jaw
- Aids chewing and closing mouth

7 **Masseter**
- Runs down and back to the angle of the jaw
- Lifts the jaw and gives the teeth strength for biting

Cheek muscles

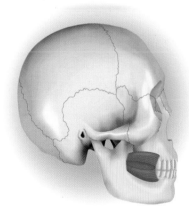

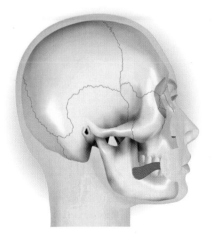

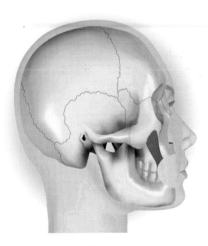

8 **Buccinator**
- Forms most of the cheek and gives it shape
- Puffs out cheeks when blowing, keeps food in mouth when chewing

9 **Risorius**
- In the lower cheek. It joins to the corner of the mouth
- Pulls back angles of the mouth – smiling and in grimace

10 **Zygomaticus**
- Runs down the cheek towards the corner of the mouth
- Pulls the corner of the mouth upwards and sideways

Mouth muscles

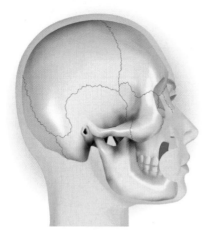

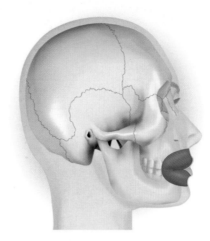

11 Quadratus labii superiorus
- Runs upward from the upper lip
- Lifts the upper lip and helps open the mouth

12 Orbicularis oris
- Surrounds the lips and forms the mouth
- Closes mouth, pushes lips forward

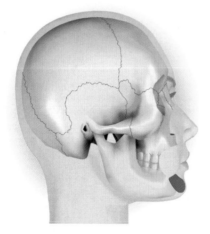

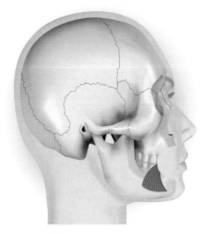

13 Mentalis
- Forms the chin
- Lifts the chin and moves the lower lips outwards

14 Triangularis
- Corner of the lower lip, extends over the chin
- Pulls the corner of the chin down

Neck muscles

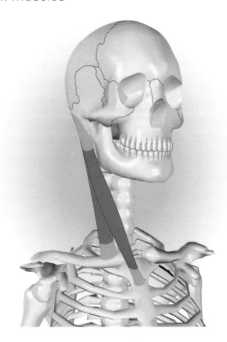

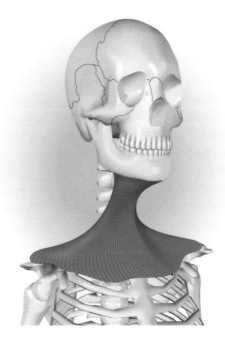

15 Sternocleidomastoid
- Either side of the neck
- Pulls head down to shoulder, rotates head to side and pulls chin onto chest

16 Platysma
- Front of throat
- Pulls down the lower jaw and angles of the mouth

Upper body or trunk muscles

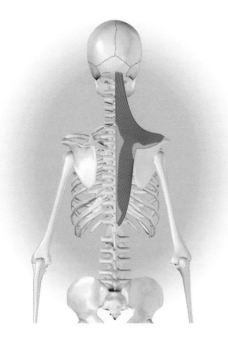

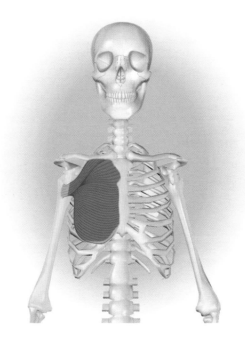

17 Trapezius
- The upper back and sides of the neck
- Rotation of shoulders, draws back the scapula bones, pulls head back, assists in rotation of head

18 Pectoralis
- Front of chest, under the breast
- Pulls arms forwards and assists rotation of the arm

Trunk

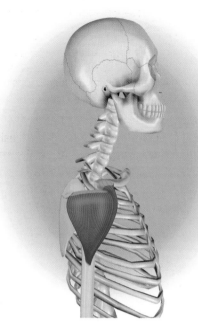

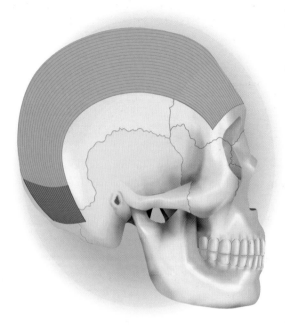

19 **Deltoid**
  - Caps the shoulder
  - Raises arm from the side, pulls it back and forward

20 **Occipitalis**
  - At the back of the skull
  - Helps with the movement of the head.

Check it out

1 Stand in front of a mirror and make faces. See if you can identify the muscles involved in making these facial expressions.
2 Can you think of any celebrities who have prominent facial muscles or bones?

The hair

Types of hair found on the body

Hair is found all over the body except on the lips, palms of the hands and soles of the feet. Different areas of the body have different types of hair. These can be divided into two types:

- vellus
- terminal.

Vellus

This is soft downy hair, covering most of the body. Normally without colour, it rarely grows longer than about two centimetres in length. Regardless of ethnic origin, vellus hair is usually straight due to the fact that the follicles are not very deep.

Terminal

Terminal hair grows from deep follicles which go down to the subcutaneous layer of the skin. They are strong hairs which contain pigment, and grow on the scalp, eyebrows, under the arms and pubic areas.

Terminal hair can be curly, wavy or straight depending on ethnic origin, hereditary factors and chemical hair treatments, such as perms! If a cross section was taken of a terminal hair for Europeans, the hair would be oval in shape, and would tend to be wavy. Asian hair would appear round in shape and tend to be straight, and Afro-Caribbean hair would appear flattened and tends to be very curly.

Hair growth

A normal hair in the body is contained in a tube-shaped pocket called a follicle. These follicles consist of an inner sheath and an outer sheath which are similar in structure to the cells of the epidermis.

The hair is made of hardened protein called *keratin*. The outside of the hair is a scaly layer called the *cuticle*. The hair grows from the bottom of its follicle by cell division, being fed by a good blood supply from the dermal papilla.

Hair growth is a continuous cycle of events, that is repeated as long as nourishment is available, or until the hair follicle is damaged through illness or the ageing process. Hair does become thinner in old age due to hormonal changes which occur within the body.

The life of a normal hair is divided into three stages:

- **anagen** – the growing phase
- **catagen** – the changing (transition) phase
- **telogen** – the resting phase.

Here is an easy way to remember the different stages of hair growth:

- **A** – active (anagen)
- **C** – change (catagen)
- **T** – tired (telogen).

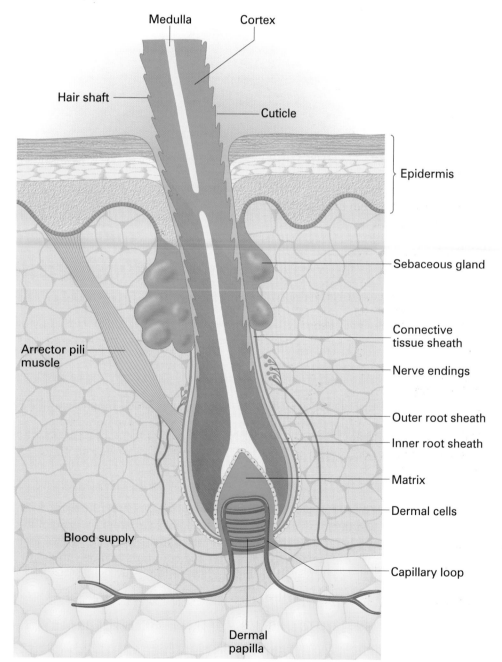

A vertical cross-section of hair in its follicle

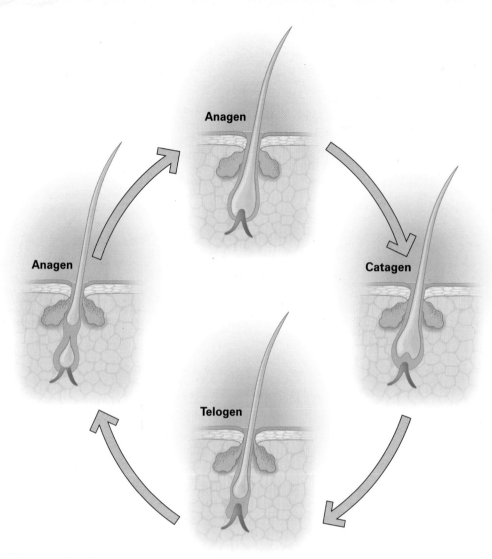

Hair growth cycle

Anagen

In the anagen stage the hair receives its nourishment via the blood supply from the dermal papilla. This enables the cells to reproduce. The cells move upwards and form the different structures of the hair shaft. Melanin cells are also produced and this forms the hair colouring.

Catagen

This is the resting or transition stage of hair growth. During this stage the dermal papilla breaks away and the lower end of the hair becomes loose from the base of the follicle. The hair is still being fed from the follicle wall and is sometimes known as a club-ended hair. The hair gradually becomes drier and continues to move up to just below the sebaceous gland. Here it is very vulnerable and can easily be brushed out.

Telogen

This is the final stage of hair growth and is the resting period. The follicle rests until stimulated by hormones to return to the anagen phase. Telogen lasts for a few weeks, with the club hair often being retained until new hair is produced – pushing the club hair out.

Check it out

1   Where would you find vellus hair?
2   What is the function of vellus hair?

Blood

Blood is the transport system for the body to deliver and remove vital ingredients needed by the cells in the body. It is pumped around the body by the heart. Arteries, veins and capillaries are the vessels that carry the blood to their destination.

Oxygenated blood flows from the heart through the arteries and deoxygenated blood flows back to the heart through the veins. Capillaries are very small vessels which form a network to get into tiny cell spaces to allow delivery (of oxygenated blood) and removal (of deoxygenated blood) to take place.

Blood is a slightly sticky fluid that is composed of:

- 55% plasma
- 45% blood cells.

Plasma is a yellow, transparent fluid made up of mostly water, with a small amount of protein present. There are three types of blood cells:

1   Red blood cells transport oxygen to the cells and take away carbon dioxide
2   White blood cells protect the body against invading bacteria and help form the immune system
3   Platelets play an important role in blood clotting.

Functions of the blood

The blood has three main functions in the body:

- transport
- regulation
- protection.

Transport

Blood transports or carries;

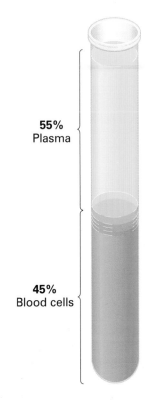

- **oxygen** from the lungs to the body cells
- **carbon dioxide** from the cells to the lungs
- **nutrients** from digestion to the cells
- **waste products** from the cells to be excreted
- **hormones** sent from the endocrine gland to regulate the cells
- **medication**, which can be passed into the cells.

Regulation

Blood regulates:

- **water** content of cells
- **body** heat.

Protection

- against **infection** and **disease**
- against **blood loss** by **clotting**.

55%
Plasma

45%
Blood cells

The structure of blood

The effects of massage on blood circulation

Massage increases the amount of blood flow into the area, which is seen as an **erythema** or reddening of the skin. The effects of this are that:

- it speeds up the flow of blood through the veins and therefore helps with the metabolic waste being carried away
- it increases the fresh blood to the area, bringing oxygen and nutrients to the cells and so helping with cell growth and repair
- warmth is created by the increase in blood flow, which is relaxing to the client
- because of the increase to the cells of oxygen and nutrients the skin will look and feel softer
- muscle efficiency and response is improved due to the increased oxygen and nutrients
- the removal of waste products gives a more toned appearance to the muscles and makes them more relaxed.

Blood flow to the face and head

Arteries of the head

The blood is pumped to the head via the common carotid artery, which has two branches. The internal carotid artery passes through the temporal bone of the skull behind the ear and takes blood to the brain. The external carotid artery remains outside the skull and divides into facial, temporal and occipital arteries which supply the skin and muscles of the face, side and back of the head.

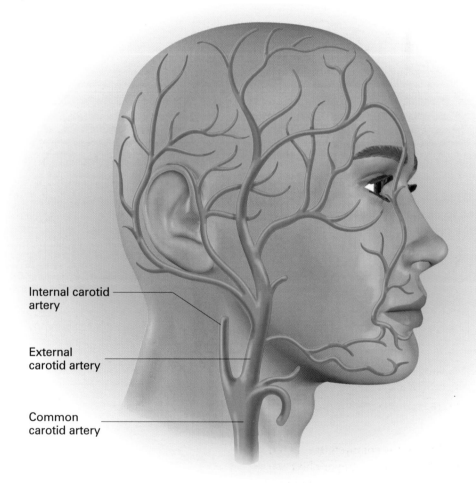

Arteries of the head

Veins of the head

Blood is collected up from the scalp capillaries by the facial, occipital and posterior veins, which run alongside the similarly named arteries. These join to form an external jugular vein behind and below the ear on both sides.

The external jugular veins go down the neck and enter the subclavian veins. An internal jugular vein brings blood from the brain, goes down on either side of the neck and enters the subclavian vein. The subclavian veins carry on towards the heart and eventually the blood enters the superior venae cavae.

> ## Check it out
>
> 1 Test your pulse rate. First take your pulse for 15 seconds and multiply by 4. This tells you your pulse rate at rest (multiplying by 4 gives you the rate per minute). Do this again after jogging on the spot for two minutes.
> 2 Has your skin developed any reddening?
> 3 What is this reddening called?

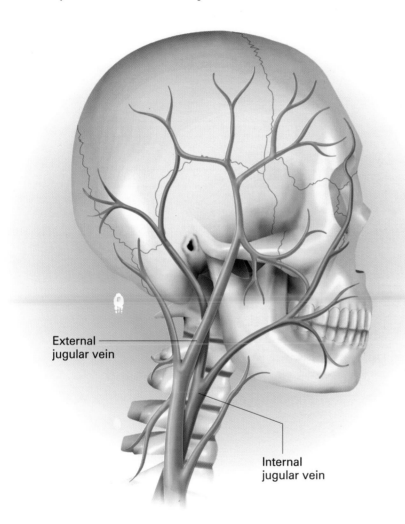

External jugular vein

Internal jugular vein

Veins of the head

The lymphatic system

The lymphatic system is the body's second circulation system for collecting waste products. It carries away waste from the tissues that the blood cannot manage to take. For example, you could think of it as a second bus that collects all the passengers the first bus left behind.

The fluid that is left behind is known as lymph and it is straw coloured. It is emptied back into the blood system via the subclavian vein which is in the upper chest. The removal of the lymph from around the body prevents the tissues from becoming clogged and swollen.

The lymphatic system also plays an important role in protecting the body against infection. At various stages along the route that the lymph travels are glands or nodes; you could think of these as bus stops. It is here that the lymph is filtered of bacteria and germs, and antibodies are produced to fight infection. When someone is ill the doctor often feels the glands in the neck and looks in the mouth. This is to find out if the glands are filtering the bacteria properly. If the glands are very swollen antibiotics may be needed to help the lymph nodes and antibodies fight infection.

Composition of lymph

Lymph is made up of:

- plasma
- proteins
- waste products
- toxins
- fats
- oxygen
- carbon dioxide
- urea
- lymphocytes.

Function of the lymph system

The purpose of lymph is to collect germs, bacteria and waste in the system, then to carry these to the lymph glands to be filtered and made harmless. The lymphatic system uses different methods to do this:

- the lymphatic system drains tissue fluid from the spaces between the cells
- it transports the tissue fluid and proteins back to the blood stream via the subclavian vein
- it transports fats from the small intestine to the blood
- it produces lymphocytes which protect and defend the body against infection and disease.

The benefits of treatments on the lymph system

As a therapist the treatments that you can perform can greatly assist the lymphatic flow. This is because:

- massage stimulates the flow of lymph so removing the toxins and fluid from the area faster
- general swelling can be reduced
- absorption of waste matter can be speeded up
- skin will be smoother and softer because cell renewal is helped.
- muscles will be relaxed and work more efficiently.

Lymphatic flow to the head and neck

Left side	Lymph from this side of the head and neck passes through the **thoracic duct** and empties into the **left subclavian vein** (the thoracic duct is situated in the upper chest under the rib cage).
Right side	Lymph from this side of the head and neck passes through the **right thoracic duct** and empties into the **right subclavian vein**.

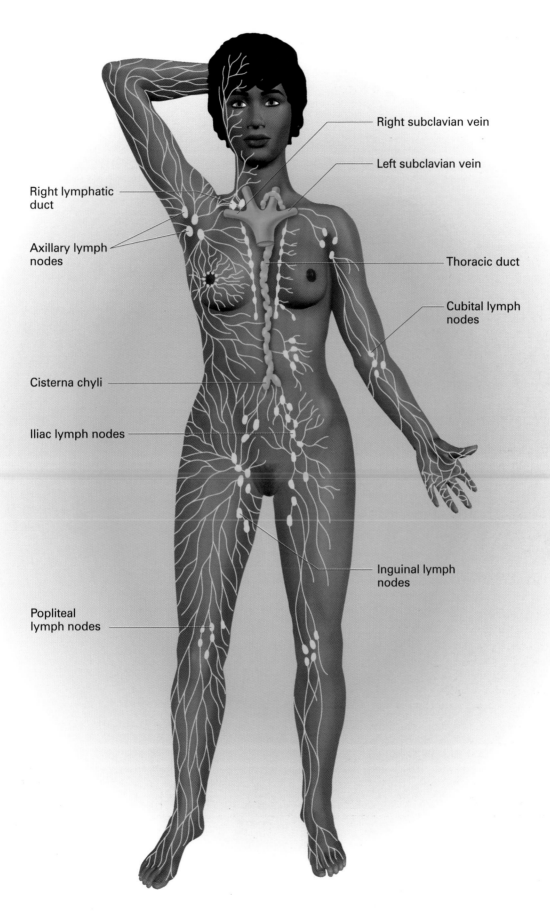

Right subclavian vein

Left subclavian vein

Right lymphatic
duct

Axillary lymph
nodes

Thoracic duct

Cubital lymph
nodes

Cisterna chyli

Iliac lymph nodes

Inguinal lymph
nodes

Popliteal
lymph nodes

Lymph nodes and vessels of the body

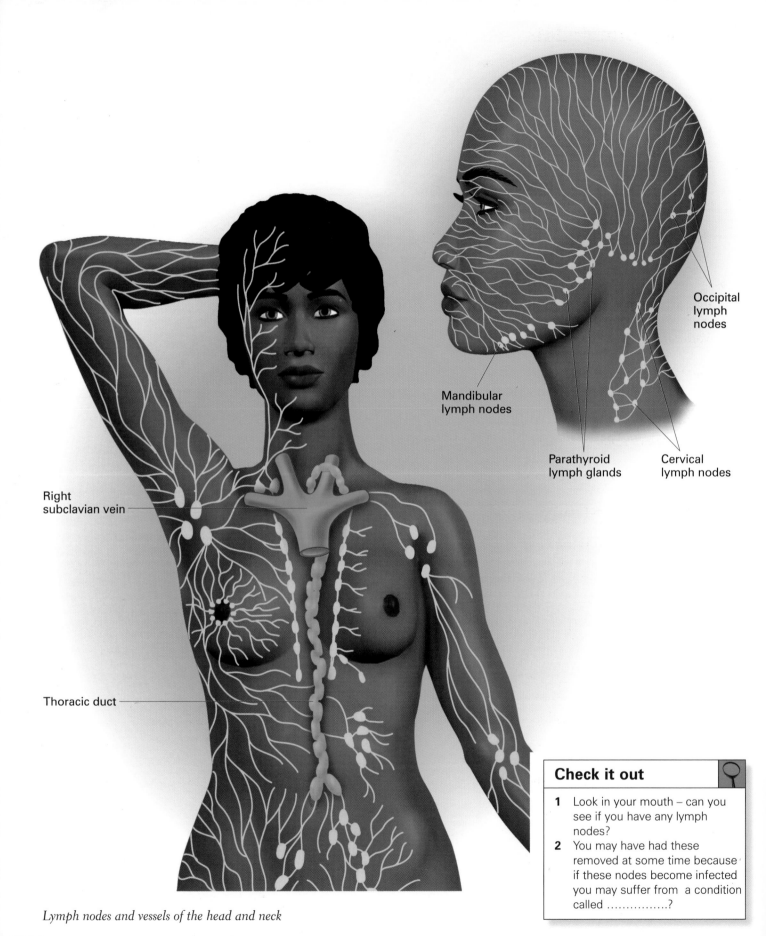

Lymph nodes and vessels of the head and neck

Right
subclavian vein

Thoracic duct

Mandibular
lymph nodes

Occipital
lymph
nodes

Parathyroid
lymph glands

Cervical
lymph nodes

Check it out

1   Look in your mouth – can you
    see if you have any lymph
    nodes?
2   You may have had these
    removed at some time because
    if these nodes become infected
    you may suffer from a condition
    called ....?

Test your knowledge

1   Name the five layers of the epidermis.

2   What is the function of the erector pili muscle?

3   What does desquemation mean?

4   What is another name for the collar bone?

5   Is the scapula fixed or can it move freely?

6   Name the bones that make up the skull.

7   What is the name of the cheek bone?

8   What is the protein that nails are composed of?

9   Name the half moon shape at the base of the finger nail.

10 Hairs have a gland that lubricates them, what is this called?

11 How many voluntary muscles does a person have?

12 Where are the pectoral muscles and what are their function?

13 List four functions of the blood.

14 Name the three vessels that carry blood around the body.

15 What colour is lymphatic fluid?

16 What vein joins lymph and blood together again?

practical SKILLS

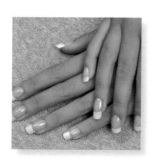 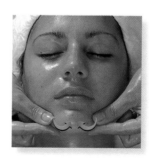 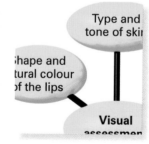

Enhance facial appearance using make-up techniques

Unit 5

This chapter contains the information that most of you will associate with becoming a beauty therapist, i.e. the application of make-up. The chapter focuses on the use of make-up to enhance the appearance, for day, evening and special occasions. Most women at some time have used make-up to enhance their appearance and have been pleased with the results – whether it was for hiding a blemish, for a special occasion or just a night out with friends. However, few people know how to use make-up to their best advantage, so it is very rewarding for a therapist to accentuate a client's best features and to enable her to disguise or minimise areas that she is not so happy with. Applying make-up correctly can help you do all this; correct application of make-up can boost confidence and self-esteem.

Within this unit you will cover the following elements:

5.1 Assess clients and prepare treatment plans
5.2 Prepare the work area and client for the application of make-up
5.3 Apply make-up to meet client requirements.

> **Remember**
>
> To carry out an effective make-up treatment you need to be able to identify and treat the client's individual skin type. Therefore, Unit 6 (Improve facial skin condition) is essential prior knowledge to ensure the best results.

Assess the client and prepare treatment plans

5.1

> **In this element you will learn about**
>
> - skin types
> - treatment planning for make-up
> - contra-indications
> - allergic reactions
> - sensitivity testing.

> **Remember**
>
> Make-up is a very personal thing. Whatever your perceptions of your client's background may be, don't make assumptions about how he or she would like to look. It's important to be sensitive to cultural differences, but never make assumptions.

Skin types

The knowledge you require to prepare the client for treatment is the same as that required for Unit 6.

Whatever tone of skin that you are preparing to make up, in order to ensure that the correct products are selected, you will need to carry out a skin analysis. This will cover:

- facial examination
- skin types
- record cards.

Treatment planning for make-up

Before a make-up can take place a full consultation should be undertaken so that an accurate assessment of the client and her needs can be made. This should be both by visual assessment of the skin and by asking a series of questions.

Visual assessment

This should be carried out on a cleansed and toned dry face, with the hair secured away from the face. You should analyse the client's skin type, facial features and bone structure in an upright position.

When carrying out an analysis for make-up the light should be falling directly onto the client's face. The light should be a combination of natural daylight and warm white fluorescent light.

Questioning the client

As well as the visual assessment, you should ask the client a few simple questions to help you both agree on a realistic treatment plan. Some useful questions to help you assess the client are listed below.

- How much make-up do you usually wear?
- What do you think are your best / worst features?
- Do you have any allergies to make-up or other related products?
- Is the make-up for a special occasion?
- Are there any colours you like / dislike?
- Are you trying to create a special look?

When you have gathered all the information you can agree a suitable treatment plan. You may both have differing views so it is important to agree on a suitable and realistic plan.

In the salon
The client comes to you with a picture of a model and wants to look like her. However, her face shape is not the same and her hair is a different length and colour. How would you deal with this client?

Remember
The facial features look very different when the client is laid flat.

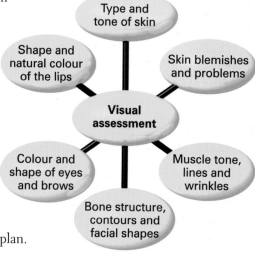

A visual assessment should include these areas

Remember
Warm white fluorescent light is the best substitute for natural light and the best for matching make-up colours.

Skin types

Skin types are usually described as belonging to one of the following four categories:

- normal
- dry
- greasy
- combination.

However, skin also falls into other categories and can be mature, sensitive, dehydrated, blemished and have broken capillaries. This all needs to be considered when choosing products for a client.

Skin can also be influenced by:

- genetic inheritance
- race and colour
- age
- hormones
- climatic changes
- central heating
- wrong products used
- prolonged illness
- medication or drugs taken – even the contraceptive pill
- poor nutrition
- smoking and alcohol intake
- stress
- allergies and reactions.

Normal skin

This skin type is recognised as soft, supple and flexible. The skin has a fine texture with no visible pores or blemishes.

Dry skin

Lacking oil and moisture, this skin type can leave the skin dry to the touch, with a tendency to flakiness. The skin is fine.

Pores and follicles are often closed and inactive and dilated capillaries may be present on the cheek area. Lines and wrinkles may also form early – especially around the eyes.

Sensitive skin

Often associated with pale or dry skin, sensitive skin lacks the protection of the skin's natural oil – sebum. This skin type may react to products and chemicals or by too much handling and may have a high flushed look.

Dehydrated skin

Any skin type may suffer from temporary dehydration due to exposure to harsh products, extreme temperature changes or due to dieting or medication. Flaking and tightness often indicate dehydrated skin.

Greasy skin

Greasy or oily skin is caused by the over-production of sebum (oil) from the sebaceous glands. It gives the skin a shiny appearance, enlarged pores form and spots and infection can be present. This skin type is often associated with puberty, when hormone levels fluctuate.

Combination skin

This is probably the most common skin type, with a combination of two or more types of skin condition. The most common is having an oily T-zone (across the forehead, down the nose and sometimes onto the chin) and dry cheeks. When carrying out a make-up treatment, products must be carefully selected for this skin type to ensure the best effect is achieved.

Congested skin

Poor removal of make-up, the wrong products and excessive sweat can all contribute to this skin condition. The pores become blocked and sweat and sebum build up, causing blackheads and whiteheads. The skin will feel lumpy and bumpy to the touch.

Infected skin

Any bacteria, fungi or virus can penetrate the skin and cause an infection. This is recognised by swelling and irritation, often with pain and tenderness, The presence of pus is also a sign of infection. Bacteria enter the follicle, causing a blocked pore, and this causes acne vulgaris. It would be advisable to send the client with acne to the GP for medical treatment before carrying out a make-up treatment.

Skin analysis for black skin

On first inspection black skins usually appear shiny, so it is often presumed that they are greasy, but this is not always the case. Black skins do have more sweat and sebaceous glands and lack the vellus hair that is found on Caucasian and some Asian skins. As black skin has a thicker epidermis the skin desquamates (loses cells) more than a white skin and this may make the skin appear grey, also an erythema (reddening) on a black skin appears only as purple patches. Therefore, a correct skin analysis requires the use of a 'wood's light'. This light should be used in a darkened room as it uses ultraviolet rays. These rays show as different colours depending on the skin type.

Skin type	Fluorescent colour
Normal	Purple / blue
Dry	Pale violet
Greasy	Coral pink
Hydrated	Deep violet
Thick horny layer	Strong white
Thin horny layer	Purple
Build-up of dead cells	Silvery white
Increased pigmentation	Brown

Black skin analysis

⚠ Contra-indications

It is important that a make-up treatment is not carried out if a contra-indication is present. Contra-indications include:

- bacterial/viral and fungal infections of eyes, lips or face
- open cuts and abrasions
- broken bones
- acute acne
- severe eczema or psoriasis.

Please refer to the **Professional basics** section (page 27) for details of micro-organisms and the diseases they cause and also how to minimise the risk of infection.

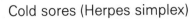

Viruses

The common cold

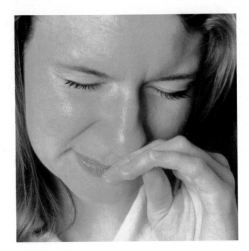

The common cold

Freely recognised. Streaming eyes and nose, coughing and sneezing easily spread.

Cold sores (Herpes simplex)

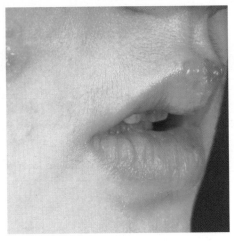

Cold sores

Found on the lips, cheeks and nose. Blisters form, the skin is broken and painful; the blisters are especially likely to spread when open and weepy and then crusts form.

Warts

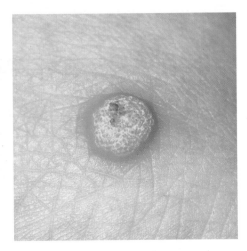

Warts

Small compact raised growths of skin – can be light or brown in colour, present on the face and neck.

Bacterial infections

Impetigo

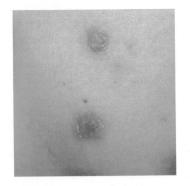

Impetigo

Highly infectious, this starts as small red spots, which then break open and form blisters. Most common around the corner of the mouth and if picked, will spread. (Some strains are particularly resistant to antibiotics.) Can be spread through use of dirty equipment.

Boils

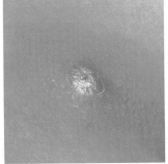

Boils

This infection forms at the base of a hair follicle. Bacteria can spread through an open scratch in the skin. The area is raised, red, and painful. Pus may be present.

Conjunctivitis

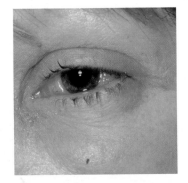

Conjunctivitis

This is a nasty eye condition. The eyelids are red and sore, with itching. Mainly caused by bacteria present, it can be irritated by a virus or an allergy.

Stye

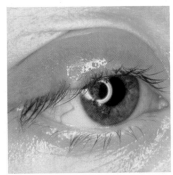

Stye

This is a small boil at the base of the eyelash follicle. It is raised, sore and red; there may be considerable swelling in the area.

Fungal infections

Ringworm (tinea corporis)

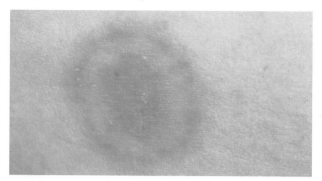

Ringworm

Red pimples appear and then form a circle, with clear skin in the middle. It is highly contagious and scales and pustules follow. It can be spread onto the face from any other area of the body. Can be passed onto humans by contact with domestic animals.

Blepharitis

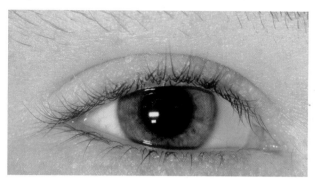

Blepharitis

An infection of the lid causing inflammation, the eye will look red and sore. Depending on the severity of the condition, it may be better to avoid eye make-up application altogether, and focus attention on the mouth, with a pretty lipstick shade.

All of the conditions mentioned would be a contra-indication to make-up application to the face. The beauty therapist carries a heavy responsibility for protecting everyone from contamination via these micro-organisms.

Conditions restricting the effectiveness of make-up

The following conditions are contra-indications that will not necessarily stop the treatment from taking place, but they may mean that make-up application has to be restricted and / or adapted. Most of these conditions are common sense, and professional judgement can be used. If the problem is not directly on the face or neck, where make-up application takes place, then just avoid the area.

Each one will depend upon the individual case, the client granting permission, and then giving **written permission** on the record card.

Cuts / abrasions / broken skin

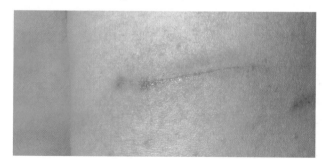

Cut

If recent, a scab will be forming, the skin may be tender and swollen in the area, and bruising may be seen. If cuts and abrasions are recent, then avoid the area altogether. If the area has healed over, and is not too recent, get the client's agreement that gentle application can take place, with careful consideration to hygiene.

Bruises or swelling

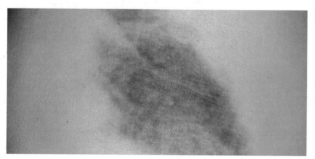

Bruise

Easily recognised as a swelling, with discoloration in varying shades. Avoid altogether if recent or painful to the touch. If healing has taken place, a gentle application of make-up will help to blend in the colour differences to the client's normal shade. Always ask for client's agreement.

Recent scar tissue

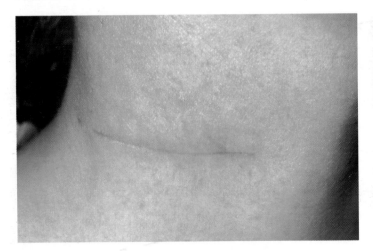

Scar tissue

Usually a different colour to the rest of the skin, following the line of injury. If the scar is recent, raised or angry looking, then avoid the area altogether. If the area is healing and not very large, gentle application with clients' permission. Scar tissue less than six months old, or over a large area, should not be touched with make-up.

Eczema

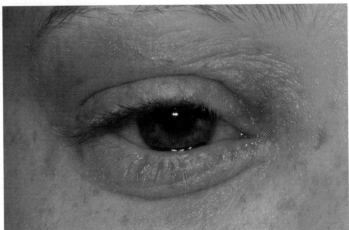

Eczema

Very dry skin, often scaly and flaky, can be red and often very itchy. If the eczema covers a large area, and is inflamed with broken skin, then leave alone, and suggest a visit to the GP. You may make it worse. If the eczema has irritated the eye area, it is unlikely the client would want make-up application. If it is only a small patch of eczema, and not angry, just exclude the area from treatment. The use of hypo-allergenic products is recommended and patch test if the client is very sensitive.

Dermatitis

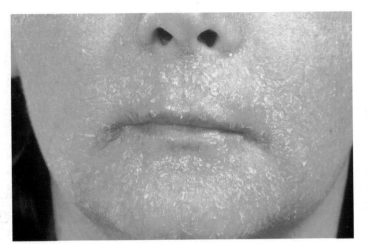

Dermatitis

This is similar to eczema in appearance, but the cause is not the same. A reaction or allergy to something in contact with the skin usually causes dermatitis. *See as above.*

Skin allergies may result in a contra-action so if the client's skin tends to react, do a skin patch test 24 hours prior to the make-up application. It may be wise to use hypo-allergenic make-up, and ask the client to bring in her own make-up if she is knows she is safe using it.

Psoriasis

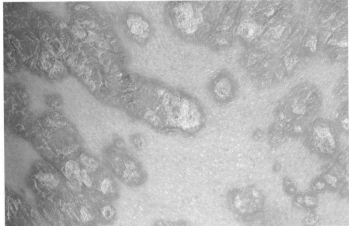

Psoriasis

Seen as scaly patches of red and / or silvery skin. This can break open and become sore. The cause is unknown but is thought to relate to the nervous system. A contra-indication would be if the psoriasis is open or bleeding. One of the common sites for psoriasis is the scalp, so the client may have a little patch visible along the hairline. If the client agrees to make-up application, and it is not directly over the area, then continue. A patch test 24 hours prior to the application of make–up is advisable to ensure that the condition is not aggravated.

Acne vulgaris

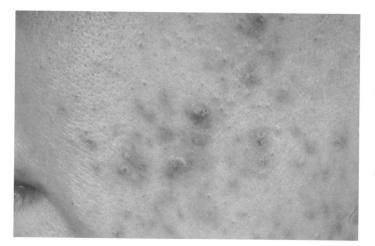

Acne vulgaris

Inflamed whiteheads, blackheads and pustules in various degrees of congestion. Mostly associated with hormones – and the presence of bacteria can make the condition infected.

Infected inflamed acne is a contra-indication. However, a client with mild acne can be treated in the salon, and a light water-based foundation applied. There may be a tendency to greasy skin, and therefore a light application of powder keeps the skin looking matt.

Acne rosacea

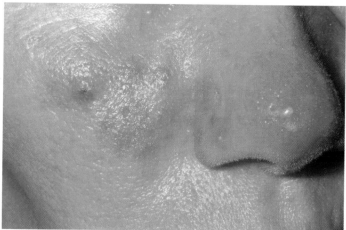

Acne rosacea

Seen as a flush of red over the nose and cheeks with a raised feel to the skin. Often those who have suffered acne vulgaris in youth are prone to rosacea in later life. If the skin is not tender and the client agrees, application of make-up can tone down the redness and therefore lessen the angry look of the skin.

Skin tags

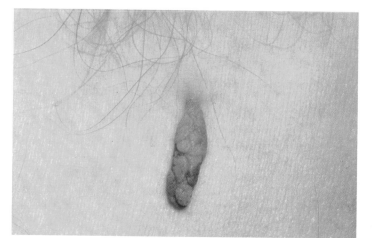

Skin tags

Usually found on the eye area or lids and / or on the side of the neck. They resemble little 'mushrooms' of skin on a stalk, which move when touched.

As these are not painful or dangerous, make-up application can take place. If they become enlarged and irritating to the client they can be removed under local anaesthetic, usually at the GP's surgery.

Milia

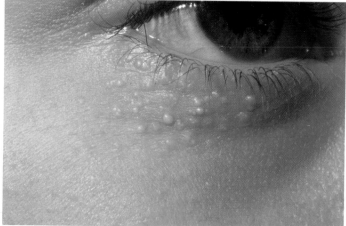

Milia

These are small white pearls under the skin, often around the eyes or on the side of the cheek, caused by a build-up of sebum. Make-up application can take place over milia, as they are not infectious.

Pigmentation disorders

These disorders are caused by irregularities in the skin's melanin production. They are not infectious and are not a contra-indication to facial or make-up treatments. Pigmentation disorders do affect the client's appearance, however, and may make the client feel embarrassed and self conscious; as a therapist, you therefore need to treat them sensitively. The use of camouflage cosmetics may help more effectively with the matching of the pigmentation than ordinary foundations and concealers.

Melanoderma

This is a general term used to describe patchy pigmentation. This is usually an increase in melanin caused by applying cosmetics or perfume which contain light-sensitive ingredients – the skin becomes extra sensitive to UV light (e.g. bergamot oil used in the perfume industry). Some drugs have a similar effect. This can also follow inflammation and is sometimes the cause of brown patches following sunburn.

Vitiligo	Chloasma	Freckles (Ephilidies)	Lentigo
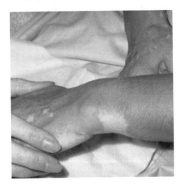	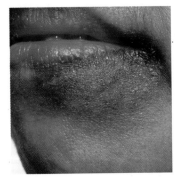	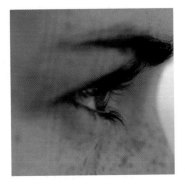	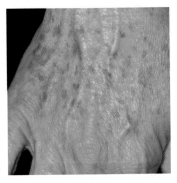
Vitiligo	*Chloasma*	*Freckles*	*Lentigo*

This is a condition in which small patches of skin have lost their pigmentation, and appear a lighter colour than the rest of the skin. These lighter areas burn easily in the sun and need to be protected. It is not raised or painful to the touch. If the discoloration is in large patches a specialist camouflage make-up should be applied to conceal and match the skin tone. This may mean referral to a specialist. If the patch is small, clever choice of foundation and careful application is acceptable. Any pigmentation disorder may require the use of specialised make-up products to ensure even coverage, and the correct colour match of the skin.

This consists of irregular patches of brown pigment caused by the over-production of melanocytes. This often appears on the face during pregnancy and is sometimes linked to the contraceptive pill. The discoloration usually disappears when the hormone balance is restored.

These are tiny, flat irregular patches of pigment on fair-skinned people, particularly blonde / redheads. They are due to the uneven distribution of melanin, and this becomes more noticeable on exposure to strong sunlight. The freckles often increase in size and join together. The skin between the freckles contains little or no melanin so burns easily. As a therapist you should recommend a good sunscreen to the client.

Larger and more distinctive than a freckle, and may be slightly raised. This pigmentation does not increase in number or darken on exposure to UV light.

Haemangioma

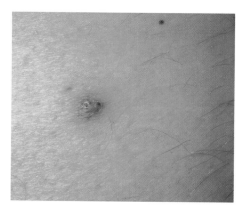

Haemangioma

This consists of various conditions caused by the permanent dilation of superficial blood vessels. Stimulating treatments will therefore be a contra-indication to treatment, but the use of camouflage cosmetics can be used.

Dilated capillaries

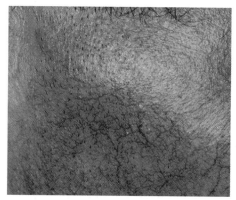

Dilated capillaries

This is the result of loss of elasticity in the walls of the blood capillaries – the cheeks and the nose are often most affected. Exposure to weather, harsh handling and lack of protection, along with spicy hot foods and alcohol, can also be contributing factors. Clients with dry/sensitive skin types are most likely to be affected.

Split capillaries

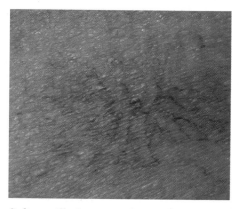

Split capillaries

Weakening and rupturing of capillary walls – clients should avoid stimulating treatments. This condition can be treated by diathermy.

Naevus

This is the term used to describe a variety of birthmarks and developmental abnormalities. It is the most common disorder involving melanocytes.

Strawberry naevus

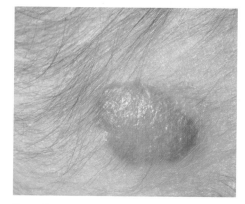

Strawberry naevus

This is a raised and distorted area, often on the face, bright pink / red. It appears a few days or weeks after birth and usually clears up completely by the age of eight.

Spider naevus

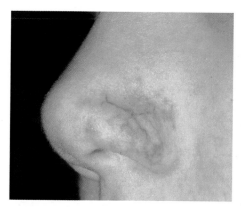

Spider naevus

A central dilated vessel with leg-like projections of capillaries. The face and cheeks tend to be most affected and this often occurs during pregnancy due to the increase in oestrogen levels.

Port wine stain

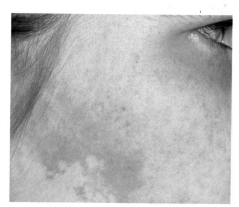

Port wine stain

This is a bright purple, irregular shaped flat birthmark that can vary in size. These birthmarks are thought to be due to damage by pressure during foetal development. These birthmarks grow with the body and can be quite disfiguring to the client. As a therapist you should always treat such marks sensitively with good cosmetic camouflage make-up.

Allergic reactions and sensitivity testing

In the European Union and the United States of America the law requires that cosmetic companies conduct very strict safety tests on materials they use to formulate products. Nevertheless, there will always be some people who are allergic to a substance which other people can tolerate without a problem. It is therefore essential that you complete a sensitivity test if you are concerned that the client may react to a product. This can be done by testing a small sample of the product behind the client's ear or in the crook of the elbow. If a reaction occurs within 24 hours the product should not be used. A reaction could include:

- redness (erythema)
- swelling
- irritation to the area.

Treat with calamine lotion and a cold compress as necessary.

Legislation

Different laws have been passed to protect both you and your clients.

The Consumer Protection Act 1987

This Act was passed following European Union directives to safeguard the consumer against unsafe products. The Act covers product liability, safety and pricing.

The Cosmetic Products (Safety) Regulations 1989

This is linked with the Consumer Protection Act and requires cosmetics and toiletries to have safe and tested formulations.

Control of Substances Hazardous to Health (COSHH) 1992

This defines the regulations for the storage and safe use of products that may be hazardous to health.

Product labelling

By law, ingredients which are known to be irritants (or sensitisers) must be listed on the packaging, together with the precautions for use. Some make-up products contain substances which cause allergic reactions in people who are hypersensitive. For example:

- lanolin – a fatty substance used as a softening agent in skin creams and lipsticks
- eosin – a red dye found in some lipsticks
- perfumes – particularly those containing bergamot, lavender and cedarwood
- alcohol – a grease solvent and astringent used in cosmetics and skin care products
- cobalt blue – a pigment used to produce eye make-up colours
- pearlising agents – ingredients which give products a shimmering effect
- gums – adhesives and binding agents in cosmetics.

Eye irritation

Although products used around the eye area are very strictly tested, and only safe pigments are used, some can still cause irritation to some clients.

Hypo-allergenic products

If your client has sensitive or allergic skin you should use this type of product, which contains no perfume as well as fewer pigments and preservatives.

How long do cosmetics last?

The European Union Cosmetics Directive 1993 states that products which contain no preservatives and natural ingredients with a shelf-life of less than six months have to be stamped with an expiry date. The cosmetics that have been tested and meet the European safety requirements are not required to be date stamped. Europe gives a shelf-life for cosmetics that is approximately 30 months from the time of manufacture, so you could calculate how long you have had a product from the day that you opened it.

Cleaning of equipment

Brushes and sponges

These need to be cleaned in hot soapy water, which should be worked into the fibres before rinsing under running water. Brushes should then be given a final clean in an alcohol solution or suitable brush cleaner before drying naturally – this will prevent the bristles from becoming misshapen. Sponges require soaking for at least one hour in a suitable disinfectant, and should then be rinsed thoroughly.

Palettes

These should be scrubbed to remove waxy deposits, then dried thoroughly.

Cleansing of products to prevent cross-infection

There is little risk of products becoming infected if good hygiene procedures are followed. However, to prevent infection by products which are normally applied directly to the face, these simple rules should be followed.

- Eye and lip pencils – sharpen before use to expose a new surface.
- Lipsticks – transfer a small amount onto a spatula before applying. Use a disposable lip brush.
- Pressed powders (eye-shadow and blushers) – either transfer products onto a palette or have a good supply of clean brushes.
- Mascara – use a disposable mascara wand for each eye.

Salon lighting

It is important to work in good lighting when applying make-up to the client, so always try to face natural light. Natural daylight is pure white light, but this light does not just fall on the face from above – it is reflected from any light coloured surface it hits. Natural daylight is the only light that shows true colours, but also the cruellest form of light as it shows up imperfections. To achieve the best from your make-up a combination of natural light and warm white fluorescent lighting gives the best effect.

Artificial lighting

Make-up colours tested in the wrong light can give the wrong effect when applied. It is therefore important to be aware of the differing effects of various types of lighting.

Standard light bulbs

These produce a yellowish colour which dulls blue tones and makes red tones appear darker. A light bulb cover with a shade directs the light down, creating unnatural shadows.

Fluorescent tubes

White tubes give out a harsh blue–white light which makes colours appear cold. If the fluorescent tube is covered by a diffuser this will soften the effect and create very little shadow. Warm white tubes with a diffuser will therefore be the best type of artificial light for matching make-up colours.

Remember

It is worth remembering that if a product is not stored properly or used is incorrectly it will deteriorate a lot faster. If a product starts to smell, change colour or separate you should throw it away.

Remember

Some salons will include the products used in the make-up in the price of the treatment, therefore they could be applied directly from the container.

Reality Check!

Look at salons in your area. Does the price of a make-up include products?

Prepare the work area and client for the application of make-up

5.2

In this element you will learn about

- preparing for a make-up treatment
- preparation and procedure
- face shapes.

Preparing for a make-up treatment

The working area should be clean, tidy and well organised. Ensure you adhere to a professional standard regarding your appearance and that your working area complies with the health, safety and hygiene regulations, and you should consult your professional body for guidelines to prevent cross-infection. The main sources of infection during make-up are usually contaminated products, dirty tools and equipment, and applying make-up over infected areas.

Basic trolley equipment for a make-up procedure

The equipment will include:

- towels
- headband – for protection of client's hair
- cotton wool pads – for the application of face powder
- damp cotton wool pads – cleansing
- bowl of cold water – for irrigating any areas and for dampening sponges
- tissue – for blotting lipstick
- palette – for decanting and mixing colours
- spatula – for dispensing products
- lip brush – application of lipstick
- eye-shadow brush – application of eye-shadow
- mascara brush – application of mascara

All brushes should preferably be disposable to prevent cross-infection.

- sharpener – to sharpen eye and lip pencils
- cleansing cream
- skin tonic or astringent
- moisturisers – all suitable for the client's skin type
- foundation
- blusher
- face powder
- eye-shadows
- mascara
- lip / eyeliner
- lipstick
- hand mirror – to view the finished result
- cape or gown - to protect the client's clothing
- selection of make-up brushes.

Make-up brushes

Often referred to as the 'tools of the trade', a good set of brushes is essential in the application of any make-up. There are individual brushes available for each stage of the make-up application. For maximum benefit it is important to understand their usage.

Remember

There should be a variety of products to suit all skin types and suitable for a varied range of clientele.

Face powder brush

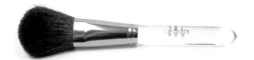

This is the largest brush as it covers the largest area. It is not restricted to defining shape, its primary purpose being to blend loosened face powder into the skin.

Blusher brush

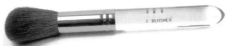

Used to apply blusher to the cheekbones. It looks similar to the powder brush but is slightly smaller in order to work on the cheek bone area.

Contour brush

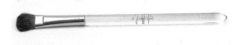

This brush has several uses: to apply contour powder under the cheek bones, to shade and highlight the face.

Eyebrow brush

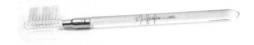

Used to shape the brows and to blend colour. It has short nylon bristles and may have a small comb on the other side to separate lashes.

Eye-liner brush

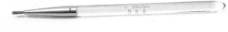

For the application of eye-liner or to blend in kohl pencils along the rim of the eye. A very thin and pointed brush is required.

Angled eye-shadow brush

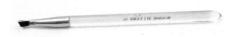

To apply and blend powder eye-shadow. The angle of the brush is important, it allows you to follow and blend into the socket area.

Eye-shadow brush

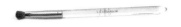

Used for general shading purposes. It is similar to the angle brush but with a straight edge.

Fluff brush

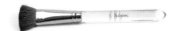

This brush is used to finish off the blending of the eye make-up. It is the largest of the eye brushes and it needs to be very soft, as it is used to soften the edges without disturbing the shape of the make-up.

Sponge applicator

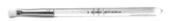

The sponge is good for applying both loose and powder eye-shadow. It is also used for blending and softening harsh pencil lines.

Lip brush

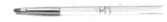

To apply lipstick, the brush must have short thin bristles to make it flat. This helps to give a clean outline to the lips.

Preparation and procedure

- Seat the client in an upright or slightly reclined position in good light.
- Remove any accessories, hair secured off the face.
- If the client wears contact lenses and has sensitive eyes remove the lenses.
- Protect the client's clothing.
- Check for contra-indications.
- Carry out a thorough skin analysis on cleansed skin.

Make-up consultation should include:

client preference
face shape
areas to be highlighted/shaded
any areas requiring corrective make-up.

- Agree a plan incorporating the above, taking into account the type of make-up required, the occasion, the colour of clothing to be worn, the client's clothing and the client's skin type.
- Agree products with client.
- Apply the make-up and explain the procedure to the client.
- Assess the results with the client, entering the colours / products used on the record card.
- Recommend products for homecare use.
- Check client satisfaction.

Face shapes

It is useful to consider some general descriptions of face shapes and some hair styles that can enhance a make-up. This will help when you are analysing the client's face shape at the consultation stage. Remember when applying make-up to clients with black skins that the entire positioning of facial features is different from European women. In African faces the jaw is more prominent, emphasising a large mouth and flatter bridge of the nose. These features can therefore provide excellent opportunities to emphasise the upper cheek bones and eyes.

Asian faces appear more oval but often need to be softened as they can appear angular. The eyes are usually the dominant feature of the face and can be enhanced by the use of a kohl pencil to give the eyes more definition.

Any corrective work on black or Asian skins should be approached in exactly the same way as for European skins, using contouring products to enhance or reduce areas.

Check it out

Look at the brushes and sponges you keep in your make-up bag. Are they clean with all bristles intact? Are the sponges caked in make-up? Even if you only use your make-up for yourself germs and infections can easily spread so get into good habits now.

Remember

Application time should be approximately 45 minutes for a make-over. A lesson should be approximately one hour.

Remember

When carrying out a bridal make-up, a practice should always be carried out in daylight to ensure true colouring before the actual wedding in order to make certain all parties are satisfied.

Oval face shape

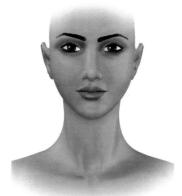

This face shape and bone structure is considered to be the ideal face shape. The chin tapers slenderly from a slightly wider forehead. The aim of make-up is to accentuate the natural shape.

Round face shape

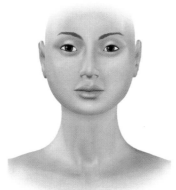

The face is usually short and broad with full cheeks and round contours. Width at the top of the head should be provided, with height from the hair, which should be worn close at the sides. The aim of make-up is to slim the appearance.

Square face shape

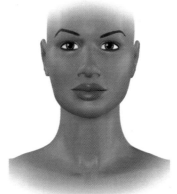

The forehead is broad, corresponding with an angular jawline. This shaped face should have a little height without width and the hair should taper well towards the jawline. The aim of the make-up is to narrow the forehead and the jawline, reducing the squareness of this bone structure.

Oblong face shape

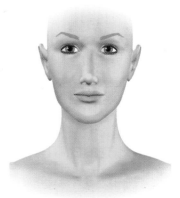

This face shape has a narrow shaped frame, the make-up aim is to create the impression of width and to shorten the face length. A fringe with short hair would be suitable.

Heart face shape

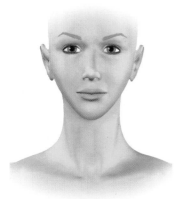

This shape usually has a wide forehead with the face tapering to a long jawline, rather like an inverted triangle. The aim of the make-up is to reduce the width across the forehead, emphasising the jawline.

Diamond face shape

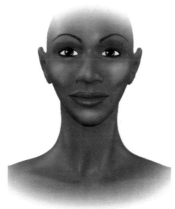

The forehead in this bone structure is narrow with the cheekbones extremely wide tapering to a narrow chin. The make-up aims to minimise the width across the cheekbones. A central fringe should be worn with hair full below the cheeks but flat at the cheekbone line.

Pear face shape

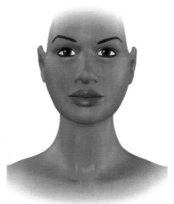

The forehead is narrow and the face gradually widens to the angle of the jaw which is broad and prominent. The make-up should aim to create the impression of width across the forehead and to narrow the jawline. The hair should be swept off the forehead to create an illusion of width with a reverse flicking fringe.

Triangular face shape

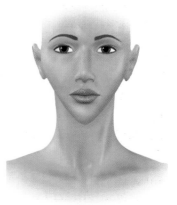

This is similar to the heart-shaped face, but not as soft. The aim of the make-up is to reduce the width of the jawline, by emphasising the forehead.

Apply make-up to meet client requirements

To achieve a successful make-up application whatever the occasion, you need to understand how and when to apply make-up products. The following pages introduce you to the main kinds of make-up products before giving step-by-step guides to make-up application for various occasions and times of day.

Sequence of make-up application

Concealer

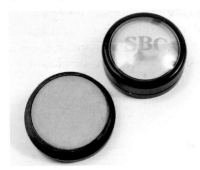

Colour-corrective concealer

This should be one or two shades lighter than the natural skin tone. Apply to the relevant area using a small brush / cotton bud. Press into the skin with a dry sponge. This applies both to the coverage of blemishes or when using colour-corrective concealer. When using colour-corrective concealer only apply to the areas that require it.

Foundation

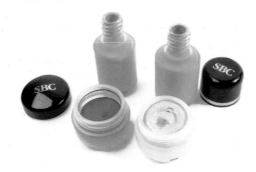

Foundation

The ideal shade will match the natural skin tone exactly – test the tone on the jawline. Work around the face using a damp sponge and fingertips, remembering to cover the eyelids and lips.

When you have finished, remove excess foundation from the hairline and eyebrows with some damp cotton wool. This stops the client's clothes from being marked.

Face powder

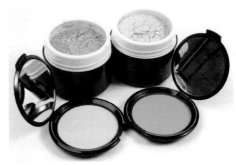

Face powder

Tip a small amount of loose powder into a bowl. If using block powder, scrape a small amount off into a bowl and apply with dry cotton wool. Work downwards, covering the eyes and all of the face, and then blend with a powder brush.

Blusher

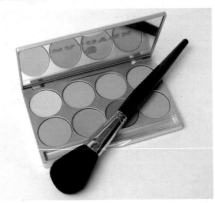

Blusher

Remove a small amount of blusher from the container and place on a make-up palette. Draw an imaginary line from the centre of the eye to the cheekbones – blusher stops here. To apply, start at the hairline and follow the line to the cheekbones. Work down the face in the same direction as the facial hair. If corrective work needs to be carried out, apply according to the face shape.

Eyebrow pencil

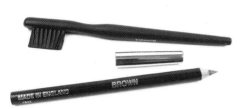

Eyebrow pencil and brush

Apply pencil if required. Brush brows to shape.

Eye-liner or kohl pencil

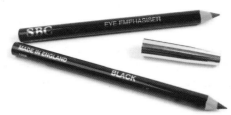

Eye-liner

This can be applied to give definition to the eyes. A pencil creates a softer look, and can be used on the top and bottom lids. A liquid liner gives a more defined look, but is not always suitable for the more mature client.

Eye-shadow

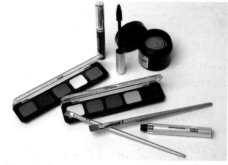

Eye-shadow

Place a folded tissue under the eyes – this will help to avoid shadow spillage onto the face. Apply individual eye-shadow colours, blend on completion.

Mascara

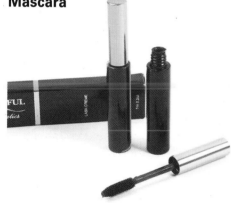

Mascara

Coat both sides of the lashes using a disposable brush. Remove any specks with a cotton wool bud.

Lipliner

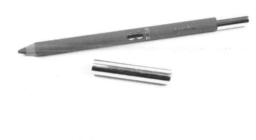

Lipliner

Apply to the outline of the lips. Ensure that colour is close to that of the lipstick, to avoid a harsh line.

Lipstick

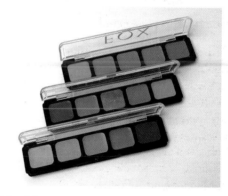

Lipstick

Use a disposable lip brush. After the first coat blot lightly and dust lips with face powder. Apply second coat.

Moisturisers

These products come in many forms and it will depend on the skin type of the client as to the one that you select. The purpose of a moisturiser when worn under make-up is to:

- even out the skin texture, and provide a smooth base for the foundation
- prolong the make-up by fixing it to the skin
- act as a barrier between the skin and the make-up by preventing pigmented products entering the pores, aiding cleansing.

Reality Check!

To minimise the risk of skin damage, you can use a moisturising product containing UVA and UVB sunscreens which protect against sunlight. These can be tinted to provide an alternative to foundation.

Concealing cosmetics

Concealer

There are few people who have a complexion that does not have some imperfections or areas they wish to change – this can be done by using a concealer. Concealer should be applied on small areas where necessary before the application of foundation. Use a colour nearest to the natural skin colour. Concealers come in various forms.

Cream concealer (camouflage)

Usually containing talc and kaolin, these creams have a thick consistency which completely covers all blemishes – including pigmentation marks, red birthmarks and dark shadows under the eyes. These creams come in a variety of colours that can be blended to match the skin.

Stick cover

These come in various shades to match the skin tone and are used to mask minor blemishes and imperfections (spots, dark circles under the eyes). They can be either oil or water based.

Medicated sticks

These are available for applying to minor spots and blemishes, containing antiseptic and drying agents. Never apply directly onto the skin or contamination or cross infection may occur.

Liquids

Liquid concealers are better for more mature skins where there are creases or wrinkles, as cream or stick concealers can clog in these areas emphasising them. When covering crow's feet it maybe best to use an anti-wrinkle product.

Correcting colour

Pigmentation creams can be used to help correct natural skin tone.

- Green is used to counteract high colour (redness).
- Lilac / pink brightens a sallow complexion.

The colour star

The colour star shows how opposite colours neutralise – for a basic corrective colour. So, for sallow yellow complexions, rather than applying corrective cream all over the face a tinted moisturiser containing lavender, lilac or mauve could be used.

Primary colours	Secondary colours
Red	Green
Yellow	Orange
Blue	Mauve

> **Remember**
>
> When using a colour corrector cream, only apply to the area of the face where it is required. Apply foundation over it, using a tapping action to prevent the corrector cream spreading and to ensure you achieve a smooth finish.

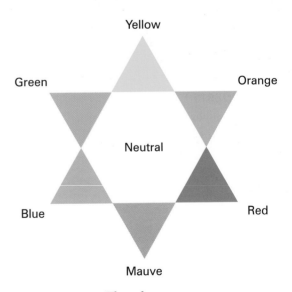

The colour star

Choosing a suitable foundation

A good foundation is probably the most important product when carrying out a make-up. The depth, tone and colour can affect all the products used. Foundations also provide a barrier to protect the skin and many now incorporate a sunscreen. A foundation is therefore used to:

- protect the skin
- conceal minor blemishes and imperfections
- provide a smooth finish
- enhance the natural skin colour.

Choosing a foundation for the client's skin colour and tone

The foundation should match the facial skin but this is not always the case when the hair has been dyed and the colour and tone have been altered.

The therapist should be aware of various tones that occur naturally in the skin. The tone of the skin is created by pigmentation in the epidermis. Skin is therefore described as:

- light
- medium (containing neutral, pink, red or blue tones)
- dark.

These simple rules can help choose a foundation colour for any skin shade:

- match or add warmth to neutral tones (honey, gold, tan)
- pink / red tones (beige, olive)
- yellow / blue (rose, gold, bronze)
- dark tones (dark bronze, sun bronze, deep peach)
- medium tones (cool beige, soft beige, tan)

It is important to get a good colour match when selecting your foundation – you don't want your client to look fake with an orange face or have a ghostly appearance. It is worth remembering that there are many different variations in skin tone so choose carefully. This may take you a little time or may require you to mix two or more colours together to achieve the desired shade and tone.

To test a foundation on your client for the first time, apply to the angle of the jawline. If the colour becomes darker or has an orange tone, you will need to choose a paler or cooler shade of foundation for your client.

Types of foundation

Foundations are available in many forms:

- cream
- liquid
- cake and pan cake
- gel
- medicated
- mousse.

Most of them are oil or water based with the addition of pigments for colouring and other ingredients to enhance and change their texture and aid the effectiveness of the product.

Cream foundations

This type of foundation blends easily on the skin because of the oil base, and contains wax, powder and a humectant (a product added to keep it moist), such as glycerol. This type of product gives medium coverage and is suitable for normal, dry, combination and mature skins. For a good finish this foundation should always be set with loose powder.

Liquid foundations

These foundations provide colour without being too heavy. They contain a higher proportion of water and give a light / medium coverage. In some products the oil is replaced with alcohol, which evaporates leaving only the powder and pigment. They are suitable for different skin types:

- oil based – normal, dry and mature skin types
- water based – combination / greasy
- alcohol – greasy.

The base of the foundation should be marked on the container.

Cake foundations

These foundations are usually applied with a damp sponge, so they can be applied as thinly or as thickly as required by adjusting the amount of water used on the sponge. Cake foundations usually contain compressed creams with extra powder for good coverage. Cake foundations give medium/heavy coverage suitable for:

- normal skin
- combination skin
- blotchy, blemished, discoloured or scarred areas
- dry or mature (cream based)
- greasy (powder based).

Pan cake foundation

This product is used a lot in the Far East as it is suitable for humid climates. The colour that appears in the compact is the colour that will appear on the skin.

Gel foundations

A gel product will provide a thin translucent colour that gives a natural look. Gels are produced like a liquid foundation but have an additional ingredient to produce a gel consistency, e.g. gum tragacanth.

Gels produce a natural tanned effect and are very popular in the summer; many now contain sunscreens. They are suitable for:

- tanned skins
- smooth skin with no imperfections, requiring a natural effect.

Medicated foundations

This type of foundation is a liquid containing antiseptic ingredients, making it suitable for greasy, blemished skins. It can be used over mild acne, but care should be taken with hygiene. It is worth remembering that severe acne is a contra-indication to a make-up application.

Mousse foundations

This type of foundation is suitable for combination to normal skin. Most are made with mineral oils, although some are made with herbal extracts. This type of foundation can be slightly more expensive to buy. If you do apply this foundation to oily skin be aware that it can be streaky if not carefully applied.

Skin type	Recognition	Suitable foundation
Normal	Small pores, fine texture Soft, supple, flexible, healthy	Cream / powder
Dry, dehydrated	Matt, uneven texture Lacks suppleness Lines and wrinkles Dilated capillaries common on nose and cheeks	Cream
Oily	Shiny, thick, blackheads Papules and pustules Open pores	Medicated liquid foundation Non-oily block / cake
Combination	Any combination of skin type – the most common is oily T-zone with dry cheeks	All-in-one fluid and powder combination
Sensitive / dry	Combination of dry areas with sensitivity Tight red appearance, broken capillaries	Hypo-allergenic products
Sensitive / allergy-prone	Reacts to products Skin flushes easily, which may appear in patches Dilated capillaries	Hypo-allergenic products

Cautions when applying foundation

Apply with a clean sponge or flat brush – these help when applying to awkward areas such as nose or eyes. Thin coverage can be achieved by using a natural sponge slightly damp. This type of sponge can, however, leave streaks because it is porous, so careful blending needs to take place. When a heavier coverage is required a latex sponge provides a smooth finish; a latex sponge is also less expensive.

Blend the foundation from the centre of the face to the hairline, this prevents clogging foundation in the hairline. You need to work quickly or the foundation will streak. Cover eyes and lips as this will provide a good base for eye-shadow and lipstick. When applying foundation to a more mature client who may have crepey skin around the neck and eyes, add a little moisturiser – this thins out the foundation and helps to prevent creases.

Check the application around the nose, hairline and chin to ensure smooth application and no visible lines.

Check it out

Look at one range of cosmetics available locally and see what types of foundation they offer. Are you able to buy suitable products for all skin types and skin colours?

In the salon

Mrs Jones comes into the salon with very dry skin and her foundation looks patchy. What could you recommend to help this client improve the appearance of her make-up?

Face powder

For a really professional appearance, most cream-based make-up products should be set with powder. Loose powder should be used for all professional make-up applications and the correct shade of pressed powder supplied for retail purchase by the client. A powder is applied to:

- 'fix' the foundation
- give a smooth matt finish
- reduce shine
- absorb grease
- protect the skin
- help conceal minor blemishes.

Loose powder

These come in two different textures – heavy and fine.

Heavy powders are often pigmented to complement the foundation and give a good cover; they contain a high proportion of kaolin and chalk.

Fine powders contain talc and a majority are translucent, which allows the colour of the skin or foundation to show through.

Some powders contain metallic particles for a pearlised effect, suitable for evening wear. If you decide to use a pearlised powder remember that it will accentuate lines and blemishes, so it will not be suitable for mature or blemished skins.

The application of loose powder should always be applied in a salon in preference to pressed powder because of hygiene. If, however, you apply pressed powder it should be decanted onto a palette before being applied, to prevent contamination.

Pressed powder

This is a product in a block that fits into a compact. The binding agent is usually gum or wax, which joins the particles together. Pressed powder is used for touching up the make-up during the day; however, this powder is not fine enough to produce an even finish on freshly applied foundation.

Always avoid areas with excessive hair growth as powder will collect there and draw attention to the area. Also avoid applying to dry flaking areas, because the area will dry out further and it will be accentuated.

Cautions when applying powder

- Dispense a small amount onto a palette.
- Firmly screw up a cotton wool pad and press into the powder, shake off excess in rolling movements, gently press into the foundation, covering all areas including eyes and lips.
- Remove any excess with a brush – firstly against the hair growth and then down the face to smooth the facial hairs and produce an even finish.
- Use a clean brush to remove any powder that has settled on the lashes or eye brows.

Contouring cosmetics

These are a range of products which are similar to foundations and powders, with the addition of coloured pigments. They come in powder, liquid, cream and gel. Contour cosmetics consist of:

- blushers
- highlighters
- shaders.

Blushers

Blushers add warmth to the make-up and give the skin a healthy glow to help define the facial features. They come in a wide range of colours. Pale colours can be used to soften and highlight areas. Bright colours can accentuate, and deep tawny colours and bronzes can shade areas. Blushers also come in a variety of forms, including gels, creams and powders.

Gels
- Best on clear skins.
- Good for the summer.
- Give cheeks a non make-up healthy glow.
- Can be applied directly over moisturiser.

Creams
- Give skins a moist dewy finish.
- Work best when applied over moisturisers and foundation.
- Good for normal or dry skin types.

Powders
- Matt or frosted finishes available.
- Applied for best results over powder with a large brush.
- Good on oily skins, but suitable for all skin types.

When choosing a blusher it should complement the foundation or natural skin tone. When applying a blusher it is best to build up the colour gradually to achieve the desired effect. It is the depth and tone of colour that needs to be selected carefully.

The use of blusher can help to alter the shape of the face. If you wish to reduce the width of the face, but give an illusion of length, keep the blusher to the side of the face, blending from just underneath the cheek bones to the temples. To create extra fullness apply the blusher to the cheeks or blend from the angle of the cheek bones to the ears. If you don't wish to change the shape of the face the blusher is usually placed on or near the cheek bones.

Highlighters

Highlighters are used to emphasise features and to create the illusion of extra length and width. The pale colours of highlighters reflect height. Use white, ivory and cream on pale skins for a subtle effect. When using a highlighter on a dark foundation it should belong to the same tone family:

- pale pink over rose shades
- pale peach over warm foundations.

The use of pearlised products are effective as highlighters, but avoid these on mature skins or hairy areas as this will draw attention to the areas.

Shaders

Shading is used to create artificial shadows or to reduce the size of areas. The colours suitable for shading contain brown pigments, which range from medium beige to dark brown. Beige is dark enough to shade when used over a pale base.

It is important to remember that the darker the foundation the deeper the shade needs to be. Warm brown colours should be avoided as a shader as they tend to look orange when applied over foundation and then act as a blusher.

Remember

To check if the colour of a product is strong enough to show up effectively, take a small amount of colour onto your finger – if the colour on your finger has the same depth as that in the compact, the colour will be suitable.

Remember

- Light colours define areas.
- Dark colours make areas recede.

Foundation may also be used to change the shape of an area, minimise or make less noticeable. To do this use a foundation two or three shades darker than the natural skin colour and blend into the ordinary foundation with either a sponge or brush.

Cautions when applying contouring products
- Use soft round-ended brushes that make blending easier.
- Tap any excess powder blusher onto a tissue or palette before applying, for a more subtle application. It is easier to build up colour in this way.
- When using a gel or cream apply with a damp sponge.
- Blusher application should start on the cheek-bones level with the midpoint of the eye.
- Regularly check you are achieving a balanced effect.
- Keep blusher and highlighter away from the corners and the lines of the eye.
- Ensure contouring is subtle for day wear for a natural appearance.
- Use corrective techniques to try and achieve a balance to the facial features. This helps emphasise the best areas and takes attention away from problem areas.

Corrective make-up

The use of contouring products to emphasise and diminish areas to achieve the perfect face shape can be used effectively. The oval face shape with almond-shaped eyes is said to be perfect, although trends change with fashion and very few people truly fall into that category. When carrying out your consultation, ensure that both you and your client have realistic expectations about what you can achieve.

Oval face shape	**Round face shape**	**Square face shape**	**Oblong face shape**
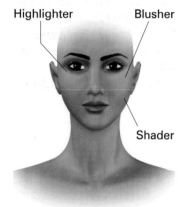	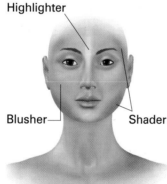	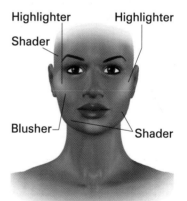	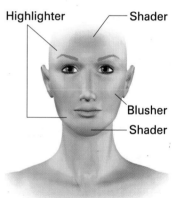
The aim of any corrective make-up is to enhance bone structure and balance contours by blending blusher along the cheek bones towards the temples, applying shader below and highlighter above.	The corrective work should create an illusion of length – to reduce the width from the sides of the face to the temples. To create length – subtle highlighter blended in a narrow strip down the centre of the face, blusher applied on the cheek – bones up to the temples, shader over angles of the jaw and temple areas.	The aim of the corrective work is to soften the jawline and reduce the width from the forehead and lower half of the face. Shader should be blended over the angles of the lower jaw and forehead. Blusher should be applied upwards from under the cheeks towards the temples or along the fullness of the cheeks.	The corrective make-up should reduce the length of the face, and create width and fullness. This can be achieved by applying shader to the tip of the chin and narrowest part of the forehead. Apply highlighter to the temples and lower jaw and blusher to cheeks to add fullness.

Heart face shape

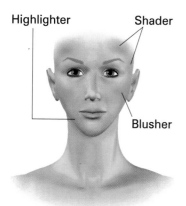

The corrective work should aim to minimise the width of the forehead and widen the lower half of the face. This can be achieved by applying shader to the sides of the forehead and temples. Highlight the angles of the lower jaw. Apply blusher to the fullness of the cheeks.

Diamond face shape

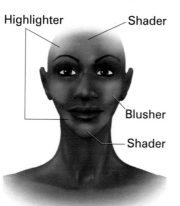

The corrective work of this face shape is to reduce the length by applying shader to the tip of the shin and the narrowest part of the forehead. To give the illusion of width, apply highlighter to the sides of the temples and lower jaw. Apply blusher to the cheeks to create fullness to the centre of the face.

Pear face shape

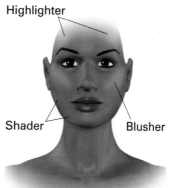

The aim of this corrective make-up is to give width to the forehead by applying highlighter to the sides of the forehead and to reduce the width of the lower face through the application of shader on the side of the shin and angles of the lower jaw. Emphasise the cheek-bones for a full appearance.

Triangular face shape

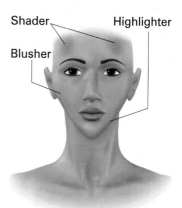

This corrective make-up is similar to that used on a heart-shaped face. The relatively wide forehead and narrow jaw line need to be balanced to prevent the face from looking top heavy. Use shader to minimise the forehead width and create the illusion of width along the jaw line by applying highlighter. Use blusher on the cheeks to balance the centre of the face and even up the whole shape.

Eye cosmetics

The eyes are the focal point of the face. People often focus on the eye make-up as the eyes are used for communicating and expressing our feelings. The trick when applying make-up is to draw attention to the eyes and not to the make-up.

The use of colour can create illusions of depth, size and alter the shape. Always remember that lighter colours enhance, darker colours recede.

Care is always needed when working around the eyes, as the skin is very sensitive and thin and can be easily over stretched. The EC Cosmetics Directive of 1976 limits ingredients which may be contained in eye make-up products and only pigments which are known to be non-toxic and non-irritant are allowed.

Eye-shadow

Eye-shadows are used to emphasise the eyes and to co-ordinate the colour of the make-up and clothing. They are available as powder, liquid, gel and cream. Creamy pressed powders are the most popular. Frosted products are available for highlighting and can be used to achieve a stunning effect when used for evening.

However, frosted and creamy products are not recommended for mature clients as they draw attention to lines and get trapped in crepey areas. Correcting the eyes by using contrasting colours and textures can be used to great effect.

Powder shadows

These are talc-based with oil for a creamy texture, available in loose or pressed form.

Creams

Cream shadow contains wax and oil pigments, not so popular with mature clients as these products settle in the creases.

Gels

Gels give a natural appearance because they produce a translucent wash of colour.

Eye-shadow colours

- Dark muted colours – use for defining and contouring. Effective on clients with dark hair and eyes. Applied with a fine brush can be used as a livening effect on people with fair colouring.
- Pastel colours – produce soft effects, particularly on people with grey / blonde hair. They emphasise the colour of the eyes when applied in the same tone.
- Pale colours – have highlighting effects when contrasted with dark shadows. When applied near the brow makes the eyes appear bigger.
- Soft muted shades – use when a more natural effect is required.
- Bright colours – use in young or fashion make-up. Some bright colours can be used as eye-liner to complement the eye-shadow, but be cautious when using bright colours on a mature client as they can give a hard and unattractive appearance.

Eyes

Small eyes

Lengthen small eyes by applying a soft eye pencil to the outer third of the bottom lid extending outward. Use a short stroke to join this line to the upper lash line, then smudge.

- Use light colours and iridescent shadows on the lid for an eye-opening effect.
- Highlight with a frosted shadow under the brow for evening sparkle.
- Curl the lashes or have them permed before applying the mascara to open the eyes even more.
- Try lining the inside of the lower lid with a soft white pencil – this will also give the appearance of the eye being more open.

Prominent eyes

Use matt shadow on the lid and blend it into the crease. Apply as darker shade to the outer half of the lid, right over the first shade, and blend so the graduation looks natural and no harsh lines are visible. Highlight under the brow with a light or frosted shade.

If you wish to achieve a sultry look, which may be suitable for evening wear, line the inner rim of the eye with a soft eye pencil. Grey, navy, plum and black are excellent depending on the eye colour, but there are many more colours to choose from.

Round eyes

Elongate the eyes by using the deepest shades on the outer edge of the eye lid, extend this to form a soft point. Lengthen the eyes even more by outlining the outer third of the top and bottom with a soft eye pencil, making sure that the outer point meets beyond the outer corner of the eye. Smudge for a softer effect, narrow the eyes by lining the inner rim with a soft pencil.

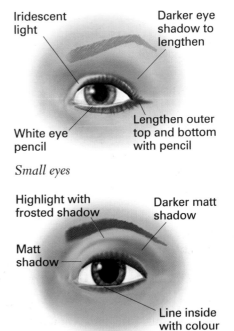

Iridescent light · Darker eye shadow to lengthen · White eye pencil · Lengthen outer top and bottom with pencil

Small eyes

Highlight with frosted shadow · Darker matt shadow · Matt shadow · Line inside with colour

Prominent eyes

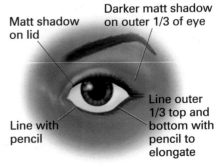

Matt shadow on lid · Darker matt shadow on outer 1/3 of eye · Line with pencil · Line outer 1/3 top and bottom with pencil to elongate

Round eyes

Deep-set eyes

Use light or frosted shadows on the lid if it is appropriate for the client and occasion. Apply a darker shade above the crease to recess this area. Apply a little shadow or soft eye pencil on the outer half of the bottom lid to balance the depth of the eyes.

Oriental eyes

Divide the area beneath the brow in half vertically. Use a lighter shade on the inner half and a darker shade on the outer half and blend well together. The application of a darker shadow creates a socket line. Apply a highlighter under the brow and blend together.

Almond eyes

Unless the eyes are set too close together or too far apart you don't have to worry about corrective techniques. Choose colours that complement the iris, ensure the brows are groomed to make application of shadows easy.

Close-set eyes

Keep all medium or dark colours on the outer half of the eye. This will draw attention outward and the eyes will seem further apart. Ensure that the brows have been correctly shaped to maximise the space between the eyes.

Wide-set eyes

Extend the shadows to the inner corner of the eye and blend inwards to the bridge of the nose to minimise the space, also ensure the brows are correctly shaped.

Cautions when applying eye-shadow

Always use clean brushes and applicators. Do not overload the applicator with shadow as excess powder could fall into the eyes or onto the face – spoiling the other make-up. It is also not cost effective to over load the applicator.

Support the skin and protect the surrounding make-up with a tissue. Beware that the skin around the eye is very delicate so don't be heavy handed and over-stretch the skin.

Ensure your client keeps her eyes closed when applying the shadow and always keep the client informed of what you are about to do.

Check the shadow is balanced on both eyes.

If applying shadow beneath the eyes ask the client to look away from the brush to prevent blinking or the eyes watering.

Eye-liner

This product is used for emphasising the shape of the eyelid and strengthening the colour of the lash line. It is good to use when strip lashes have been applied to give a more natural appearance. Liners are available in a number of colours and types. Like all make-up, eye-liner follows fashion trends and was very popular in the 1950s and 1960s.

Cake eye-liner

This is the most versatile product but the most difficult to apply. It is applied with a fine brush that is wet before applying to the eyes.

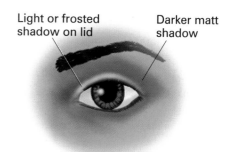

Deep-set eyes

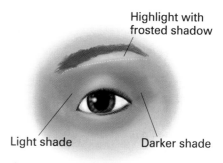

Oriental eyes

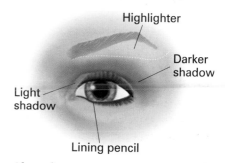

Almond eyes

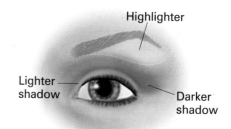

Close-set eyes

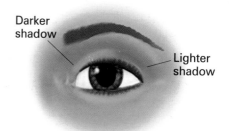

Wide-set eyes

Liquid eye-liner

This is a gum solution containing pigments, which gives a heavier effect.

Pencils

These are available in a range of colours, usually soft enough to blend with the shadows because of their wax formulation. Ensure they are sharpened between each eye to get an even application and to prevent cross infection occurring.

Kohl

This is a soft waxy black pencil which is applied to the inner rim of the lower eyelid to enhance the white of the eye. A kohl pencil is not recommended for use on a mature client.

Cautions when applying eye-liner

- Gently lift the skin from beneath the brow so the line is drawn up to the base of the lashes.
- Ensure the client keeps the eyes shut when liner is applied to the upper lid.
- Always apply liner outwards towards the corner of the eye.
- Check that the thickness and angle of the eye-liner are the same for both eyes.

Mascara

Mascaras are available in a variety of colours – including a clear mascara. Mascara is used to accentuate the eyes by darkening and thickening the lashes. Many now contain moisturisers and lash building ingredients which include filaments of nylon and rayon. These fibres temporarily lengthen the lashes. Clear mascara enhances the natural features of darkened lashes and is especially useful after the lashes have been tinted.

Cake mascara

A mixture of waxes and pigments in a soap base, this is applied with a brush. This type of mascara is gaining popularity again in salons as the brush applicator can easily be cleaned and sterilised.

Liquid mascara

Applied with a brush or wand, this type of mascara is contained in a water or alcohol and water base with extra features e.g. waterproof, thickening, and protein enriched. Read the packaging to find out what exactly the mascara contains. When applying this type of mascara to a client, disposable brushes should be used for each eye to prevent any contamination of the product.

Cautions when applying mascara

- Ensure that the client is relaxed as this makes the application of mascara easier – especially to the upper lashes.
- Apply mascara downwards on upper lashes and then upwards for maximum coverage.
- Place tissue under lower lashes, before applying, to prevent mascara marking the skin.
- Instruct the client to look away from the wand when applying the mascara to the lower lashes.
- Build up the mascara in fine coats to prevent clogging. Allow to dry between applications.

Remember	

When using the lash building mascara, caution should be taken with clients who have contact lenses as the fibres can cause damage to the lenses. Check that the product is suitable.

Eyebrow pencils

These pencils are used to strengthen the colour of the brows and define shape. They should be applied to the brow in light feathery strokes for a natural look. The use of an eyebrow pencil is good for filling in bare areas if the brows are sparse. Use short strokes in the direction of the hair growth and blend into the natural brow shape with the aid of a brow brush.

Eyebrow pencils are produced in a limited range of colours to complement the natural brow colour. As with other pencils they should be sharpened between eyes to prevent cross contamination occurring.

Cautions when using eyebrow pencils

- Brush brows into shape.
- Check the colour tone and shade of the pencil – this should look natural and complement the rest of the make-up.
- Ensure the pencils are sharpened after doing each brow, to prevent cross contamination, and ensure feathery strokes are used rather than one harsh line
- for a natural look.

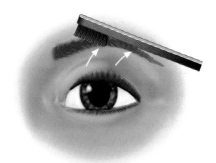

a Separate brow hairs

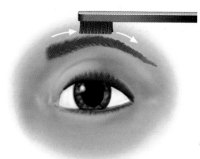

b Smooth them into shape

> ### In the salon
>
> Mrs Patel is preparing for her daughter's wedding, and comes in for a pre-wedding make-up practice. Her eyebrows are thick and her eyes are quite small – what can you recommend?

Lip cosmetics

There is a variety of cosmetics on the market for lips, in a range of colours and forms. There are lipsticks, glosses and pencils. These are used to define the mouth, by adding colour, and to protect the lips from the environment. The use of lip cosmetics can, as with other forms of make-up, be used as corrective make-up to enhance shape. All lip products contain the same ingredients of oils, fats and waxes, with the addition of safe pigments for colour.

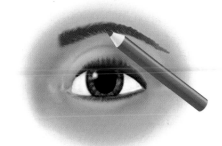

c Fill in the gaps and extend the length of the brow by using fine strokes that follow the natural hair growth

Lipsticks

These contain a high wax content that makes them hard. Some products also contain sunscreens to protect the delicate skin of the lips from ultraviolet light. Lipstick should be applied with a brush to outline the mouth and spread colour over evenly.

Lip gloss

This product can be used over lipstick or on its own for a natural look. It is usually of a gel consistency and is available in either lipstick form or as a gel.

Lip pencil

This is used for outlining the lips before applying lipstick and contains a high proportion of wax, which means it is less likely to smudge. It is useful to prevent lipstick colour from 'bleeding' into the fine lines around the mouth. It is also helpful for correcting lip shapes.

Lipstick sealer

Usually produced as a liquid, this is a colourless sealer, designed to prevent lipstick fading and to keep it in place. Applied with a brush.

Lip primer

This is used mainly for mature clients to prevent 'lipstick bleeding'.

Choosing a suitable lipstick

When selecting a lipstick it should be used to balance the colour scheme and co-ordinate with the clothing. Strong and vibrant colours draw attention to the mouth, so avoid them if you are trying to take the emphasis away from the mouth or jaw area. Strong colours look best with subtle and muted eye make-up colours

Deep colour lipstick or pencil should be used when outlining a corrective lip make-up. Pale, pearlised lipstick or lip gloss give lips a fuller appearance.

To reduce fullness, bronze, purplish pinks and blue-toned reds are useful.

Cautions when applying lip cosmetics

- Apply foundation and powder to the lips before applying lip cosmetics. This gives a good base and makes lip cosmetics last longer.
- Outline the mouth first and then fill in the colour.
- Blot the first application with a tissue as this helps to fix the colour.
- Apply a second coat for a final finish.
- Never apply lip cosmetics to any infected area or if the lips are excessively chapped or cracked.

Corrective lip make-up

Thin lips

The thickness of the lips can be increased by drawing a line slightly outside the natural lip shape.

Full or thick lips

Use dark colours to make the lips recede and create a new lip line inside the natural one by blotting out the natural line with foundation and powder.

Thin or straight upper lip

Create a new bow to the upper lip by pencilling just above the natural line to add fullness.

Thin lower lip

Create a new lower lip line slightly below the natural lip to give balance to the mouth.

Asymmetric lips

These lips are unbalanced so create a lip line where required to achieve balance.

Droopy mouth

Build up the corners of the lower lip, slightly extending upwards at the corners to meet the upper lip line.

Facial problem areas

Jawline shapes

Broad jaw

A broad jaw can be minimised by the use of a darker shader, starting from the temple area down and over either side of the angle of the mandible, bringing the centre of the face into sharper contact and so creating a more balanced width.

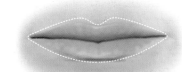
Thin lips

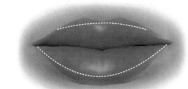
Full or thick lips

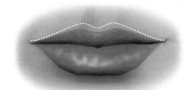
Thin or straight upper lip

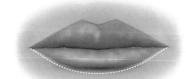
Thin lower lip

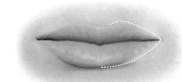
Asymmetric lips

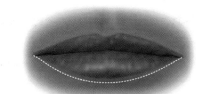
Droopy mouth

Narrow jaw

Narrow jaws are highlighted to create an illusion of width.

Round and square jaws

These can be shaded with a darker foundation applied to the width, to appear more rounded.

Chin and neck shapes

Prominent chin

A dark foundation or shader should be used on the chin, and sometimes a touch of blusher can be just as effective.

Receding chin

A lighter foundation or a highlighter will make a receding chin appear more prominent.

Double chin

A double chin or loose skin should be shadowed, with a dark foundation or shader.

Thin neck

This should be highlighted to create the illusion of roundness and prominence.

Thick neck

This requires shading to make it appear smaller.

Nose shapes

Large or protruding nose

This is made smaller by applying a dark foundation or shader, blending it smoothly into a lighter foundation on the sides of the cheeks. Blusher should be kept away from the nose.

Thin short nose

This is made narrower by shading the sides of the nostrils.

Long thin nose

This can be broadened by applying a highlighter foundation down its centre to above the tip, which is to be shaded.

Colour and skin pigmentation

Freckles and moles

These can be faded with the use of a good foundation or cream which is slightly thicker. It must be toned into the rest of the foundation, otherwise it will stand out.

Age lines

Creases round the mouth and crow's feet around the eyes can be softened by making the eyes appear fuller. This is achieved by the use of a lighter coloured foundation applied over the area. The crevices appear to be lifted out and less noticeable, but do not apply too heavily or you will make the areas more noticeable.

Clients with contact lenses or glasses

The effects that glasses have on the appearance of the face and make-up will vary according to the:

- colour of frame
- frame size
- lenses.

Frames

- Heavy frames – can take strong lip colour and eye make-up to help balance the facial features.
- Lightweight frames – ensure the colours are soft, using liner or mascara. Eyebrow pencil to define the brows and lashes will look more subtle with this colour frame. Bold colours will make light frames recede.
- Coloured frames – make-up should complement them. Muted shades should be used if the frames are very bright.

Lenses

- Short sighted – these make the eyes appear smaller.
- Long sighted – these lenses make the eyes look larger.
- Tinted lenses – these lenses may change the colours of the make-up.

Contact lenses

Some clients are quite happy to have their lenses in place when the make-up takes place, but you should always take the following precautions to prevent irritating the eyes.

- Work gently.
- Avoid heavy creams that could smear the lenses.
- Avoid creating dust that could land on the contact lenses and irritate the eye, always ensure the client keeps the eyes closed when applying powder shadow.
- Use eye make-up shadows with a creamy pressed texture.
- Use mascara without alcohol and added fibre filaments.

Bridal make-up

Many brides have their make-up applied professionally so that they can be confident of looking their best. Therefore, to ensure you give the best advice, a preliminary consultation is essential. During the consultation you need to find out the following details.

- The date and time of the wedding. The final appointment must be scheduled within the overall preparations, as ideally make-up should be applied before the hair is dressed and the dress put on.
- Details of the dress – design, colour and material. Colours will look stronger if the dress is white. Lightweight fabrics need softer make-up than heavier fabrics
- Hair style and headdress – this can affect the facial features.

Remember that lipstick and nail colours need to tone with the colour scheme of the dress and flowers. Pearlised products will emphasise flaws and defects and eye-make-up will lose definition in photographs.

When carrying out a wedding make-up, avoid stimulating the skin for 48 hours before the wedding. Shape eyebrows and apply individual lashes one or two days prior to the wedding. Apply fake tan one or two days prior to the wedding if the dress is low cut and reveals paler areas of the body.

Remember

The bride wants to look beautiful and radiant, but she also wants to be recognised – it is not the time for dramatic change.

It is important to promote waxing, manicure and pedicure treatments before the wedding for a truly well groomed appearance and for honeymoon preparation. Many salons include wedding packages in their price lists that include these treatments.

Photographic make-up

Many large photographic studios now employ a make-up artist to help clients get the best from their photographs. This service is included in the cost of the photographic package. You need to consider the following points.

- Lighting can be hot and make-up may melt, so do not apply a heavy make-up and cool the skin if possible during application.
- Avoid greasy products and creamy textured products as these emphasise shine, creases and open pores.
- Re-apply translucent powder to achieve a matt finish.
- Pearlised products can cause glare and emphasise flaws.
- Ensure that all products are well blended. This is particularly important around the jaw and hair lines.
- Highlight under the eyes, chin and sides of the nostrils before applying foundation, to prevent discoloration and shadow created by skin folds.
- Use highlight and shadow techniques to create facial contours and define bone structure. Foundation should be as light as possible to enhance the contour cosmetics.

Step-by-step daytime make-up

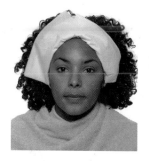

Prepare the client, in an upright position, fully covered and the skin lightly moisturised. Headband and tissues protect the hair. It is best to apply daytime make-up in natural daylight.

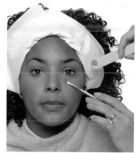

Apply concealer / colour corrector, if needed, followed by suitable foundation for the skin type with a damp sponge or clean fingertips. Work from the centre of the face outwards, using light movements.

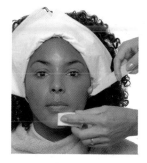

Using dry cotton wool, lightly pat on loose powder to set the foundation, remembering the eyelids and the lips, to make a dry base for eye shadow and lipstick.

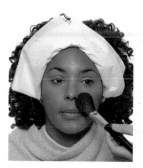

Using a large round brush, remove any excess powder, using downward strokes.

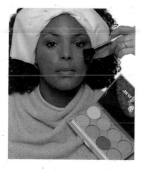

Shader, blusher and highlighter can now be applied to contour the face, as discussed in the treatment plan. Always decant product – this palette just shows the colours available.

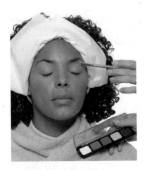

Apply eye shadows, remembering to use disposable applicators and to decant the colours onto a pallet, to avoid contaminating the remaining eye shadow.

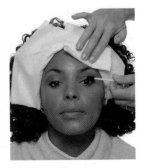

Apply eyeliner or pencil, without dragging on the eye, and remember to sharpen the pencil between clients, for hygiene.

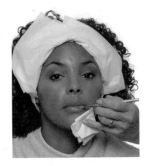

When applying mascara, remember to support the eye with a tissue, ask the client to look down, and stroke upwards, with the eyelash growth. A disposable wand is always used.

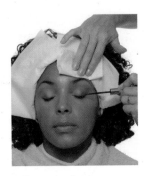

Lip liner and lipstick are next. Remember to sharpen the lip pencil, and to decant the lipstick onto a pallet, applying it with a clean brush.

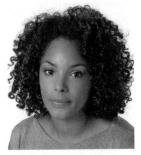

Show the client the finished result with all covering removed. Her own hair and clothes will give a natural look. Hold the mirror upwards for a flattering result.

Step-by-step evening make-up

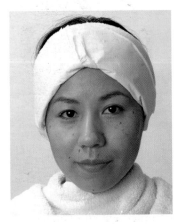

Begin with the client fully prepared, covered and with moisturised skin.

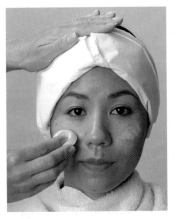

Concealer and foundation can be applied, with a damp sponge. For evening make-up, the shade can be a skin tone darker than for daytime.

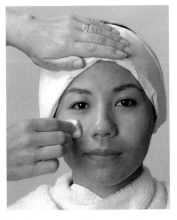

Pat loose powder over the foundation, remembering eyelids and lips. This will help the eye shadow and lipstick stay on throughout the evening.

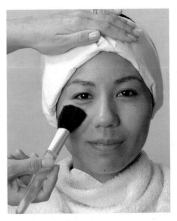

With a fat brush, sweep downwards to remove any excess powder, which may be clinging on to the tiny facial hairs.

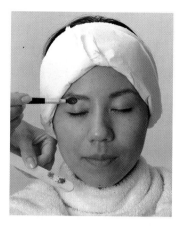

Decant your chosen eye shadow colours onto a wooden spatula. For evening make-up choose sparkling or iridescent colours, to complement the eyes and / or outfit.

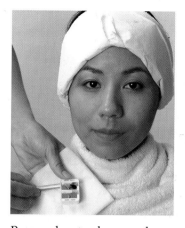

Remember to sharpen the eyeliner pencil before applying. Not all clients like an inner kohl line, so remember to ask, before attempting to apply.

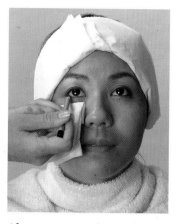

Always protect the make-up by using a tissue barrier to rest your hands on; this stops you from transferring any grease from your hands onto the skin.

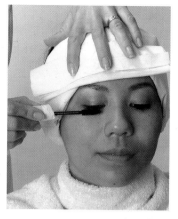

Apply mascara with a disposable wand, in light movements from base to tip. It helps if the client looks down. Try not to let your hand shake.

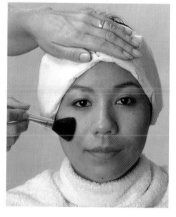

Evening blusher and shaders can be applied. A slightly sparkling blusher gives the cheeks a glow. Sweep from the plump part of the cheek upwards to create a high-cheeked appearance.

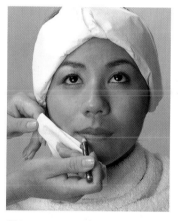

Sharpen pencil and apply lip liner along the natural lip line, unless correction is required. Using a tissue to rest upon, draw a subtle light line.

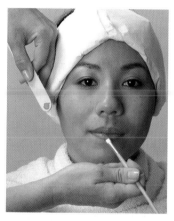

Decant the chosen lipstick onto a wooden spatula and apply, just inside the lip liner. A gloss can be applied over the top, if suitable and agreed with the client.

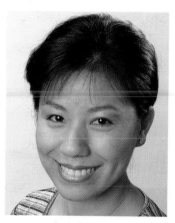

The finished look should complement and enhance the client's features. Make sure her clothing and hair are restored before revealing the finished result.

Step-by-step special occasion make-up

Special occasion make-up can be a little more individual than day make-up, but not quite as heavy as evening make-up. The key to making the whole look glamorous but not overdone is to co-ordinate the make-up colours with the outfit and add a touch of sparkle, with a lip gloss or shiny eye shadow. Ask the client what she will be wearing; see the outfit, if possible, and definitely have a trial run before the event.

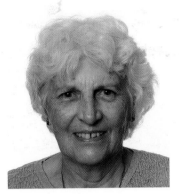

Study the client's natural skin and hair colouring, to avoid choosing make-up colours that clash. Research the type of special occasion and what the client will be wearing.

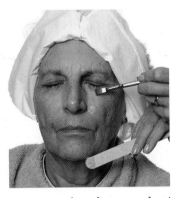

Decant and apply concealer / colour corrector, if required. Take into account that your client may or may not be used to wearing much make-up usually. Keep application and colour light, particularly when applying make-up to mature skin.

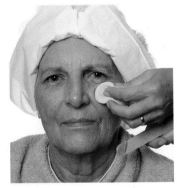

Apply foundation with a sponge or clean fingertips, blending from the centre of the face, outwards. Ensure foundation chosen is suitable for skin type – foundation for mature skin should be light in texture and colour.

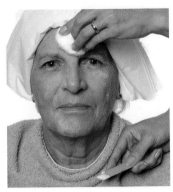

With a dry piece of cotton wool, pat loose powder all over the face, remembering eyelids and lips. Translucent powder is suitable for mature skin.

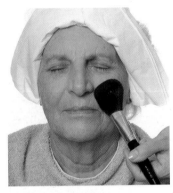

A light stroke with a large blusher brush will remove any excess powder. Stroke the brush all over the face, in a downward motion, to avoid a powdery look to the face.

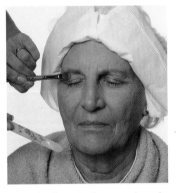

Eye shadow is decanted and applied lightly over the lids. If the client wears glasses, or has quite lined eyelids, make the colour and application fairly light.

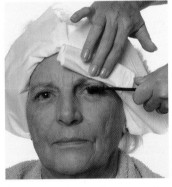

Apply a light application of mascara using a disposable wand. Soft shades of navy, grey or brown mascara are less harsh than black on mature skin.

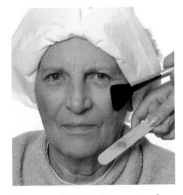

Decant the blusher onto the wooden spatula and apply lightly to the cheeks. Soft corals, peaches or pinks usually suit mature skin.

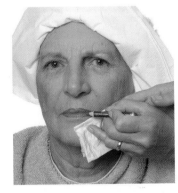

Sharpen the pencil and apply a light lip liner, which prevents the lipstick bleeding into the lines around the mouth.

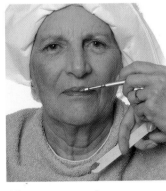

Choose a complementary lipstick and decant, then apply.

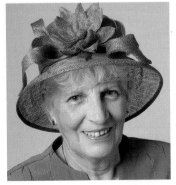

You gain the whole effect for special occasion make-up if you have a complete dress rehearsal – including the hat!

Children's face painting

Although not strictly a salon treatment, from time to time clients may request children's face painting for parties and birthday treats. No special skill is required – you just need some water-based face paints (child friendly for easy removal) and a flair for invention.

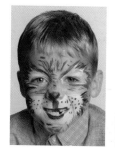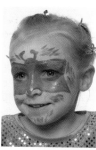

Aftercare advice

To enable the client to gain the most from the make-up treatment and subsequent make-up applications, the client should be given the following information.

- Correct preparation for applying make-up, including the cleansing and toning routine, and the correct application of moisturiser suitable for the client's skin type.
- Correct choice and application of cosmetics – colours, textures and types suitable for the features of the client and her skin type.
- Effective and hygienic use of products and equipment.
- How to keep make-up fresh by: applying pressed powder; applying a fine spray of water to keep the make-up from drying and cracking; applying more lipstick.
- Removal of make-up with products suitable for the client's skin type.
- In the event of an allergic reaction, remove all make-up, soothe with damp cotton wool and apply a soothing substance, e.g. calamine lotion.

Link selling and retail products

Many therapists work on a commission basis for the sale of retail products and a make-up treatment is a good opportunity to carry out such sales. These can include:

- sale of other treatments within the salon
- regular facial treatment
- eyebrow shape
- eyelash and brow tints
- application of false lashes for special occasions
- eyelash perming
- manicure and pedicure treatments
- waxing.

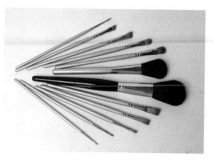

Make-up brushes are an example of products that can be purchased by clients for use at home

Retail products

These can include:
- cleanser, toner and moisturiser to suit skin type
- foundation and powder
- matching lipstick and varnish
- make-up brushes and applicator
- eye cream
- throat / neck cream.

It is therefore important that you have a good knowledge of the products that you are recommending for home use and can demonstrate how to use these effectively. This will give the client confidence in you as a therapist.

Your questions answered

Why is it important to do a skin analysis prior to carrying out a make-up application?
It is important so that you can fully assess the client's skin type and select suitable products. This should be carried out on cleansed dry skin.

What action should be taken if the foundations are not the correct shade?
You can blend your own shades by mixing two or more colours together on a palette to obtain the correct shade.

Do I have to use a colour corrector, if a concealer has been used?
Colour correctors do just what they say – they neutralise the colour to make a more even shade – so they should only be applied where they are needed.

Is the lighting really that important when applying make-up?
The more natural the lighting and the closer to daylight, the better the finished results will look. Different coloured light bulbs and shades on light fittings can give a false appearance and you may find that that the application is too sparing or too heavy handed.

Why is it important to use the correct products on black/Asian skins?
Because of the different colours and pigmentation of the skin, specialist products should be used so the correct skin tones and a natural and realistic look can be achieved.

Test your knowledge

1   How would you select the correct foundation colour?

2   What is the purpose of foundation?

3   What type of powder is recommended for touching up make-up?

4   When applying eye make-up to more mature clients what type of product should be avoided?

5   What is the difference between day and evening make-up?

6   What should you do between each eye when using a pencil to line the eyes?

7   Why is the position of the client important when applying make-up?

8   What type of mascara is best to use on a client who wears contact lenses?

9   How would you contour a client with a round face shape?

10   What is the purpose of a highlighter?

Applying make-up

Ensure all products and equipment are close to hand.

Carry out a consultation, checking for contra-indications, and a skin analysis to determine the products to use.

Apply moisturiser.

Apply concealer and colour corrector if required.

Apply foundation, check the colour on the jaw line. Apply powder to set the foundation.

Apply shaders and highlighters to minimise or emphasise areas as discussed with the client.

Apply eye shadow (hold a tissue under the eye to prevent flaking shadow).

Apply eye-liner or pencil (sharpen between eyes).

Apply mascara (using disposable mascara wands).

Apply lip pencil or liner. Apply lipstick.

Show client the finished result. Record details, including products used and where applied, on client record.

Improve facial skin condition

Unit 6

A facial is a lovely treatment to offer any client as it is both extremely relaxing and very beneficial. In fact, for a professional beauty therapist, a facial can be as relaxing to give, as it is to receive. Many clients even fall asleep during a facial, as the relaxation is so deep.

A facial makes a perfect present to give someone, and vouchers for the treatment can be purchased in most salons. For many women a facial is the height of luxury; for a beauty therapist it will rate very highly on the scale of favourite treatments to give.

Unit 6 helps you achieve the skin care part of a facial treatment. Make-up and eye treatments are covered in Units 5 and 8.

Within this unit you will cover the following elements:
6.1 Assess clients and prepare a treatment plan
6.2 Prepare the client and work area for treatment
6.3 Improve skin condition using skin care and massage techniques.

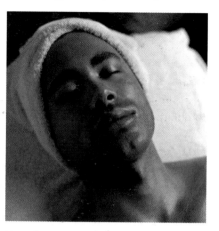

Facial massage is relaxing and improves skin condition

Assess clients and prepare a treatment plan

6.1

A full consultation is required before the treatment can begin – please refer to **Professional basics** for detailed information on how to conduct a consultation. The facial anatomy and physiology related to the head and face is covered within the anatomy section (see page 84).

A facial is a treatment, which helps the therapist to do a number of things – as shown in the diagram.

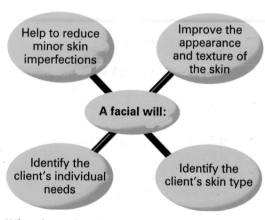

What does a facial involve?

In this element you will learn about:
• facial examination • mask treatments
• skin types • massage techniques.
• facial products

Facial examination

When examining the face and neck it is important to consider the following points.

• Check the skin prior to the treatment for any contra-indications that would prevent treatment, or any adaptation that may be necessary.
• Correct identification of the client's skin type is essential, both to enable the therapist to give the correct treatment, and to recommend the most suitable products.
• Look for any minor skin problems that can be given specific treatment for improvement.
• Take into account the client's age, lifestyle, nutritional intake and general health, as this will be reflected in: the colour and texture of the skin, muscle tone in the facial muscles, elasticity, the amount of wrinkles present and skin discoloration. Record the client's colouring and skin pigmentation, as well as any facial features;

this will help with a make-up application and for recommending other treatments, such as eyebrow shaping.

There are three necessary parts to a facial examination:

- questioning
- visual examination
- manual examination.

Questioning the client before her facial will establish the factors that contribute to the skin's condition:

Gentle questioning will help to identify the client's normal skin care routine and products used. It helps you identify the client's expectations of her treatment – they do need to be realistic. It is important that the client understands that a skin condition may take several treatments to clear and a realistic treatment plan for both a time-scale and cost should be discussed, prior to the treatment taking place.

Visual examination should be done under a strong light, using a magnifying glass, with a clean skin, that is free of make-up. Any areas of sensitivity or problem areas, such as comedones (blackheads) or an oily T-zone, can be recorded on a facial record card.

Manual examination should be gentle, and will give some indication about the elasticity of the skin, its warmth and texture. A gentle pinch of the skin in the main facial areas should allow the skin to spring back into its original shape. Poor elasticity of the fibres will mean that the skin takes longer to recover from the pinch test and this could be due to age.

The warmth of the skin will indicate how good the circulation is to the face, and the texture will be felt as smooth, coarse or rough; any lumps under the skin may need further investigation.

Preparation of the client for examination

The client's position and preparation are the same as for a full facial; refer back to Unit 5 and **Professional basics** to refresh your memory, if you are unsure.

The client's modesty needs to be preserved, and behind a closed cubicle ask the client to remove all her top clothes and put on a gown. Her tights and half-slip may be kept on, but shoes should be removed.

Assist the client onto the couch and remove the gown. Depending upon the time of year, wrap the client in either a blanket with towels or just towels, so that she is comfortable and warm. It is distracting for you both if the client is feeling insecure or cold! The client should remove all jewellery, accessories, and glasses or contact lenses. Clients who wear contact lenses may prefer to remove them during the written consultation stage, if they have suitable storage for them. Some clients prefer to keep them in, even though make-up will be removed. Be guided by the client's choice, as she knows which is most comfortable for her.

A headband or turban should be used to remove all hair from the face.

The bra straps need to be tucked under a small towel placed over the chest area, as cleanser may get in contact and make them sticky.

Before beginning the examination:

- wash your hands thoroughly
- remove all make-up and cleanse, deep cleanse, tone and pat dry the skin, using a tissue.

Remember

Facials do instantly make the skin look cleaner, fresh and feel softer, but a skin problem, such as mild acne, will definitely take more than one treatment for a good result to be seen.

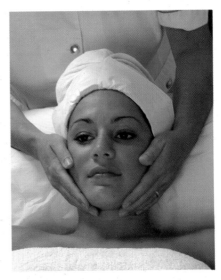
Preparation of the client

The texture of the skin can be felt as the cleansing movements are used, and the muscle tone will be felt under the hands.

What to look for in a facial examination

Contra-indications

The general contra-indications to a facial treatment are:

- cuts and abrasion of the skin's surface
- scar tissue of less than six months old
- recent sunburn
- any undiagnosed lumps or swellings
- severe eye infections
- any bacterial, fungal or viral infections present
- conjunctivitis
- bruising to the area
- a known allergic reaction
- the presence of an unrecognizable lump or bump.

Risk of infection

There is a risk that if a treatment is given in the presence of some of these conditions it could put the therapist and other clients at risk, from cross infection.

The condition could be made worse by treatment, or it could be prolonged. The client could experience pain and discomfort if the treatment went ahead and the therapist could be found negligent by her insurance and professional body, if the client decided to take legal action. Any client with a suspected infection should be referred to her GP. But be careful – it is not a therapist's job role to presume medical diagnosis.

If no contra-indications are present you can continue your analysis.

Recognising skin types

Skin types are usually described as one of four categories:

1 Normal
2 Dry
3 Greasy
4 Combination.

As well as these four basic types, skin can also be mature, have blemishes, be sensitive, be dehydrated, have broken capillaries, have comedones or milia.

The true skin type may not be very easy to diagnose at first, as all skins react to the environment, to products used, and to different lifestyles.

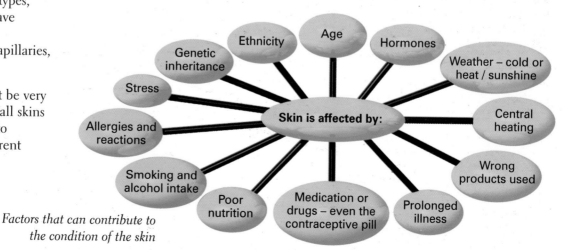

Factors that can contribute to the condition of the skin

Skin analysis

Problem areas / abnormalities noted	Area	Colour	Texture	Type	Sensitivity
	T-zone				
	Eyes				
	Cheeks				
	Chin				
	Neck				
	General elasticity: Firm ☐ Loose ☐				
	General colour				
Overall skin type	Treatment recommendations / adaptions				

Products used

	In salon	At home
Cleanser		
Toner		
Moisturiser		
Mask		
Night cream		
Eye cream		
Specialist products		

Analysis conclusion

Cause of skin problems	Product recommendations / homecare

Client agreement:
The treatment has been fully explained to me. I do not knowingly suffer from any medical conditions to prevent me from having a facial treatment.

Signed:	Date:
Products purchased:	

A facial analysis sheet

Normal skin

This exists when the oil and sweat glands are working in harmony. This skin has a good balance of moisture content and oil to keep the skin soft, supple and flexible. It is an ideal skin type, but rare. The skin is fine textured with no visible pores and smooth to the touch.

Normal skin will sometimes have a tendency to go either slightly on the dry side or slightly on the greasy side. It should never be assumed that it is always normal. The skin should feel warm to the touch, and it heals well if damaged.

Questions to ask your client

1   Is your skin generally in this condition?
2   Do you feel you have any problem areas?
3   Have you had problems in the past?
4   What skin care routine and products are you currently using?

Dry skin

This type of skin is oil- and moisture-deficient, leaving the skin dry to the touch. There may be some loss of elasticity depending upon the client's age, and a tendency to flakiness. The texture of the skin is fine; dry skin can often be thin and small red veins (dilated capillaries) may be present on the cheek areas. Pores and follicles are often closed and inactive. The skin chaps easily and can be inclined to be sensitive. Lines and wrinkles may form early on with dry skin, especially around the eyes.

Questions to ask your client

1   Does your skin feel tight and drawn?
2   Does your skin sometimes flake?
3   Does exposure to cold and wind make your skin sore?
4   Do you burn easily?

Oily skin

Greasy or oily skin is caused by an over-production of sebum from the sebaceous glands. It looks shiny; it can be slightly thicker in consistency than normal skin, sallow, coarse and have problems associated with it. This skin is often referred to as **seborrhoeic**.

Enlarged pores, congested pores, comedones and infection may occur on greasy skins, so care must be taken. A greasy skin often develops during puberty, when there is a surge of glandular activity under the influence of hormones. It often corrects itself when the hormone levels settle, and the use of the correct skin preparations can certainly help.

Questions to ask your client

1   Is your skin prone to pimples and blackheads?
2   Does the skin shine?
3   Is it difficult to keep make-up on?

Combination skin

Some skins are a combination of two or more skin types, and the most common one is a greasy T-zone along the forehead and nose, with normal or dry skin on the cheek area. This is because there are more sebaceous glands along the T-zone which may therefore show all the characteristics of greasy skin.

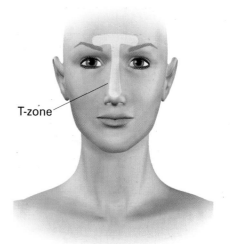

T-zone

The T-zone is commonly found in combination skin

Questions to ask your client

1 Is your nose shiny?
2 Are you prone to blackheads in the T-zone area?
3 Does the skin on your cheeks ever feel tight or dry?

Sensitive skin

All skin needs to be sensitive for good health, but in beauty therapy a sensitive skin is really one that is super sensitive, i.e. it reacts to even mild stimulus. This condition is often associated with pale skins or a dry skin that lacks the protection of enough sebum. Sensitive skins have a highly flushed look, with a tendency to colour easily, and can react to beauty products or chemicals used within the salon.

Questions to ask your client

1 Is your skin prone to allergic reactions?
2 Do you have a high cheek colour often?
3 Does your skin show signs of being dry but slightly red?

Dehydrated skin

Skin may have the normal sebaceous secretions and still suffer from flaking and tightness due to loss of surface moisture – a condition of dehydration. Any skin can suffer temporary dehydration, which may be caused through using products that are too harsh on the skin or through exposure to extreme temperatures, central heating or over-stringent dieting.

Questions to ask your client

1 What skin care products are you using on the skin?
2 Have you altered your diet recently?

Mature skin

In a fine-textured, older skin the slower rate of the sebaceous secretions, accompanied by loss of elasticity are contributory factors in the aging process, leading to a mature skin type. Wrinkles begin to form; the epidermis may become thinner, with a lack of springiness and loss of support from underlying muscles.

Congested skin

Congestion occurs because the pores become blocked and sweat and sebum cannot escape onto the skin surface which can be seen and felt as lumpy and coarse. Whiteheads and blackheads can build up and the epidermis may harden. Poor removal of make-up, using the wrong products and excess sweat building up all contribute to this skin condition.

Infected skin

Any bacteria, fungi or viruses can penetrate the skin and cause infection. This is easily recognised as swelling or irritation, with pain and tenderness. The presence of pus is also a sign of infection.

Bacteria entering the follicle, causing pore blockage to occur, causes **acne vulgaris**.

For a further breakdown of skin conditions and how to recognise them, refer to **Professional basics** (pages 116–121).

Reasons for skin damage	How to recognise the signs or symptoms
Excessive exposure to the sun, artificial sunlight (sun beds), excessive lines and wrinkles from alcohol intake and smoking	The skin ages prematurely, causing a breakdown in collagen and elastin, which supports the skin; uneven pigmentation can also occur
Pollution from chemicals, traffic and thinning of the protective ozone layer	Contamination of the skin leads to clogged and blocked pores, irritations occur and a tendency to comedones and allergic reactions. This causes dehydration and over-activity of the sebaceous glands, which causes further problems
Heat and steam	Overstretching of the skin, causing damage
Incorrect use of skin care products	Inappropriate products can cause comedones to form or lead to an over-sensitive skin
Excessive heat	Chapped and dehydrated skin

Skin damage – reasons and recognition

The best way of caring for the skin is:

- to avoid skin damage
- to take care of the skin internally with good nutritional habits
- to use correct skin care products
- to avoid unnecessary stress.

Prepare the client and work area for treatment

6.2

Facial products

To improve the facial skin condition, there are many products available on the market that can be used to good effect within the facial treatment. These can include:

- cleansers
- toners
- moisturisers
- exfoliants
- masks
- massage products
- specialist skin preparations.

The cosmetic and skin care preparation market is huge. The range of different manufacturers producing good quality products both for salon use, and for retailing, is ever-growing. Your salon or teaching establishment may have their own particular favourite, which through experience they prefer to use.

Remember

There are many moisturisers on the market, with differing prices and with varying promises to work wonders on the skin. The brand name, the packaging and the promotional skills that go with the cream can dictate the price. Also affecting the price is the quality of oil used and whether other key selling ingredients are included, such as vitamins.

Procedure	Action on the skin	Products available
Cleanse am & pm	Removes dirt, sweat, sebum and make-up from the skin's surface	Cleansing creams, lotions and milks, facial wash-off bars, gels
Tone am & pm	Tightens the skin, stimulates the circulation, and eliminates any trace of remaining cleanser from the skin	Toning lotion, astringent, skin tonic, bracers and fresheners
Exfoliate Once a week	Sloughs off the dead cells from the top layer of the epidermis to improve the texture and colour whilst stimulating the circulation	Cleansing grains that form a paste when mixed with water, ready mixed granular paste, fruit acid peels
Day cream am & pm	A protective film to keep the skin soft and supple. It restores the oil to the skin after toning, helping to keep the outer layers hydrated	Moisturiser creams or milks
Night cream pm	An absorbent intensive rich cream to restore the skin's well-being without leaving the skin feeling oily	Rich moisturisers in cream form
Face mask Once a week	Deep cleanses, soothing and balances the skin	Clay masks, peel off masks, thermal masks, fruit masks, biological masks
Eye make-up remover pm	A very gentle eye make-up remover, finer than a cleanser, for the delicate eye area	Lotions and creams, wash-off gels
Eye balm When needed	A delicate balm for upper and lower lid area. Soothing and refreshing, reduces puffiness	Moisturising lightweight creams or lotions

A good skin-care routine

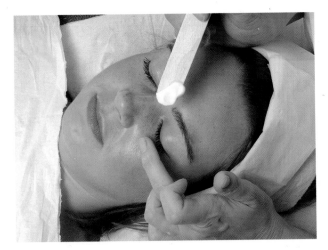

Applying special eye cream / balm

Check it out

All beauty therapists need to use a variety of different products from manufacturers until they find their own personal preference. You need to attend the various trade shows and exhibitions to experiment and try the vast range available. Go to your nearest large perfumery and approach the various cosmetic houses for free samples of products, until you find one you most like. Try at least three each of cleansers, toners and moisturisers. Collect price lists and advertising leaflets for your portfolio.

Facial products and their functions

Cleansing creams

Key ingredients

- An emulsion of oils, usually mineral oil.
- Waxes, usually beeswax or paraffin.
- Water and water soluble ingredients.
- Emulsifiers.
- Fragrance.
- Preservatives.

What they do

- Waxes provide a creamy firm texture to the product.
- The water content cools the skin and provides slip to allow easier spreading.
- Emulsifiers prevent the ingredients separating, i.e. oil and water.
- Fragrance makes the cream smell nice and gives appeal.
- Preservatives provide the product with a good shelf-life and prevent deterioration.

Summary of action

- A deep efficient cleansing action, removes even heavy make-up application.
- Leaves skin smooth and supple.
- Ideal for dry or normal skin types, too rich for an oily skin.

Method of use

- Decant a small amount onto a spatula, close lid, spread from spatula onto fingertips and massage over face and neck area using upward circular movements.
- Remove with tissues or damp cotton wool.

COSHH considerations

- All ingredients commonly used in cosmetic products, non-hazardous, non-inflammable.
- If ingested drink milk or water.
- If in contact with eyes wash well with water if irritation occurs.
- If spilled use absorbent towels to clean the area, wash with detergent and water to avoid slippery floors.
- No special handling and storage precautions necessary.

Cleansing milks

Key ingredients

- An emulsion of oils, usually mineral oil.
- A smaller proportion of waxes, than in a cleansing cream.
- Higher proportion of water and water soluble ingredients, than creams.
- Detergent.
- Emulsifiers.
- Fragrance.
- Preservatives.

What they do

- A mineral oil will dissolve grease and oil-based products on the skin, i.e. make-up.
- Waxes provide a creamy firm texture to the product.
- The water content cools the skin and provides slip to allow easier spreading.
- Detergent will act as surface-active agent, which helps emulsify and create foaming action.
- Emulsifiers prevent the ingredients separating, i.e. oil and water.
- Fragrance makes the product smell nice.
- Preservatives provide the product with a good shelf-life and prevent deterioration.

Summary of action

- A light cleansing lotion, which is easier to remove than a cleansing cream.
- Some cleansing milks can be worked into lather with water to wash off the skin.
- Ideal for most skin types except the very dry.

- Preferred by people who like a lighter feel to their cleanser.
- Also ideal for younger or greasier skins.

Method of use
- Either apply directly onto the skin on damp cotton wool pads, stroking in an upward motion, or apply with the fingertips in small circular movements.
- Remove with tissues or damp cotton wool.

COSHH considerations
- All ingredients commonly used in cosmetic products. Non-hazardous, non-inflammable.
- If ingested drink milk or water.
- If in contact with eyes wash well with water if irritation occurs.
- If spilled – use absorbent towels to clean the area, wash with detergent and water to avoid slippery floors.
- No special handling and storage precautions necessary.

Cleansing lotions

Key ingredients
- Detergent solution in water.
- Emulsifiers.
- Fragrance.
- Preservatives.
- Anti-bacterial ingredients.

What they do
- The water content cools the skin and provides slip to allow easier spreading and the detergent will act as surface-active agent, which helps emulsify the lotion.
- Emulsifiers prevent the ingredients separating, i.e. oil and water.
- Fragrance makes the lotion smell good and gives appeal.
- Preservatives provide the product with a good shelf-life and prevent deterioration.
- Anti-bacterial ingredients help a greasy or problem skin.

Summary of action
- A light cleansing lotion which can be applied on cotton wool pads.
- Ideal for most young skins, especially problem or blemished skins.

Method of use
- Apply directly onto the skin on damp cotton wool pads, stroking in an upward motion.

COSHH considerations
- All ingredients commonly used in cosmetic products.
- Non-hazardous, non-inflammable.
- If ingested drink milk or water.
- If in contact with eyes wash well with water if irritation occurs.
- If spilled – use absorbent towels to clean the area, wash with detergent and water to avoid slippery floors.
- No special handling and storage precautions necessary.

Facial washes / gels

Key ingredients
- A mixture of cleansing and wetting agents (often derived from palm oil).
- Water and water-soluble ingredients.
- Fragrance and foaming agents.
- Preservatives.
- Conditioners and colour.

What they do

- The water content cools the skin and provides slip to allow easier spreading.
- Cleansing agents will absorb the oil particles of dirt.
- Fragrance makes the product smell good and gives appeal.
- Preservatives provide the product with a good shelf-life and prevent deterioration.
- Conditioners will match and balance to the natural pH of skin, while colour will give appeal, for example tea-tree oil may be added to give an anti-bacterial, healing property to the wash and that is enhanced with a colour additive.

Summary of action

- Use a small amount on a moist skin – this method of cleansing can be used with a facial soft bristle brush, for added stimulation.
- This is ideal for use with a brush cleanser unit (a small motor rotates the brush) and can be applied to the chest and back – this makes a very good treatment for a congested skin, and is very popular with male clients who suffer with problem skin.
- Some gels can also be used as a shaving foam, cleansing at the same time (check individual manufacturer's instructions for use – there are many preparations that can be bought over the counter).

Method of use

- Apply directly onto moist skin in circular motions and massage lightly over face and neck; avoid contact with the eyes.
- Rinse off with water.
- Foaming properties will vary, depending on the hardness or softness of water.

COSHH considerations

- All ingredients commonly used in cosmetic products.
- Non-hazardous, non-inflammable.
- If ingested drink milk or water.
- If in contact with eyes wash well with water; if irritation occurs seek medical advice.
- If spilled use absorbent towels to clean the area, wash with detergent and water to avoid slippery floors.
- No special handling and storage precautions necessary.

Toners / skin fresheners

Key ingredients

- Alcohol, usually ethanol.
- Water and fragrance.
- Astringents, such as witch-hazel.
- Antiseptic, such as hexachlorophene.
- Humectants, such as glycerine.
- Additives, such as cucumber, althea extract (from plants).
- Preservatives, colour and perfume.

What they do

- The alcohol removes traces of grease on the skin and helps with the drying action while the water content cools the skin and dilutes the alcohol content.
- Fragrance makes the toner more attractive and hides the alcohol smell.
- An astringent tightens the skin and makes pores appear smaller.
- Antiseptic properties help heal a congested skin.
- Additives such as cucumber and plant extracts will soothe and soften skin.
- Humectants attract water and help re-hydrate the skin.
- Colour and fragrance will give appeal, for example cucumber may be added to give a soothing property to the toner and that is enhanced with a colour additive; blue or green are associated with cooling and calming properties (the preservatives provide a good shelf life and prevent deterioration).

Remember

- Skin toners contain between 20–60 % alcohol.
- Skin fresheners 0–20 % alcohol.
- Some gentle toners for use on dry / sensitive skins do not contain any alcohol.
- Skin toners with more than 25% alcohol can only be used on an oily skin.

Summary of action

- Toners cool and refresh the skin, and are available in differing strengths, depending upon skin type: strong toners for oily skins contain more alcohol, which dissolves grease, and the astringent properties tighten the skin.
- All toners contain mostly water and humectants which help with moisture retention.
- Fresheners are available, which contain only soothing agents, such as azulene or camomile; as no alcohol is present they are not as good at removing grease from the skin, but are ideal on a sensitive skin.

Method of use

- Apply to the skin with damp cotton wool pads, stroking in a firm but gentle rhythm all over the face and neck.
- Toners can help smooth, soften and heal skin, increasing cell regeneration.
- They prepare the skin to receive a moisturiser, by removing any trace of grease left by the cleanser.

COSHH considerations

- All ingredients commonly used in cosmetic products.
- Non-hazardous.
- Non-inflammable if less than 10% alcohol ratio.
- If ingested drink milk or water.
- If in contact with eyes wash well with water, if irritation occurs seek medical advice.
- If spilled – use absorbent towels to clean the area, wash with detergent and water to avoid slippery floors.
- No special handling and storage precautions necessary.

Exfoliants

Key ingredients

- Abrasive powders such as finely ground olive stones, nuts, oatmeal, corn cob powder or synthetic micro-beads.
- Detergent.
- Water and water-soluble ingredients.
- Kaolin, or other clay based ingredients.
- Sodium lactate.
- Added moisturisers / vitamins.

What they do

- An abrasive will act as a gentle buffer to remove the dead skin cells, felt as small grains on the skin.
- Detergent continues the cleansing process.
- Water and water-soluble ingredients help provide slip, so that the cream or paste flows over the skin easily and does not pull or drag the skin.
- Kaolin or other clays will absorb grease and dirt particles, gently cleansing and bleaching the skin slightly.
- Sodium lactate is an excellent humectant to regulate moisture content within the skin.
- Added moisturisers and vitamins impart a light smooth feel to the exfoliant without it being sticky or greasy.

Summary of action

- The definition of exfoliate is to peel, flake or scale – in this case the skin's cells.
- As the top layer of the epidermis is constantly shedding, an exfoliant helps the process along.
- It brightens the complexion, softens and makes the skin very receptive to receiving moisture.
- Exfoliants come in many commercial forms as a powder, which must be mixed with water, a ready-made paste or in a suspension (with water) that can also be

Remember

A guide to the appropriate level of alcohol in toners / fresheners for each skin type is:

10%	sensitive skin
0–20%	dry skin
10–25%	normal skin
25–50%	greasy skin.

Remember

- Exfoliation can be done on the body, in the shower, and is an ideal preparation for a lasting false tan application.

- Exfoliants can increase the effectiveness of all other skin preparations and treatments by up to 30%.

- Many commercial salons do not use steamers for skin preparation, an exfoliant is a quicker way of removing the dead skin cells and old make-up.

left on to form a face mask – exfoliating face masks usually have a higher proportion of clay, to make the mask dry and set on the face.
- All skin types benefit from exfoliation providing care is taken in choosing a suitable type for the skin problem.

Method of use
- Apply a thin layer onto damp, cleansed skin, in circular motions, avoiding the eyes.
- Work upwards with light pressure – care must be taken over the delicate cheek area.
- Don't let it drag the skin – add more water if necessary, without soaking the client.
- Rinse off.
- Follow manufacturer's instructions, as some exfoliants can also be left on the skin as a face mask, which is left to dry, then rinsed off.
- Some face masks double as a peel, and the mask is removed by using dry fingers in a circular motion to slough off the remaining cream, before rinsing.

COSHH considerations
- All ingredients commonly used in cosmetic products.
- Non-hazardous, non-inflammable.
- If ingested, drink milk or water.
- If in contact with eyes, wash well with water; if irritation occurs seek medical advice.
- If spilled use absorbent towels to clean the area, wash with detergent and water to avoid slippery floors.
- No special handling and storage precautions necessary.

Fruit acid peels
Key ingredients
- Available as lotions or masks containing Alpha Hydroxy Acids (AHA).
- AHAs are fruit acids from citrus fruits, bilberries and sugar cane.

What they do
- The fruit acids help dissolve the surface skin cells whilst stimulating the blood supply.
- They soften the skin cells and give the skin an appearance of being smoother and brighter.

Summary of action
- The products come as a mask or a lotion to be applied to the skin in an upward smooth motion.
- Ideal for a dry, mature skin.

Method of use
- AHA treatments can cause a slight contra-action after treatment: the skin may go pink, with a tingling sensation and mild itching – this is a normal reaction and the client should be warned to expect it.

COSHH considerations
- All ingredients commonly used in cosmetic products.
- Non-hazardous, non-inflammable.
- If ingested, drink milk or water.
- If in contact with eyes, wash well with water; if irritation occurs seek medical advice.
- If spilled – use absorbent towels to clean the area, wash with detergent and water to avoid slippery floors.
- No special handling and storage precautions necessary.

Moisturising creams

Key ingredients

- An emulsion of oils and waxes, such as coconut or jojoba oil.
- Water and water-soluble ingredients.
- Emulsifiers.
- Preservatives.
- Fragrance and colour.
- Humectants such as glycerine or sorbitol.

What they do

- Oils and waxes condition and improve the skin's natural water barrier – some oils such as jojoba oil prevent water loss, so are ideal to add to a cream.
- Creams contain approximately 60% water, which re-hydrates the skin.
- Emulsifiers prevent the ingredients separating, i.e. oil and water.
- Preservatives provide the product with a good shelf life and prevent deterioration.
- Colour and fragrance will give appeal – for example coconut oil has a very distinctive smell, which appeals to most people.
- Humectants attract water and help rehydrate the skin.

Summary of action

- Moisturising creams can be used morning and evening, depending upon skin type and cream used.
- Moisturising creams are recommended for dry skins that need the softening effects of the oil and wax – cream is especially good for skin in dry conditions, such as hot sun, or with central heating, and with temperature imbalance such as very cold weather.
- Make-up application is made easier with a moisturiser underneath it.
- Be careful about applying cream too near the delicate eye area, which may absorb the cream and become puffy – only eye cream should be used in the eye area.

Method of use

- Apply a light film to create a natural protective layer and prevent dehydration of skin.
- To avoid too much cream sitting on the skin surface, check the amount applied by pressing a clean tissue to the face one minute after application – if grease is present on the skin too much cream has been applied, or the cream is too rich for the skin type.

COSHH considerations

- All ingredients commonly used in cosmetic products.
- Non-hazardous, non-inflammable.
- If ingested, drink milk or water.
- If in contact with eyes, wash well with water, if irritation occurs seek medical advice.
- If spilled – use absorbent towels to clean the area, wash with detergent and water to avoid slippery floors.
- No special handling and storage precautions necessary.

Face masks

Key ingredients

Varies depending upon type of mask used – refer to pages 171–177.

What they do

- Masks are deep cleansing and draw any impurity to the surface of the skin.
- They may be slightly astringent to help dry up an oily skin, or rehydrating to help a dry skin.
- Please refer to specific mask information.

Summary of action

- Please refer to specific mask information.

Method of use

- Please refer to specific mask information.

COSHH considerations

- Health hazard: inhalation of fine particles can cause irritation if mixing up powder.
- Use / handling care should be taken when mixing powders.
- Avoid inhalation.
- If inhaled move to fresh air, if coughing persists seek medical advice.
- If mixing up large quantities a face guard is advisable.
- Storage should be in a cool dry place in a closed container.
- If in contact with eyes rinse with plenty of water – seek medical assistance if irritation continues.
- If ingested seek medical advice immediately.

Eye make-up removers

Key ingredients

- Varies depending upon whether it is an oil, a gel or a lotion preparation.
- Most of them are prepared from a mild cleaning agent in a cosmetic base.
- Typical ingredients may include:
  - horse chestnut extract
  - hydrolysed wheat proteins
  - vitamins
  - organic alcohol, e.g. PEG 200.

What they do

- Horse chestnut is used for a decrease in swelling and reduces puffiness to the eye area.
- Wheat proteins moisturise lids and lashes.
- Vitamins such as B5 increase cell regeneration.
- Organic alcohol is a solvent, which cleanses water and oil-based dirt.

Summary of action

- Eye make-up remover should be light, non-greasy and easily used without dragging the skin.
- Always ask the client if she is wearing contact lenses or false eyelash extensions – both may require specialist removers, certainly one that is non-oily.
- It is very irritating to the client to have a film left over the eye after removal of eye make-up. It must be thoroughly removed and not leaked into the client's eye.

Method of use

- Pre-soaked pads bought over the counter are usually lint pads soaked in remover.
- In a salon, damp cotton wool pads are normally used.
- Gently move over the eye area with an upward and inward movement, always supporting the eye area.
- Be careful to check that the client is not allergic to the metallic fibres present in cotton wool before commencing the treatment.
- A good eye make-up remover dissolves make-up immediately.
- Specialist oil-based remover may be needed to remove waterproof mascara.

COSHH considerations

- All ingredients commonly used in cosmetic products.
- Non-hazardous, non-inflammable..
- If ingested, drink milk or water.
- If in contact with eyes, wash well with water, if irritation occurs seek medical advice.

- If spilled – use absorbent towels to clean the area, wash with detergent and water to avoid slippery floors.
- No special handling and storage precautions necessary.

Eye creams / balms / gel

Key ingredients

- Ingredients vary depending upon cream or gel but may include:
  - oil in water emulsions
  - vitamins
  - methyl cellulose
  - collagen
  - plant and herb extracts
  - essential oils
  - azulene, witch hazel, cucumber and camomile.

What they do

- Oil-in-water emulsion is easily absorbed by the skin and is a good moisturiser, so it forms a good base for a daytime cream under make-up.
- Water-in-oil is a heavier solution and therefore only really good for the eyes at night.
- Vitamins help with cell regeneration.
- Methyl cellulose thickens the suspension to give it its gel-like consistency, which dries on the delicate eye area firming and tightening the skin.
- Witch hazel and cucumber are mildly astringent and cooling to the eye, usually found in eye lotions.

Summary of action

- Eye creams should be used regularly to delay the formation of fine wrinkles and lines appearing with age.
- Ideally prevention is better than cure, so eye protection should begin prior to lines forming.
- Lotions are better for oily skins and the richer thicker textured creams are really suitable for dry or lined skin.

Method of use

- Less is more with eye creams: application of too much is a waste of product and may cause swelling in the eye area if the soft tissue around the eye area has absorbed it.
- A small blob of cream should be warmed between your fingers before gently massaging the cream around the eye area – the ring fingers, i.e. the third fingers of each hand, have the lightest pressure, to avoid damage to the area.
- Work in small circular motions from the bridge of the nose, outward to temples across the top of the eye, just under eyebrow and then underneath the eye towards the nose.
- Any excess can be blotted, but try not to waste any of it.

COSHH considerations

- All ingredients commonly used in cosmetic products.
- Non-hazardous, non-inflammable.
- If ingested, drink milk or water.
- If in contact with eyes, wash well with water; if irritation occurs seek medical advice.
- If spilled – use absorbent towels to clean the area, wash with detergent and water to avoid slippery floors.
- No special handling and storage precautions necessary.

Neck creams

While a lot of attention is given to the face, the neck area is a very clear mirror reflecting age and / or neglect of the skin. All facials should include the neck area, and there are some very good preparations available to use on the neck area.

Unfortunately many clients do not bother with their neck until signs start to show; it is worth encouraging younger clients to pamper the neck area to prevent damage occurring.

Most neck preparations are very rich in formula, with a high oil content to nourish and moisturise.

Hydrolysed collagen, elastin and vitamin E are common ingredients, which will moisturise, increase suppleness and firm the neck.

Advise the client to apply a light film after toning at night, and encourage the client to include the neck area in the morning routine of cleanse, tone and moisturise, even though make-up application will not go onto the neck. The neck still needs protection from pollution, the environment and the sun, and from the danger of dehydration.

Hand care

Yes, this is still the facial section! Another area to show signs of neglect and of ageing, like the neck area, is the hands. Encourage the use of hand creams and again, prevention and protection are better than cure.

The client should rub in any excess moisturiser into her hands, rather than waste the product, and a hand cream should become part of a night-time routine. Please refer to the manicure section for further reading.

Lip care

Again, a sadly neglected part of the face, until cold sores and chapped lips become a problem.

When removing the client's eye make-up the lipstick can also be removed, and the cleansing medium and massage motion if removing, will help keep the lips moist. Lip balms, flavoured lip-gloss and lip creams are available to help dry or sore lips. Remember that the lips need protection against the sun, as they have no melanin of their own, and while most lipsticks contain a sunscreen, naked lips will not be protected.

When recommending products to the client it is important to take into account the client's personal preferences. If the client likes the feel of a cream on her skin, but you recommend a milk cleanser, a compromise might be a fluffy cream with a high water content.

Sun preparations

Although sun preparations do not come under the normal facial routine in a salon, lots of clients need the right information for homecare advice and use of the correct products, especially if going on holiday, whether in this country or abroad.

Wise health education means that people are now more aware of the damage that the sun does to the skin, and the ever-present risk of skin cancer, which is on the increase. The sun is damaging to the skin but because a tan has been fashionable since the 1950s some clients like to keep a high colour.

Sun protection can come in lotion, cream, or milk form, and some large manufacturers have now designed a spray-on application for sun protection.

Remember

Some clients have been using the same make of product for years and although you may advise a change that the skin will benefit from, old habits are hard to change.

Sunscreens filter the harmful ultraviolet rays, UVA and UVB, for a period of time. Most are water resistant and contain moisturisers to help nourish the skin. They come in various strengths, measured by a sun protection factor (SPF) ranging from 2–35. The higher the SPF number the greater the protection.

The SPF number allows the wearer to stay out in the sun that length of time longer, e.g. SPF 6 permits skin exposure six times longer than unprotected skin, before burning. A SPF of 30 allows 30 times the sun exposure.

The choice of SPF depends upon the skin type and the strength of the sun. The nearer the equator, the hotter the sun, so a higher protection factor would be needed in the Mediterranean than in southwest England. The sun's rays are also reflected so there is a risk of getting sunburnt when sailing or skiing, even when the temperature is low.

Sun blocks are total blocks and will screen out all the sun's rays. They have become essential in some countries, such as Australia, where there is a high incidence of skin cancer. Sun blocks are also available as coloured strips of cream that sit on the nose and forehead — very popular with cricketers.

Skin type	Recommended sun preparation
Fair skin or redhead with pale skin, burns easily after 30 minutes' exposure	20–25 SPF or sun block for complete protection
Sallow skinned person who is pale, will tan, but feels sore after 30 minutes	10–15 SPF
Darker skins that tan easily but tend to get sore initially	2–10 SPF

Skin products for different skin types

See individual products and follow individual recommendations, as products do vary. As sun on the face will accelerate the ageing process, clients can be advised to wear a hat or cover the face liberally with the correct SPF factor cream.

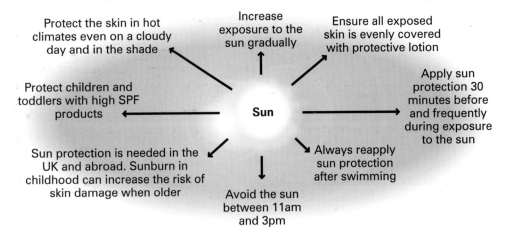

Safe sun advice

Check it out

Buy several samples of self-tanning preparations and try them out at home. Remember to exfoliate first and then apply moisturiser, before applying the tan. Follow the manufacturer's instructions and apply to your legs. Note the different textures and smells – which one did you prefer? Which one gave the most natural colour?

(Do remember to scrub your palms if not wearing gloves, otherwise they will be tanned too.)

Self-tanning creams

This is a very popular salon treatment for both face and body, and the safest way to get a tan. After exfoliation and moisturising, the tanning lotion is applied and will develop over several hours and last for several days. Most large cosmetic houses make 'false' tan for the face, which is not as strong as the body self tan.

The active ingredient is a chemical called dihydroxyacetone which reacts with the keratin in the skin to produce a golden colour through oxidation. This has become a very popular salon treatment to offer clients. It looks very natural and lasts about a week, depending upon the depth of the application.

Skin type	Products most suitable	
Normal (depending on personal product preference)	Eye make-up remover lotion Light cleansing cream or lotion Facial wash if preferred	10–20% alcohol content toner Light moisturiser cream or lotion Eye lotion
Dry	Eye make-up remover oil or cream Low alcohol content toner or no alcohol if sensitive too Paraffin wax mask Non-setting mask Eye cream Cream moisturiser	
Greasy	Eye make-up lotion Cleansing lotion or cleansing milk Facial wash / foaming gel 25–50% alcohol content toner	Cleansing grains / peel Clay-based masks Moisturiser milk Light eye gel
Combination	T-zone – follow greasy skin recommendations Dry cheek areas – follow dry skin recommendations Normal cheek areas – follow normal skin recommendations Young congested T-zone – follow congested skin with normal recommendations on cheeks	
Sensitive	As for dry skin If hyper-sensitive then specialist products are available Check for known allergies to products Check for allergies to cotton wool	
Dehydrated	As for dry skin Specialist treatments are available in most salons using advanced techniques, such as galvanic facial (NVQ level 3 work). Be aware and read the salon price list to recommend to the client. Another therapist may be able to help the client's skin.	
Congested	Eye make-up lotion Cleansing lotion and cleansing milk Facial wash / foaming gel 25 – 50% alcohol content toner	Cleansing grains / peel Clay-based masks Moisturiser milk Light eye gel

Summary of products for different skin types

Improve skin conditions using skin care and massage techniques

6.3

Step-by-step facial cleanse

Ensure that the client is correctly prepared for the treatment.

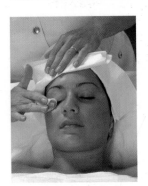

Using damp cotton wool apply eye make-up remover, working around the eye, over lid, underneath and over lashes. Work from inner to outer area. Remove with damp cotton wool.

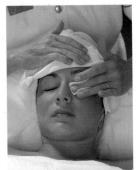

Follow the same routine with the other eye. Be careful to support the eye area, and do not drag, or apply any pressure.

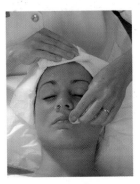

Apply a small amount of cleanser, using damp cotton wool and remove the lipstick, in small circular motions.

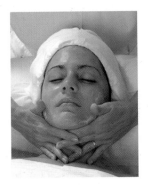

Apply dots of cleanser over the entire face. Working from the neck upwards, use upward movements towards the jaw line.

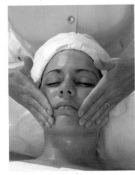

Work from the jaw line; use alternate hand movements to cover the entire cheek area.

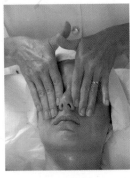

Using the index fingers, work into the nose, with small circular motions, without blocking the nostrils in! Use light pressure only.

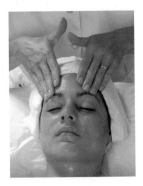

Travel over the bridge of the nose, onto the forehead working out towards the temple areas. Using index fingers, apply a little pressure to the temples.

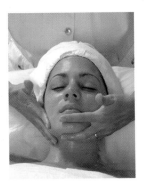

Sweep back down to the chin, working over the jaw line with alternate hand movements, to finish the cleanse routine.

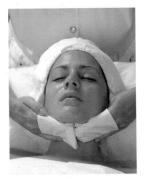

Remove cleanser, following the same routine direction as for the application of cleanser, with tissues, damp cotton wool or sponges.

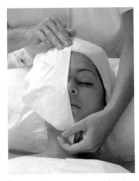

Blot the face with the tissue folded in a triangle. Pat gently with the hand, turn tissue over and repeat on the other side of the face.

Face masks

There are many different types of face mask available, both over the counter and in salons. They can be divided into two categories – setting masks and non-setting masks.

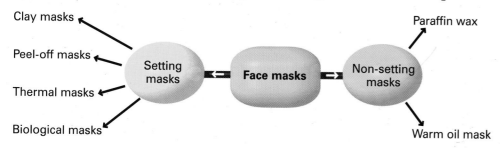

Masks can have different actions depending upon their formulation. The choice of mask depends on accurate skin analysis and knowledge of the effects of basic mask ingredients.

Some masks come already mixed and some need mixing: generally the pre-prepared types tend to be more expensive. The ones which have to be made up as needed take more skill and knowledge of the ingredients and portions required, but the basic ingredients can be purchased in bulk and stored.

Natural ingredients can also be used for a face mask and provide great variety and fun.

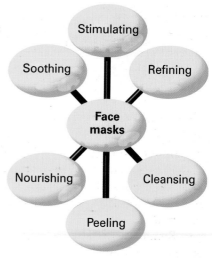

Actions of a face mask

Properties of face masks

1   They should be smooth, free from gritty particles and unpleasant odours. In powder form, they should be easily dispersed in water to produce a paste.

2   They should be easily removed from the face after use without causing pain or discomfort.

3   They must be harmless to the skin and non-toxic.

Contra-indications to the application of face masks

These can include:

- skin disorders and diseases
- excessively dry or sensitive skin
- loose, crepey skin
- cuts and abrasions
- recent scar tissue.

Note Clients who are claustrophobic may prefer a non-setting mask.

Materials required for a face mask treatment

- Bowls
- Spatulas
- Mask brush – flat and sanitised
- Damp cotton wool
- Headband
- Tissues
- Skin tonic
- Moisturiser
- Couch roll
- Client record card
- Scissors for eye pads

Clay masks

These could be classed as natural ingredients because they are usually clays found in the earth – which makes them very good at drawing out impurities, and deep cleansing. Some can be quite stimulating and are good for improving the circulation, others are mild and soothing on the skin.

The key is to know which ingredients are suitable for which skin type.

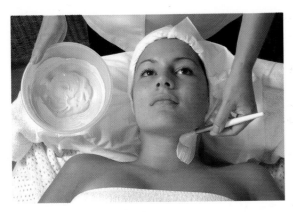

Calamine face mask application

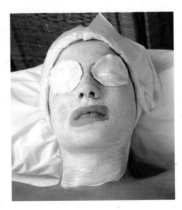

Calamine face mask

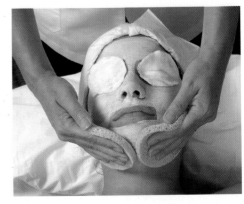

Removing a calamine face mask

Skin type	Clay powder	Benefits	Mixed with
Dry skin	Calamine (a pink powder)	Contains zinc carbonate to soothe the skin and calm down a high colour	Rose water, orange flower water (or distilled water for sensitive skin)
	Magnesium carbonate (a white powder)	Refines and softens the skin, mildly astringent	A couple of drops of vegetable oil, almond oil or glycerol can be added
Greasy skin	Fuller's earth (a grey / green powder)	Deep cleansing. Not suitable for sensitive skin as it can be quite stimulating	Distilled water with a drop of witch hazel if required
	Sulphur (a pale yellow powder)	Drying action so can be used on individual blemishes	Distilled water with a drop of witch hazel if required
Normal (balanced)	Magnesium carbonate (a white powder)	Refines and softens the skin, mildly astringent	Mix with equal proportions of rose water, orange flower water or witch hazel
	Calamine (a pink powder)	Contains zinc carbonate to soothe the skin and calm down a high colour	Mix with equal proportions of rose water, orange flower water or witch hazel
	Fuller's earth (a grey / green powder)	Deep cleansing. Not suitable for sensitive skin as it can be quite stimulating	Mix with equal proportions of rose water, orange flower water or witch hazel
Combination skin	Follow the dry/normal skin for cheek areas and greasy skin for T skin zone, depending upon the severity of each area		

Types of face mask

Active ingredients

A clay mask needs to be mixed with active ingredients to turn the powder into a liquid paste. The liquids are selected to complement the skin type and mask to be used — they reinforce the action of the mask.

* **Rose water:** gives a mild toning effect, which increases the toning action of a mask. Made from rose petals. Recommended for dry, normal and mature skin types.
* **Orange flower water:** gives a stimulating tonic effect. This is natural plant extract, from the fruit of the tree.

- **Citrus dulcis:** very fragrant. Recommended for normal, dry and mature skin types.
- **Witch hazel:** this has a drying, stimulating effect, so is contra-indicated on fine sensitive skins; it is much better suited to greasy or combination skins. It is made from the dried leaves and bark of the Hamamelis Virginia tree: It has a tissue-firming action on the skin.
- **Almond oil:** can be used on dehydrated or neglected younger skins or on the more mature skin. It is a natural oil obtained from the kernels of the seeds of whole almonds. It improves the condition of the skin.
- **Distilled water:** this is ordinary water that has had the chemicals, such as magnesium bicarbonate or calcium carbonate, removed from it. These can be removed by boiling the water or chemically removed by water softeners.
- **Calamine lotion:** this liquid contains zinc carbonate to soothe and heal the skin. Iron oxide produces the pink colouring.

Skin type	Recipe	Time on face
Normal skin	1 part kaolin 1 part fuller's earth Mix with water and a few drops of witch hazel to form a smooth thin paste	8–12 minutes
Dry skin	1 part kaolin 1 part magnesium carbonate Mix with rose water or orange flower water to form a smooth thin paste	10–15 minutes
Oily skin	Fuller's earth Mix with witch hazel to form a smooth paste	5–15 minutes
Sensitive skin	1 part calamine 1 part magnesium carbonate Mix with rose water to form a smooth paste	5–10 minutes
Sulphur mask	1/2 tsp Epsom salts 1 tsp oatmeal 1 tsp magnesium carbonate (for acne) 1 tsp precipitated sulphur Mix with hot water to form a paste	Apply over gauze, leave for 15 minutes – keeping warm with infrared lamps
Stimulating mask (for open pores, capillaries and contracting the tissues)	6 parts magnesium carbonate 2 parts fuller's earth Mix with rose water or almond oil according to the moisture content of the skin	5–15 minutes
Astringent mask	6 parts magnesium carbonate 1 part calamine Pinch of alum Mix with witch hazel	Apply over gauze Apply one coat until almost dry then apply second coat 10 minutes

Setting masks

Peel-off masks

Peel-off masks are gel or latex based. (Paraffin wax masks also come into a peel-off category, although they are classed as non-setting.)

Because perspiration cannot escape from the skin's surface, moisture is forced back into the epidermis. Some peel-off masks also create heat, so could come under the thermal category.

The gel masks are purchased as a ready-made suspension containing starches, gums or gelatine, to allow the correct consistency. Synthetic non-biological resins are commonly used as well.

The mask is applied over the skin and when it makes contact it immediately begins to dry. It can be peeled off over the face as a whole facial mould, when sufficient technique has been mastered.

The gel mask can be used on most skin types, depending on the ingredients used, so check with individual manufacturer's instructions.

A **latex mask** is an emulsion of latex and water. The water evaporates leaving a rubber film to form the mask. Alternatives include synthetic PVC resins. These have a firming, tightening effect on the skin and can be used on a dry or mature skin.

Biological / natural masks

These include the following.

- **Fruit extracts**
  e.g. avocado – mashed to a smooth paste.
  Action: helps stabilise skin's pH and acid mantle.
- **Herbal and vegetable**
  e.g. cucumber – sliced and placed over skin.
  Action: calming or astringent effect.
- **Biological**
  e.g. natural yogurt applied in bought state.
  Action: refines skin's texture, helps rid waste from skin, counteracts possible infection.
  e.g. egg – use with almond oil for dry skin, or lemon for oily skin.
  e.g. honey – use on dehydrated or mature skin for a softening effect.

Warm oil mask

The skin is cleansed, a piece of gauze is soaked in warm olive or almond oil. Eye pads are placed over eyes, and the gauze carefully put onto the face. An infrared lamp is placed in position for 10 to 20 minutes. The distance of the lamp is determined prior to application to suit client's skin type.

Indications

- Crêpey fine lined skin.
- Premature ageing.
- Dehydration or dry skin.
- Younger skin as a preventative measure.

It is important to prepare client and couch adequately to protect all areas.

Effects:
- Cleanses and aids desquamation.
- Increases smoothness, softness and elasticity.

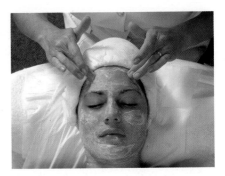
A peel-off face mask

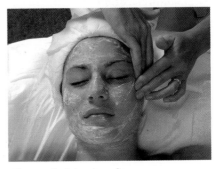
The mask dries very fast

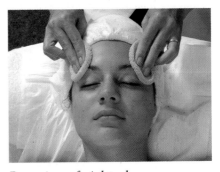
Removing a facial peel

Remember

A gel mask does adhere to the facial hair, and can be painful during removal – rather like a plaster coming off! If the client has a lot of facial hair you should offer an alternative mask.

- Due to the mask working on heat penetration, the skin will absorb cosmetic preparations more. Massage oil into skin after application for maximum benefit. Ensure toning and moisturising is thorough without over-stretching or over-touching skin.
- Client should be advised skin may have an uneven appearance directly after application for up to 3 or 4 hours.

Paraffin wax mask

Preparation

A small amount of clean sterilised paraffin wax should be poured into a small clean bowl lined with foil. (Wax heaters may be too large to be mobile.) The working temperature is 49°C.

The wax treatment may be applied within the facial routine in place of a setting mask. Disposable paper should cover normal towels for protection.

Application

Eye pads are put in place. Wax should be applied in a firm layer build-up, over the neck, cheeks, chin, nose and forehead, using a small brush. The wax can be applied over gauze for easy removal. Your client should have complete confidence in you; your presence should be known so she may relax.

Depending upon the skin type, the time on the face may vary from 10–20 minutes. Then remove eye pads, gently slide fingers under the edges of mask, place hands under mask at throat, pulling the mask up a little at a time, taking care that any bits of mask are stuck to the main bulk. Pressure toning with water may be suitable, but usually it is best to leave.

Effects

- Natural perspiration cleans the skin.
- Circulation is improved.
- Dead cells removed, improves desquamation.
- Increased elasticity, smoothness and softness of texture.
- Removes cellular matter.
- Moisturising (perspiration cannot escape, so moisture is forced back into epidermis).
- Local increase in temperature.

Indications

- Dry, dehydrated.
- Mature skin, where regeneration is needed without over-stimulation.
- Crêpey, finely lined skin.
- Uneven textured skin (unstable pH) to promote desquamation, and refine texture.
- Seborrhoea conditions, to remove oily blockages and surface adhesions.

Contra-indications

- Highly nervous, tense clients, claustrophobic.
- Extreme vascular conditions.
- Sepsis, skin infection and irritation.

Step-by-step paraffin wax face mask application

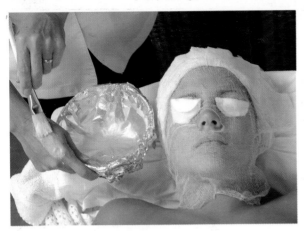

Cut gauze to fit face, with eye and nose holes. Use damp cotton wool to cover eyes. Decant hot wax into a bowl lined with tin foil. Test on self.

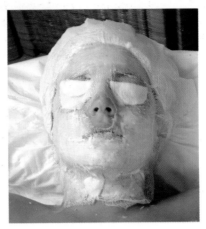

If the wax is a comfortable temperature, quickly apply a thick layer all over the face, starting on the neck, using a mask brush, avoiding the eyes, lip and nose areas.

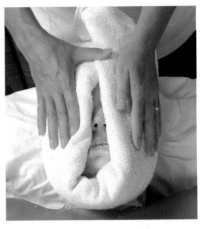

To keep the heat in, and maximise the treatment, place a wrapped warm towel over the face, avoiding the nose and mouth. Leave on for max. 15 mins.

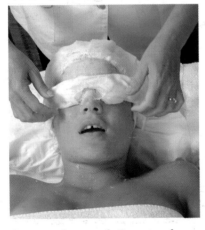

Remove the towel. Because the mask will have hardened, removal can be completed in one upward movement, rolling up the gauze from the neck.

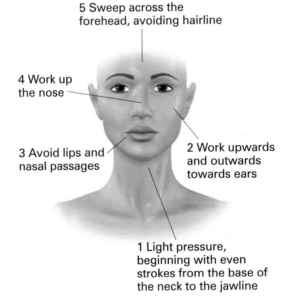

5 Sweep across the forehead, avoiding hairline

4 Work up the nose

3 Avoid lips and nasal passages

2 Work upwards and outwards towards ears

1 Light pressure, beginning with even strokes from the base of the neck to the jawline

Applying the face mask – sequence of hand movements

Remember

Be sure to leave enough gap around eyes, nose and mouth for client comfort.

Basic mask formulation

As every facial diagnosis differs slightly, no exact formulation can be assumed to be suitable for all skin conditions. **No rules can apply in mask therapy** due to the variety of mask products and to the different actions they are capable of producing. Observation and client discussion regarding tolerance to the mask will increase your knowledge of the skin's reaction to certain ingredients.

Final tips for face masks

- Follow manufacturer's instructions.
- Always use a mask that complements the range of products being used. e.g. René Guinot or Clarins, or whichever range the salon is using.
- Always do a thorough facial analysis in order to be able to decide the correct mask for the client.

Facial massage

All massage is extremely therapeutic – for the face, scalp or body. It is very satisfying to give a facial massage as well as to receive one. A good therapist knows her massage movements so well that she doesn't have to think about what to do, and she can also enjoy the experience.

Massage movements can also be incorporated into a cleansing routine, and most other facial and cleansing treatments.

To be truly relaxing, a good massage has continuity, rhythm and the correct depth, appropriate to the area being treated, and the needs of the client.

Benefits

The benefits of facial massage include the following.

- Dead surface cells are helped to loosen and shed. This helps the natural exfoliation process, and produces a clean-looking, fresh complexion.
- Facial muscles are relaxed, and they receive more blood supply because of the stimulation to the circulation. This improves the tone and strength of the muscles, giving a firmer facial appearance.
- As the blood circulation is improved the face area is warmed, which is very relaxing for tense muscles, especially in the jaw and forehead, which tends to be clenched and tense.
- An increase in lymphatic drainage to the face (massage always flows in the direction of the lymph nodes) produces an increase in cellular activity and the removal of toxins. The sebaceous glands are stimulated to increase sebum production, and this keeps the skin protected and supple.
- To make the treatment doubly effective, and help the massage medium penetrate deeper into the skin, try the application of heat onto the skin with either hot towels or steaming (see page 187), or exfoliation by brush cleansing.
- Psychologically, massage is very beneficial. Some clients drift off into sleep, it is so relaxing. The gentle rhythm is soothing and calming, both to the nerve endings and to the soul. The atmosphere within your working area should enhance this calm and tranquil haven; relaxing music helps the process along, and encourages the client to let go of conscious thought and drift away.

> **Remember**
>
> A good tip is to cover the edge of the turban or headband with tissue. It means you can throw the tissue away if your application is less than perfect.

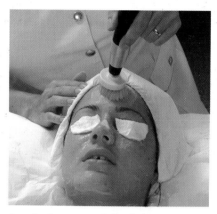

Brush cleansing of the face

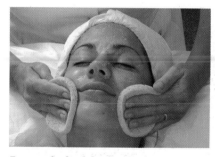

Removal of gel for brush cleanse

> **Remember**
>
> The way in which you approach a massage also affects your client and the mood of the treatment. If you are rushed and hurried, no benefit will be gained and it is almost as if you are cheating your client out of what should be a relaxing experience. Be calm, fully prepared and collect your thoughts before you begin. Giving a massage should be like a little bit of meditation for the therapist – it should be a quiet, soothing time for you both.

Facial massage movement

Massage movements are performed with the hands, over the neck, shoulders and chest, as well as the facial area. The movements require practice in order to perfect the skills and outcomes required.

Movements are adapted according to the needs of clients and relate directly to the facial analysis or the consultation. It may be that your client has specific areas of tension, or that her skin is particularly dry and therefore needs an oil, rather than cream. The basic massage movements are classified by their names (in French) and their particular effects and benefits to the skin.

The movements are:

- effleurage
- tapotement
- petrissage
- vibrations.
- frictions

Effleurage

There are two types of effleurage: superficial and deep.

Superficial effleurage

This is a light flowing pressure used at the beginning and the end of most treatments. It introduces your hands to the client, spreads the massage medium and can be a great linking movement to help the massage flow.

So how do I do it?

Use the entire palmer surface of the hands, keeping the fingers together and the thumb either close into the side of the hand, or open and out of the way. The area being massaged is covered by all or part of the palmer surface. Pressure should be light and even, with good contact with the skin, with the hands warm and relaxed. Superficial effleurage does not normally affect the circulation, as it is not a deep movement, so it can be used in any direction.

Benefits of superficial effleurage include:

- relaxation of tense muscle fibres
- a general feeling of relaxation
- stimulation of sensory nerve endings and a feeling of pleasure
- introduction of the massage medium onto the skin
- soothing and calming.

Deep effleurage

This is the same type of movement as superficial effleurage but with more pressure applied – not too much to make the sensation uncomfortable, but enough to encourage muscular relaxation and for you to feel the tension knots.

Maintaining contact with the skin helps avoid over-stimulation of the nerve endings. This is because when contact is broken and then re-established, this sets up a reflex response in the nerve endings, which prevents the muscles from relaxing.

Benefits of deep effleurage are that it helps:

- venous return
- arterial circulation by removal of congestion from veins
- desquamation.

Remember

Make sure you have enough of the massage medium on the skin: too little and the hands become sticky and the movements don't flow, too much and it will run down the client's face! If in the first application you can judge that the client's skin is dry and soaking up the cream or oil, then apply a little more, at the beginning, rather than having to stop the massage, to apply more – not very relaxing!

Petrissage

There are four different categories:

- kneading
- wringing – mostly used on body
- rolling – mostly used on body
- picking up.

Petrissage **always** follows effleurage.

It is a compression movement, performed using intermittent pressure with either one or both hands using different parts. Most petrissage movements work on all or part of a muscle and it is important that, as a muscle is slowly released from application, pressure is reduced.

Petrissage movements must be applied rhythmically and not in a hurried way. Too much pressure may result in damage to the skin – adaptation to your client's needs is vital.

Benefits of petrissage include the following.

- Aching, hard muscles are relaxed, helping to prevent the formation of tension nodules.
- Skin regeneration is stimulated.
- It has a toning effect on muscle tissue.
- It helps eliminate muscular fatigue by aiding in the removal of lactic acid.
- It helps removal of waste products and lymphatic flow.

> **Remember**
>
> Always use effleurage to link petrissage movements.

Frictions

Frictions are classified within the petrissage group, but their purpose differs. Friction movements will loosen adherent skin, loosen scars, and aid in absorption of fluid around the joints.

The pressure is firm and the movement is usually applied in circular directions, and on the face; fingertips or thumbs are mostly used in small areas.

Benefits of frictions include the following.

- Adhesions and loose skin are freed.
- Scar tissue can be stretched and loosened.

Tapotement

This is a percussion movement and is achieved very much as its name implies, i.e. tapping. The tips of the fingers are used to create very light tapping movements, which in turn stimulate the skin.

It is very important that sufficient adipose tissue is present to perform the treatment. Sensitive skin must not be treated in this way due to possible over-reaction and the risk of skin damage occurring.

Benefits of tapotement include the following.

- It increases localised blood supply.
- It increases nervous response due to stimulation.

Vibrations

Vibrations are fine trembling movements performed on or along a nerve path by the fingers. The muscles of the operator's forearm are continually contracted and relaxed to produce a fine tremble or vibration that runs to the fingertips.

Benefits of vibrations include the following.

- It can be used at occipital region in facial massage.
- It can relieve pain and relax client due to its sedative effect.

Step-by-step facial massage routine

Each movement should be done six times. The massage should last for 20 minutes.

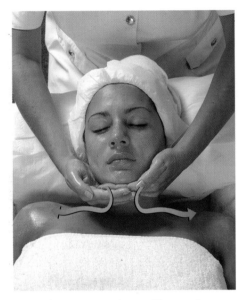

Apply massage medium all over the face, neck and shoulders and spread evenly. With both hands together, start at chin, and move down either side of neck towards shoulders.

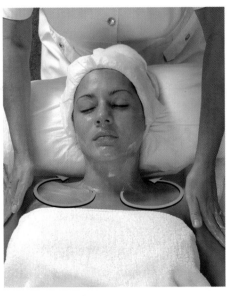

Apply pressure over the chest and go over the shoulders, working along the upper back towards the spine.

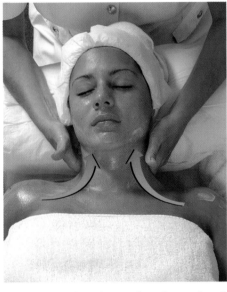

When your hands reach either side of the spine, work upwards and gently stretch the neck, lifting the head slightly off the couch.

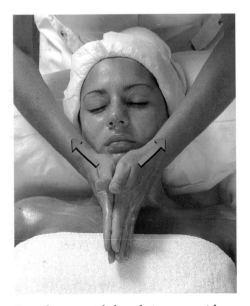

Face brace: with hands in an upside-down prayer position, begin under the chin, with heels of the hands resting lightly on the chin.

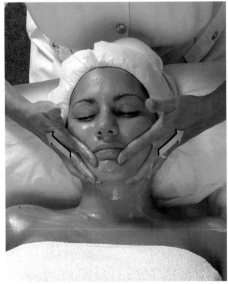

Work upwards, over the cheeks, lifting quite firmly The cheeks will move slightly, as the client is relaxed.

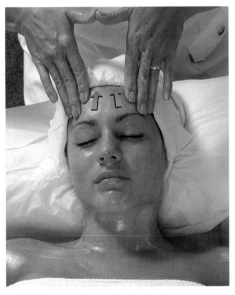

Finish with a firm, lifting movement on the forehead.

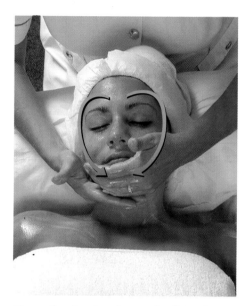

From the forehead, gently slide the hands back to the jaw line.

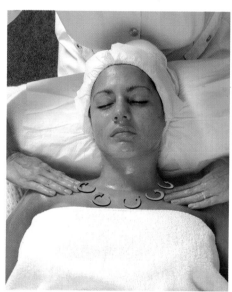

Perform rotaries of petrissage, starting from the chin and moving down either side of neck towards the shoulders and beyond, paying special attention to the arm and deltoid muscle.

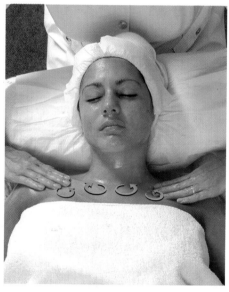

Use small circular motions across all of the chest area. You may only be able to use your fingertips if the client is small. No long nails for this movement!

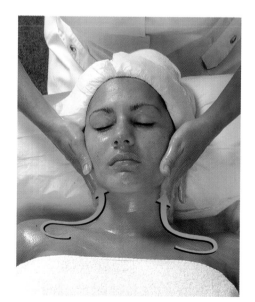

Continue your circular massage up the sides of the neck, ready to begin another movement.

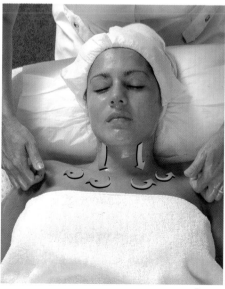

Turn your hands into loose fists and rotate your fingers to form knuckling. Come down from the neck and across the chest, over shoulders and back to the occipital cavity.

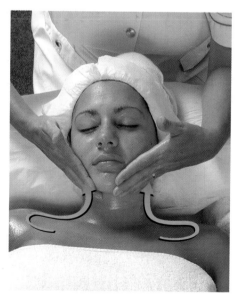

Finish the movement at the jaw line ready to begin alternate triangular sweeping.

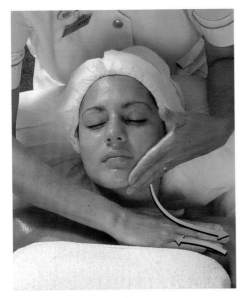

Support the jaw with your left hand; with the right hand, stroke down the right side, to the shoulder. Stroke across the chest to the other shoulder.

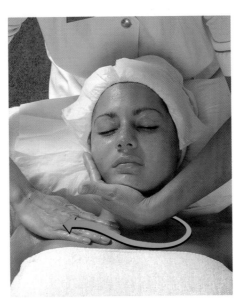

Take your right hand behind the shoulder.

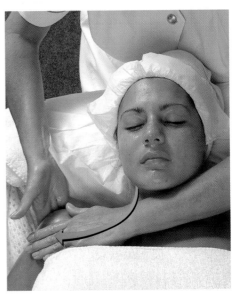

Stroke your left hand across the chest to meet the right hand at the right shoulder.

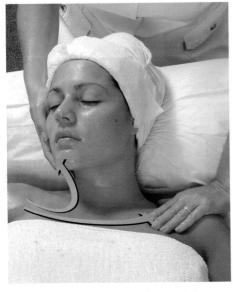

Bring the right hand back up to the jaw and left hand back across the chest.

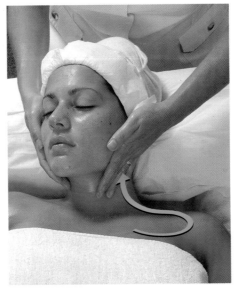

Bring the left hand back up to meet at the jaw.

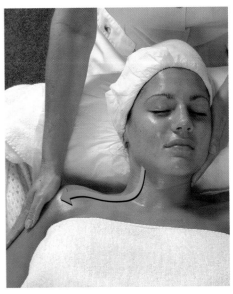

Bring the right hand back down at the shoulder.

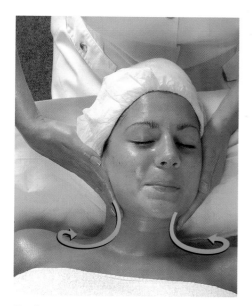

Perform trapezius rolling –work hands together on one side, then the other.

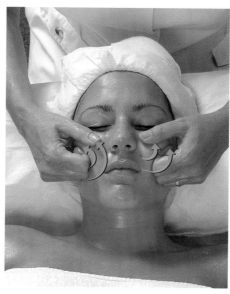

Cheek lift – index finger to little finger – turn and twist off.

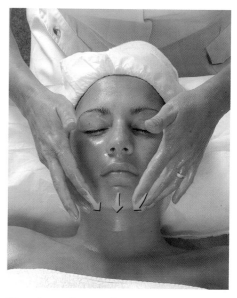

Tap along the jaw line.

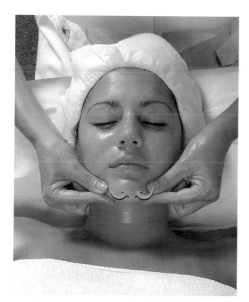

Perform rotaries along jaw line – thumbs abducted – centre outwards.

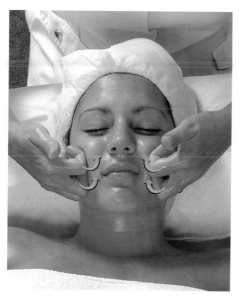

Knuckle over chin and cheeks.

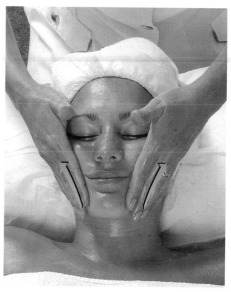

Facial lift –work hands along each side of the face – lift and join hands together over the forehead, then divide off.

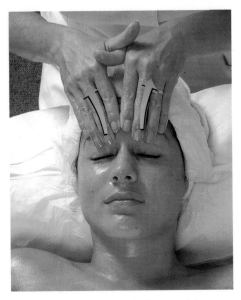

Forehead brace – both hands lift up the eyebrows to the hairline.

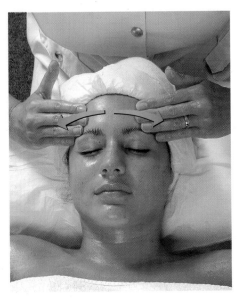

Turn hands sideways and gently pull the forehead from the centre, smoothing out the temples.

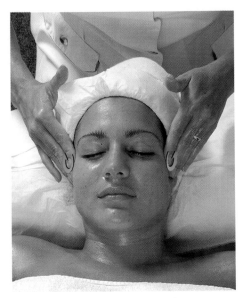

Finish with slight finger rotation pressure at the temples.

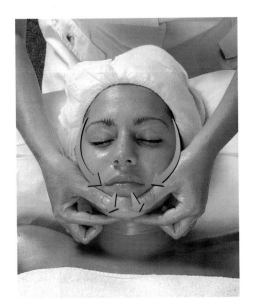

Slide hands down to the jaw. Pinch along the jaw line, using thumb and forefinger.

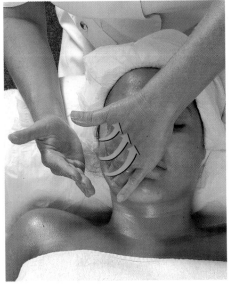

Using alternate hand movements, begin roll patting over cheeks and forehead.

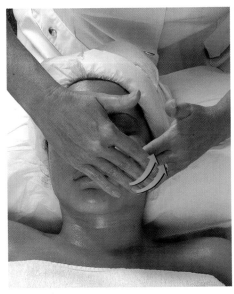

Repeat this movement over both sides of the face.

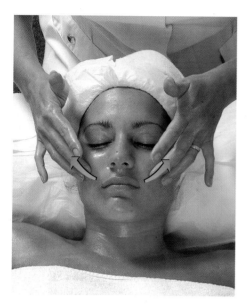

Tap over cheeks, using light pressure – fingertips only.

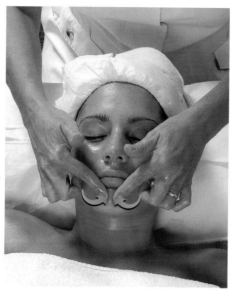

Apply frictions, using index fingers, around mouth and chin.

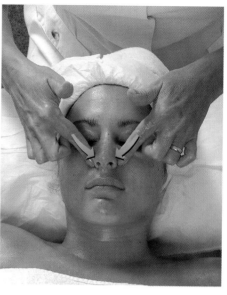

Apply frictions, using index fingers, around nostrils.

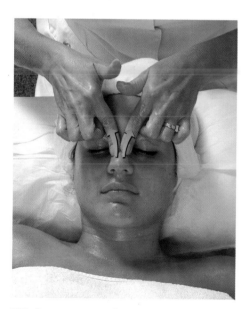

Work up nose with index fingers.

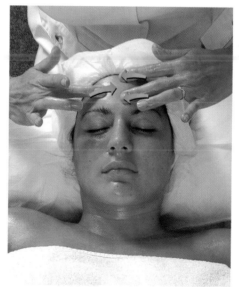

Zigzag with middle fingers going into a V created by the other hand over forehead.

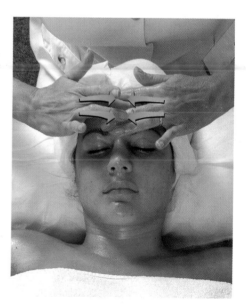

Working right across and down the forehead, cover all areas – this movement is especially appreciated by clients who suffer from headaches.

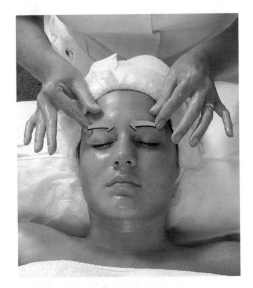

Do small circular pinching movements along the length of the eyebrows.

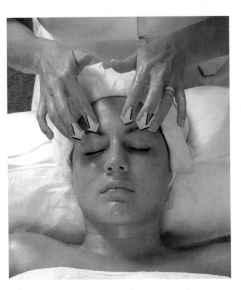

Piano playing across brow: circle eyes and bring all fingers across the brow. Start with little finger and finish with index finger.

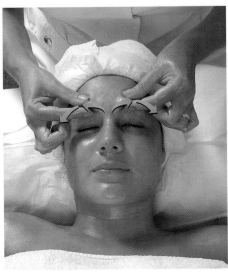

Pinch brows – centre to sides. Slide back and repeat.

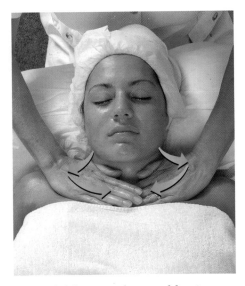

Come back to jaw line and begin superficial effleurage down either side of the neck.

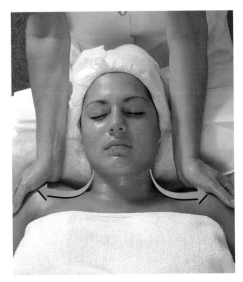

Perform superficial effleurage over shoulder area, gradually slowing down as you finish the massage.

Pre-warming the skin

Applying warmth to the face is a good way to help maximise the effects of the treatment. Warmth will help to relax the muscles, open the pores and soften the skin, in preparation for further treatments. Extraction (e.g. of comedones) and nourishing the skin are extremely effective after warming.

There are several ways to warm the skin:

- hot towels
- facial steaming
- self-heating products such as thermal masks.

Hot towels

Hot towels are a very convenient method of warming the skin. They can be applied without equipment and are ideal for the mobile therapist who does not have the use of a facial steaming unit.

Hot towels were always used in the old fashioned barber shop when a close shave was offered with the haircut. A hot flannel would have the same effect, but may make a client claustrophobic.

How do I do it?

- Fold a hand-size towel into four and immerse in hot water – leaving an edge for the hands to grip on to.
- Remember health and safety - if the towel is too hot to wring out with the hands, it is too hot to go on the face. It needs to be hand hot.
- Wring out and fold over the client's face, with the towel ends at the forehead. This will allow the nose to remain uncovered for claustrophobic clients.
- Press gently into the contours of the face until the towel cools. Do not allow the face to become cold again – this will negate the benefits of the treatment.
- The hot towel procedure can be repeated if needed.

Further treatments can now be carried out on a beautifully clean, receptive skin.

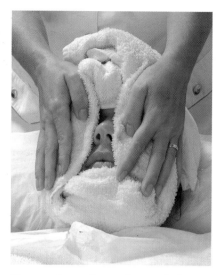

Hot towels can be used to apply heat

Facial steaming

Face steamers work in the same way as a big kettle, boiling the water to create steam, to benefit the skin by opening the pores and deep cleansing. They are nearly always used in conjunction with face masks and are classed as a special treatment.

Contra-indications

- hypersensitive skins
- open cuts – infection could set in
- acne rosacea
- split capillaries – where increasing the circulation and heat will put extra strain on these delicate blood vessels, and in some cases makes them worse
- bad streaming colds or hay fever
- severe bronchial conditions or asthma
- excessive high blood pressure or where the client suffers from dizzy spells
- any eye infections, such as conjunctivitis, which could spread in the warm conditions ideal for diseases
- diabetes – the metabolic rate of diabetics must not be increased
- sunburn or previous ultraviolet exposure
- claustrophobia suffers.

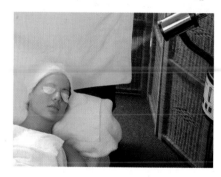

Facial steaming

Benefits of steaming

- The circulation is increased – causing the pores to open and the skin to sweat, getting rid of impurities, such as dirt and grime, old make-up, and dead skin cells, leaving the skin with a fresher, glowing appearance.
- The oil glands are stimulated, improving moisture content to the skin.
- Blackheads (comedones) are more easily removed with less risk of scarring or marking the skin.
- It aids the process of shedding old skin cells – called desquamation.
- It helps with regeneration of skin cells in a dry, mature or dehydrated skin.
- It is a relaxing and restful treatment for the client, due to the warmth, especially if essential oils are used.

Preparation for steaming

Items required

1 Distilled water (required for refilling machine).
2 Cotton wool rounds (damp) for eyes.
3 Tissue (this is used to wipe the client's face during treatment, avoiding drips which can lead to client's discomfort).

Preparation of couch

1 Check that the couch is stable and will not move during treatment.
2 Place ready in semi-reclining position.

Preparation of client

1 Prepare client, as you would do for any facial treatment, paying special attention to the head and ensuring that there are no stray hairs around the face and neck.
2 Ensure the client is comfortable and relaxed and all jewellery has been removed.
3 Lay a towel across the neck area (if doing neck and face then lay the towel across the chest). Tuck towel in at either end.
4 Explain treatment to client - to allay any anxieties she may have. Commence treatment with facial cleanse.

Safety precautions

1 Check machine, e.g. wires, flex, plug, on / off switch.
2 Check correct level of distilled water.
3 Check machine is functioning correctly and producing ozone (prior to client's arrival).
4 Ensure the couch is stable and in correct position.
5 Always ensure that the flex does not trail across the salon floor, which would endanger the safety of the other clients and your colleagues.
6 When machine is not in use, make sure it is unplugged and kept in a safe area away from the main bulk of activity in the salon.
7 During treatment the therapist must be in attendance at all times.
8 Eye pads must be used throughout this treatment.
9 Whilst machine is in use, ensure that it is the correct distance away from the client to avoid scald and spitting from the machine.
10 Take care when re-positioning the machine, as it gets very hot during use.
11 Always ensure you have steam before placing over your client.

Pre-treatment to facial cleaners

1 Manual cleanse.
2 Brush cleanse (depending on skin type).
3 Facial vacuum (depending on skin type).

Steaming procedure

1 Check tank is full and switch machine on 5 to 10 minutes before it is required to permit water heating to commence. The vapour switch is only required at this stage.
2 Ensure the client is well protected with towels and that her hair is covered.
3 Prepare client for facial treatment by cleansing the skin, and at the same time discuss and explain the treatment and its effects. Inform her that the machine will make a noise and that an unusual smell will be present – all of which is perfectly normal.
4 Ensure client is in a semi-reclined position.
5 Place damp eye pads over client's eyes to avoid irritation.

6   When client is fully prepared, position steamer approximately 30–45 cm (12–18 inches) from client's face, using at this stage only vapour.

7   Once client is settled then inform her you are switching over to ozone; this is done by switching on the ozone control. The steam then changes its consistency, becomes ionized, cloud-like and very fine in appearance.
(**Note** Refer to your professional body for directives about using ozone.)

8   Stay in attendance at all times and regularly check client's skin reaction. *Points to note are hot spots, erythema, or client's discomfort – if necessary, discontinue treatment.*

9   Remember to wipe away with tissue any drips that might cause client discomfort.

10 Do not exceed treatment time. This will vary from 10–20 minutes according to skin type.

11 On completion of treatment return to vapour then switch off completely. Unplug machine and place in a safe area of the salon.

12 Dry the skin with tissue before starting other treatments.

13 If necessary use a metal eradicator (comedone extractor) for blackheads.

14 Complete treatment with massage and face mask or continue with other electrical apparatus – depending on client's skin type or treatment plan.

Recommended application of time and treatments

1   General cleanse and tone:
  - 5 minutes on lower neck
  - 5 minutes on lower face
  - 4–5 minutes on full face.

2   Disinfecting and anti-bacterial effect on oily and blemished skin:
  - 10 minutes on lower face and neck
  - 10 minutes on full face.

3   Regenerating effect on dry / dehydrated / mature skin:
  - 2–3 minutes on lower face and neck.
  - 1–3 minutes on full face to achieve erythema.

Conclude this treatment with a nourishing massage to prevent irritation and over-dryness.

Note After treatment, surface moisture should be removed, then other treatments, or a mask should be applied.

Salon after-treatment

1   Extraction of blackheads (if required/oily skin).
2   Massage - all skin types.
3   Massage including audio sonic – dry/dehydrated skin.
4   Mask – appropriate mask used according to client skin type.
5   High frequency:
  - direct – oily skin
  - indirect – dry / sluggish skin.
6   Galvanic – iontophoresis – dry/dehydrated skin.

From this short list and from the pre-treatment to facial steaming list (above), you can see that a treatment plan with variety can be compiled, offering maximum benefits to the client.

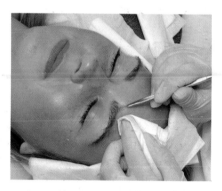

Using a sterilised comedone extractor, gently apply pressure to the comedone centre and ease the comedone out. Do not apply too much pressure, or squeeze, as this can cause scarring.

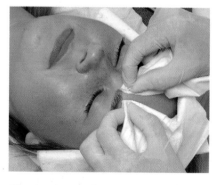

If a metal comedone extractor is not available, cover the fingertips with tissue and gently roll the skin around the comedone, to ease it out.

Face steaming – suggested routines

A	B	C	D
Cleanse	Cleanse	Cleanse	Cleanse
Facial steam	Brush cleanse	Facial steam	Brush cleanse
Manual massage - either normal/dry or oily skin	Facial steam	Massage including audio-sonic – dry / dehydrated skin	Facial vacuum
Mask	Use of comedone extractor – oily blemished skin	Mask	Facial steam – oily / blemished skin
Tone, moisturiser	Mask	Tone, moisturiser	Mask
	Tone, moisturiser		Tone, moisturiser

E	F	G	
Cleanse	Cleanse	Cleanse	
Facial steam	Facial steam	Facial vacuum	
Direct high frequency	Massage	Facial steam	
	Galvanic iontophoresis – dry/dehydrated skin	Indirect high – dry / dehydrated skin	

Examples of treatment plans

Awarding body code of ethics on the use of ozone

The use of ozone can be very beneficial when administered in small quantities and under supervision, but it may also be a destructive element when used incorrectly.

Some public health authorities and beauty examination boards believe that the use of ozone can be bad for your health, especially when inhaled in great strength, leading to respiratory infections.

Most awarding bodies are among those who do not recommend that ozone is used under any circumstances.

Thermal masks

Refer back to the section on masks for use of thermal masks to pre-heat the skin.

Aftercare advice

After a facial it is important to recognise that the immediate aftercare is as important as the long-term aftercare in order to gain maximum benefit from the salon treatment.

Immediate aftercare

- The skin has been deep cleansed, stimulated and nourished. No further aftercare is required except to leave it alone.
- Avoid the temptation to apply make-up for 12 hours, where possible.
- Ideally, evening cleansing is not necessary, but if the client prefers, a light cleanse, tone and moisture should be recommended.
- Suitable and compatible homecare products should be recommended and will complement the good work of the therapist in the salon.

Long-term aftercare

- Regular use of homecare products will help the skin.
- Regular facials will help to regulate a problem skin. Timings and intervals must be decided on by the therapist and client and may depend on cost.
- A booking of six regular facials could have a complementary eyelash tint or manicure included, as an added incentive.
- Future treatment needs may be discussed with regards to specialist help for specific problems, such as facial steaming for comedone extraction or regular paraffin masks for a dry skin. Targeting a problem and then giving intensive treatments to help that condition is very rewarding. The client is pleased and the therapist has job satisfaction and a happy client.
- A treatment plan should make allowances for timing intervals, the cost involved and how convenient it is for the client to get to the salon.

The client should be given a price list and all relevant information for her treatment.

Your questions answered

Can I use any old face mask on the client's skin, if it's the one we have in the stock room?

No – if you cannot use the correct type for the client's skin, do not apply one at all. Using the wrong type of mask can dry out the skin, or over-stimulate it. Do, however, remember that you can use natural face mask ingredients, such as cucumber slices, which may be available. The same rule applies to face masks as it does to cooking – the ingredients must be fresh!

Why do I have to cut my nails and not wear any nail varnish for facial work?

This is important for hygiene, health and safety and for the client's comfort. Short nails allows you to relax your fingers and give a smooth massage, without worrying about stabbing the client with your long free edge, especially around the delicate eye area. It is possible that the client has an allergy to nail varnish, and therefore a reaction may occur – again, especially important around the eye.

How important is it to use the correct products for the skin type?

It is very important. To give the most professional treatment and to be honest with your client you really need to give the best and most suitable products for the skin. Using a toner that is too strong can dry out the skin; using a moisturiser that is too light can leave the skin not looking or feeling as good as it should. The client may not come back to you, if she feels her treatment has been compromised.

Can I offer other treatments with a facial?

Of course you can, and you should. If you client would like her eyelashes tinted, you could do that while her face mask is drying. If the client's eyebrows are bushy, you can suggest a reshape and include this in a facial treatment. Some clients like to have nail varnish applied while their facemask is drying.

Should I always use this recommended facial massage routine?

It is a good idea to stick with one routine when you are first learning, especially for assessments – you will get to know the routine so well that your hands do the routine automatically. When you are a little more experienced, and you see other therapists doing different movements, you can mix and match your routine and adapt your massage to suit your clients' needs. There are many effective massage techniques, and if you go further with your training and go on to aromatherapy, Indian head massage or manual lymphatic drainage techniques, you will come across different movements and want to try them.

Test your knowledge

1   *A skin analysis should be carried out:*
    a   *after a superficial cleanse*
    b   *before removing make up*
    c   *after the deep cleanse*
    d   *after the face mask.*

2   *An excess of sebum produces:*
    a   *dry skin*

b oily skin
c sensitive skin
d normal skin.

3 The skin type, which has oily and dry areas, is known as:
a unusual skin
b problem skin
c combination skin
d sensitive skin.

4 Facial massage is carried out:
a after a deep cleanse
b after a face mask
c after coffee break
d after eye make-up removal.

5 Massage is good for the skin because:
a it helps bring oxygen to the skin surface
b it soothes the nerve endings
c it smoothes out wrinkles
d it makes you thinner in the face.

6 The most suitable cleanser for dry skin is:
a cream cleanser
b milk cleanser
c wash-off cleanser
d baby lotion.

7 Dilated capillaries and milia are a feature of:
a dry skin
b oily skin
c normal skin
d sensitive skin.

8 Moisturisers are designed to:
a rehydrate the skin
b make the skin feel nice
c prepare the skin for make-up application
d fill up all the wrinkles.

9 Face masks should be of a smooth consistency so that they:
a can be applied evenly
b look nice on the skin
c set quickly
d retain moisture.

10 Fuller's earth is a clay which is used in a face mask for:
a dry skin
b oily skin
c normal skin
d sensitive skin.

Preparation of full facial, including massage

Couch and working area tidy and prepared.
Couch prepared with blanket and towels.
Couch roll on headrest and foot area, and on the floor for client to stand on.

Trolley fully prepared with:
- products
- spatulas
- tissues
- wet and dry cotton wool
- sponges if preferred
- jewellery bowl for client
- headband.

Record card and pen. Client record number if known.

Make sure there are two chairs, a magnified mirror and a bin with bin liner.

Short nails. No jewellery.

You are now ready to greet your client.

Full consultation and contra-indication check.

Position client onto couch with headband on and jewellery off.

Wash hands prior to treatment.

You are now ready to begin your treatment!

Remove and lighten hair using temporary methods

Unit 7

This unit focuses on ways to temporarily remove unwanted hairs from the body, disguise hairs, or temporarily lighten darker hairs found on parts of the body.

The unit covers these elements:

7.1 Assess clients and prepare treatment plans
7.2 Prepare the work area and client for removing and lightening hair treatments
7.3 Remove unwanted hair to meet client requirements
7.4 Lighten hair using bleaching techniques.

The process of removing unwanted hairs (particularly by waxing and sugaring) is called depilation. This is a popular salon treatment as it provides a quick and efficient way of removing unwanted hairs in both small and larger areas.

Superfluous hair is the term used if the hair growth is normal but the client feels it to be unattractive and is very aware of it, especially dark-haired clients who may feel that their hair growth is visible, e.g. on the upper lip.

There may be no medical reason for a strong, or dark, growth, but many clients find facial or body hair that is noticeable rather embarrassing and are delighted to have it removed, using various methods.

Some clients are happy not to have the hair actually removed, but lightened by bleaching, and that too is acceptable. Other clients will wish to have a permanent removal of the hair using an electrical current, and this is called epilation.

(Epilation is taught in NVQ level 3 and is a specialist treatment. It is permanent removal of the hair and requires considerable skill and therefore considerable training.)

There are many hair-removing creams available that can be bought over the counter, as well as electrical shavers for women and disposable razors that women can use with adapted shaving foams – so that the skin is kept soft and moisturised. Therefore, there are many choices for the client to make.

Hair removal is very much a matter of personal choice and the client should be given full information available, to make an informed decision. The client needs to know the various methods of hair removal available, and their advantages and disadvantages, and to be given the therapist's professional advice on the particular problem she has, especially regarding the cost and time involved in the treatment.

Why the human body has hair

The human body evolved with hair all over it in order to keep warm – just as the body laid down fat deposits to keep warm. It was part of survival.

We still retain hair for the purpose of warmth, such as terminal hair on the head, but now hair has become more a fashion accessory and can be styled and changed depending on the current trends.

Through the ages, facial hair on men has been considered to be a sign of virility, strength and masculinity. In recent times there has been a big change in fashion towards clean-shaven faces, except of course for the 'designer stubble' trend of pop stars.

Types of hair

- **Terminal hair** offers protection and therefore grows long and often is coarse in texture.
- **Scalp hair** protects the head and helps keep in the heat.
- **Eyelashes** protect the eyes by catching particles that may fall into the eyes.
- **Underarm / pubic hair** protects the delicate skin and cushions against friction caused by movement.
- **Body hair** protects against heat loss.

Hair growth

Both men and women have terminal hairs, but the hair growth is determined by several factors.

The amount of hair follicles

Lots of follicles mean lots of hair, which will look very thick. This tends to be genetic, which means it has been inherited from the parents. (If a male has baldness running in his family, there is a strong possibility he will develop the same hair growth pattern too.)

Cultural influences

Hair growth patterns and strength, texture and amount of hair is also determined by geography and ethnic background. There is a higher proportion of blonde and fair-skinned people in countries such as Norway and Sweden, and so excessive face or body hair is fair and not noticeable. However, the nearer the equator, and hence the nearer the sun, skin and hair colour becomes darker, e.g. Italians, Spaniards and Greeks are recognisable by their dark hair and skin. So, their facial hair or excess body hair may be more noticeable. The British colouring can be a mixture of light and dark – certainly the Celtic (e.g. Scottish and Irish) peoples tend to have darker colouring. Generally, it is darker-haired clients who are more concerned with superfluous hair than those with a light growth or colour, mostly because it shows more.

Hair strength and texture

Again, this tends to run in families. People with a thick, strong hair growth may also have lots of follicles and have a really thick head of hair. Others may have lots of follicles, but the hair itself may be very fine in texture and therefore look fine.

Some people have a combination of few follicles with fine hair texture which doesn't present much of a problem, and so they may never need to use depilation; however, this is not so good if the fashion is for a thick head of hair.

Illness

This can have a great effect on hair growth, usually making the hair lank and lifeless. This would not generally affect hairs to be removed, but certainly could affect hair styling.

Medication

Some drugs have a strong effect on hair growth, either:

- producing lots of coarse thick hair, which can be depilated, with a doctor's permission
- or, causing the follicles to weaken and wither, and the hair to fall out. For example, some forms of chemotherapy for the treatment of cancer cause baldness. Often this is only temporary and the hairs will re-grow.

> **Remember**
>
> In some European and Mediterranean countries body hair on women is considered the norm. Many women are quite happy with strong underarm hair or other body hair, so be careful not to be too hasty in giving treatment advice, as a client may not wish to have full hair removal.

Hormones

Hormones can also have an effect on hair growth, e.g. women going through the menopause, when hormone levels may be erratic, may find they develop 'whiskers' of coarse hair on the face.

Emotional

A sudden shock, accident or death of a loved one, can cause hair loss, which may re-grow, or may not. This is called alopecia, which can occur as patches of hair loss, or total baldness.

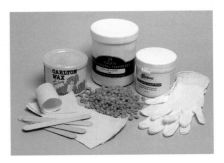

In our society excessive hair growth on women is considered masculine and many ladies feel unfeminine, regardless of how light the growth is. Some women feel the same about hairy legs and body hair.

Some men have hair removed from their body. For example, some professional sportsmen, e.g. cyclists and Olympic swimmers, reduce their body hair to enhance their performance. Don't be surprised if you get a booking for waxing body hair from a 'Mr' rather than a 'Miss' or a 'Mrs', as it is quite common.

Various wax products

Assess the client and prepare treatment plans

7.1

Before you can effectively assess the client and decide on her waxing or lightening needs, and draw up your treatment plan, you need to have a thorough background knowledge of all the products. This will help you form a professional assessment and give the best treatment, tailor-made to suit your client's requirements.

Therefore, the information in this element will not necessarily be in the same order as the following element titles; however, this is to your advantage, as you will be highly informed before you begin the practical application.

Advantages and disadvantages of depilation and hair lightening

Method of hair removal	Advantages	Disadvantages
Warm wax	• Quick, cost effective • Efficient over large areas • Once mastered, easy to apply	• Sticky • Can cause skin damage if reapplied over the same area • Can leave a residue, which if not fully removed can leave the client feeling sticky
Hot wax	• Good for strong hair growth • Suitable for ethnic hair types, which may have bent follicles (Refer to anatomy section)	• Skilled technique of application may take some time to master • Because of the temperature control needing to be accurate, application needs to be quick • Not suitable for some skin types • Can be messy when learning application
Strip sugaring	• As warm wax • Water-soluble	• Can be less efficient than warm wax • Tricky technique to master

Method of hair removal	Advantages	Disadvantages
Manual sugaring	• Water-soluble • Applied at body temperature, so less likely to burn the skin • Cost effective as no paper / material strips are necessary	• Difficult technique to master • More time-consuming to perform
Hair-removing creams	• No skill needed • Less pain involved • Home treatment • Minimal costs • Less bristly regrowth	• Not suitable for all skin types • Messy application • Regrowth short term • Hair only removed from just below the skin's surface
Cutting	• Quick • No skill involved • Home treatment • No pain involved	• Short term only • Blunt regrowth, as hair removed only to skin level • Risk of cutting the skin
Shaving	• Quick • No skill involved • Home treatment • No pain • Equipment cheap to purchase	• Not suitable for all skin types • Blunt regrowth • Risk of skin damage • Not hygienic • Short term only • Only removes surface part of the hair
Plucking	• Precise • Ideal for small areas i.e. on the face • Equipment cheap to purchase	• Only suitable for small areas • Risk of skin damage (bruising or pinching the skin) • Breakage of hair may occur • Can be time-consuming • Not ideal for clients who wear glasses for a DIY treatment
Threading	• Cheap • No equipment needed • Suitable for Mediterranean and Asian clients • As effective as plucking	• Skill needed to apply • Possible breakage of the hair
Impregnated cold wax strips	• Minimal skill needed • Less messy for home use • No specialist equipment needed • Quick	• Bruising or skin damage may occur as the strips stick to the skin and not to the hair • Painful to remove • Unsatisfactory results • Can be costly for large areas
Abrasives (gloves / pumice stones)	• No skill needed • No specialist equipment needed • Improves the skin texture as dead skin cells are shed (desquamation) • Cheap treatment for home use	• Hair breakage may occur • Hair is only removed at skin surface level • Could result in skin damage • Not terribly effective on strong dark hair growth
Electrical appliances (e.g. electric razors, etc.)	• No skill needed • Re-usable • Ideal for home use • Clean and quick	• Only removes surface hairs • May damage the skin • Some can be expensive • Regrowth produced is blunt and growth stubble

Method of hair removal	Advantages	Disadvantages
Bleach	• Little skill involved in application • Quick results • Suitable for facial hairs • Suitable for clients having epilation • No distortion of the follicle takes place, so no problems occur if epilation is done at a later date	• Not suitable for all skin types • Patch test required • Not suitable for large areas, e.g. the legs • Regrowth is more noticeable when it does come through • Skin irritation can occur

Prepare the work area and client for removing and lightening hair treatments

7.2

The products used for hair treatment

Wax

There are many excellent types of wax available, with various ingredients for different effects. Wax is classed according to its working temperature.

Type of wax	Working temperature
Hot hard depilatory wax	Works best at 48–68°C
Warm soft depilatory wax	Works best at 40–43°C
Cream depilatory wax	Works best at 35–43°C
Organic wax	Organic wax varies – refer to suppliers
Cold wax	Needs no heating

Type of wax and its working temperature

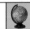

Reality Check!

These temperatures are supplied courtesy of Bellitas Ltd, Beauty Suppliers, known for their 'Strictly Professional' waxes. Manufacturers' instructions will vary with different products, so always refer to the recommended temperatures and heating units for maximum benefit and safety.

Ingredients of wax

The working temperature is determined by the wax's ingredients. These will vary among manufacturers, but the higher the proportion of good quality resin (and the type used) to beeswax, the more heat is required, to get the wax to a manageable working consistency.

Resins are organic polymers that may be naturally occurring or synthetic. A polymer is a compound such as starch, or perspex, and forms most of the basis for all our plastics and man-made fibres.

Natural resins occur when certain plants and trees are injured – the fluid that oozes out from the wound hardens into a solid resin, to protect the plant's injury. The balsam tree, pine tree, the gum tree as well as the rubber tree all produce resins. The gum tree is actually where chewing gum resin comes from. Resins are used in the making of perfume, waxing and some cosmetics.

Chemists can now artificially make synthetic resins to avoid using up more of the world's resources of plant life. Large quantities of resins are produced as a by-product of the petroleum oil business, and are extracted from crude oil, when it is pumped out of the ground.

The following health and safety data complies with EEC directives 88/379 and provides all precautions, correct handling, storage and first-aid measures.

Hard depilatory wax

What is it?

A hard depilatory wax, sold in solid pellet form, which becomes molten when heated.

What is it made of?

It is a mixture of natural resins, beeswax and microcrystalline wax. It is insoluble in cold water, but soluble when hot. It has a low chemical reactivity and is stable.

Warm wax

What is it?

This is a soft, thick liquid. It may vary in colour from warm honey to amber / light brown. Soft wax is supplied in a tin or plastic tub, which fits into a specially fitted heating unit. There are many soft waxes on the market, and it is recommended that the wax is only heated in the correct heater, following the manufacturer's instructions, as the temperatures for best performance may vary slightly.

What is it made of?

Composed mainly of refined gum resin and hydrocarbon tackifiers. This gives the wax its sticking properties.

Cream wax

Many manufacturers now produce good quality cream wax. Cream wax contains ingredients such as moisturisers and azulene that condition the skin. Azulene is anti-inflammatory and soothing, suitable for more sensitive skin types. (Azulene is the ingredient that turns the cream a blue colour.) Cream wax also works on slightly lower melting and working temperatures, thereby enhancing client comfort during waxing. Cream waxes have enhanced sticking properties, which means that they can be spread thinly and are therefore very economical to use.

Please follow soft waxing information in the COSHH regulations.

Organic wax

Organic waxes are very popular, as they contain natural ingredients such as honey. They do, however, contain chemical ingredients to keep them stable. Organic waxes do not set when cold but they become more liquid when heated.

Cold wax

Some cold waxes are available to buy as an over-the-counter purchase, as pre-coated wax strips, as well as being produced and sold by some manufacturers to beauty salons.

Retail strips

These can be purchased from most large chemists and come in packs of 6–10 strips, usually made by the same companies that produce hair-removing creams. These pre-coated strips are double-layered, one piece of wax paper being a non-stick backing

Reality Check!

Non-recoverable waste should be disposed of via a licensed waste contractor; a set fee is charged for a regular collection. Waxing waste should be put into a separate lined bin, ready for picking up by the disposal company. For example, a company called Rentokil will operate a weekly collection for a set fee.

strip, from which the coated strip peels away, to be placed on the skin. They contain hydrocarbon resins so are sticky, but as they are cold the adhering properties are not as effective as warm or hot wax. Most manufacturers recommend that the strips be warmed between the hands before splitting and applying. The wax coating is also quite fine, and may not be sufficient to grip a strong hair growth. Therefore, the strips are only really suitable for light hair growth, and are not normally recommended for facial use, the elderly, diabetics and people with skin irritations.

They can be used as a stopgap for quick removal for a light growth between waxing, and special occasions, and should the client not be able to visit her usual salon for a warm waxing.

Roller waxing

Many manufacturers provide complete systems with disposable roll-on heads, which are very popular in salons and with therapists offering a mobile beauty therapy service.

The applicators look a little like a roll-on deodorant stick, and come in various roller head sizes for different parts of the body. They can be disposed of after use, or the refill cartridges alone can be purchased and the head attachments of the roller taken off for cleaning and sterilisation. Some salons favour the client purchasing the whole roller applicator, which the salon then keeps for only that client, to avoid cross-contamination.

Other products used in waxing

For the health and safety of using these products, see the information on pages 201–204.

Pre-waxing lotion
What is it?

This is a cleansing lotion applied to the area before treatment, to cleanse and remove any grease or dirt on the skin that may prevent good hair removal.

What is it made of?

The product usually contains ethanol and camphor oil in a cosmetic lotion. The ethanol is an alcohol for cleansing, and the camphor has anti-bacterial and anti-inflammatory properties, and is anti- viral and a counter irritant.

Purified talc
What is it?

It is a dry powder, used as a light dusting over the area to be waxed, to ensure the hairs have a covering for the wax to adhere to, and that the hairs stand away from the skin.

After-wax lotion
What is it?

This is a soothing lotion used after treatment to help cool and calm the skin, and prevent irritation.

What is it made of?

The product contains an emulsion of oils, waxes, water, water-soluble ingredients, emulsifiers, fragrance and preservatives.

Remember

Always follow instructions on the individual packaging.

Wax equipment cleaner

What is it?

This is a powerful cleaning liquid that is used on waxing equipment – it has a very strong smell.

What is it made of?

It is a hydrocarbon solvent.

Health and safety relating to the use of waxing products

Hard depilatory waxes

Hazards

- Classed as non-hazardous if used in correct professional circumstances.

First aid procedures

- If used at the correct temperature and in the correct procedure for hair removal this wax poses no hazard.
- High temperatures should be avoided, as this will cause thermal burns.
- If an overheated wax has solidified on the skin, leave it on, in place, and consult a doctor.
- In the event of wax entering the eyes, the eyes should be flushed immediately with water for 15 minutes and medical attention obtained.

Fire-fighting measures

- This wax is stable, but it has a flash point greater than 220°C – make sure that the thermostat controlling the temperature on the heater is working.
- Although not strictly classed as flammable this wax will burn, so avoid contact with flammable fabrics, e.g. placing it near the curtains.
- In the event of a small fire, foam, carbon dioxide, dry chemical powder, sand or earth may be used to extinguish it. For a large fire use foam or water spray.

In the event of an accident

- In the event of a large spillage, any wax entering the drains will solidify and cause blockages. The local health authority will need to be notified if this happens.
- Allow spilt hot wax to cool and solidify and scrape up for disposal.

Storing

- Hard depilatory waxes in tightly closed jars can be kept for up to six months in cool dry conditions, away from possible sources of contamination.

Handling

- Adequate protective clothing must be worn when handling wax in a molten state.
- It is recommended that advice be sought from the individual awarding body and professional organisation that is favoured by your training establishment. To ignore their recommended guidelines may make any assessments taking place null and void, but more importantly, it may invalidate any insurance protection.

(Refer to the legislation covered in the Professional basics section, page 33.)

Warm wax

Hazards

- Classed as non-hazardous if used in correct professional circumstances.

First aid procedures

- If used at the correct temperature and in the correct procedure for hair removal, this wax poses no hazard.
- High temperatures should be avoided, as this will cause thermal burns.
- If an overheated wax has solidified on the skin leave it on, in place, and consult a doctor.
- If the eyes are affected, irrigate immediately with copious quantities of cold water for at least five minutes. Obtain medical attention.
- If inhaled remove from exposure to fumes from the molten products. If irritation persists obtain medical attention.
- If ingested no special treatment necessary.
- If there is hot contact with the skin, cool the affected area by plunging into cold running water for at least 10 minutes. DO NOT REMOVE ADHERING MATERIAL. Obtain medical attention. If a limb is completely surrounded by wax, the wax should be split to avoid a tourniquet effect.
- If there is cold contact, wash thoroughly with soap and water.

Fire-fighting measures

- Although not strictly classed as flammable, soft wax will burn above 200°C.
- Avoid contact with flammable fabrics, e.g. do not place near the curtains.
- Check that the thermostat on the heating unit is in working order, by regularly maintaining the equipment.
- In the event of a small fire, use carbon dioxide, dry powders or foam fire extinguishers.

DO NOT USE WATER ON SOFT WAX.

In the event of an accident

- When soft wax is molten, care must be taken to prevent burns from molten products by ensuring that application temperatures are kept to the minimum necessary for adequate product performance.
- At no time is it necessary to heat the product above 60°C.
- Ensure good ventilation in the working environment.
- Where accidental overheating occurs the source of heat should be disconnected and the molten product left undisturbed until cool. Make sure that everyone is aware of the potential hazard.

Storing

- Soft wax may be maintained as a cool liquid within its own container, or be heated within the unit on a daily basis, and may be kept for up to six months in cool dry conditions.

Handling

- The same handling as for hard wax.
- Adequate protective clothing must be worn when handling wax in a molten state.
- It is recommended that advice be sought from the individual awarding body and professional organisation that is favoured by your training establishment. To ignore their recommended guidelines may make any assessments taking place null and void, but more importantly, it may invalidate any insurance protection. (Please refer to the legislation covered in the Professional basics section, page 33.)
- Soft waxes are unlikely to cause any environmental hazards, but do remember that all waxes are generally non-biodegradable in the short term.

Pre-waxing lotion

Hazards

- If used properly this product has no hazards.

First aid procedures

- If ingested, drink milk or water.
- If it gets into the eyes, wash well with water; if irritation persists seek medical advice.

In the event of an accident

- If spillage occurs, clean up with an absorbent material, followed by washing with detergent and water to avoid a slippery floor.

Storing

- No special precautions considered necessary.

Handling

- No special precautions considered necessary.

Purified talc

Hazards

- All dry powders can give respiratory problems if precautions are ignored.
- It is non-flammable.
- Avoid excessive use, especially near the nose and mouth.

First aid procedures

- If ingested, drink milk or water.
- Avoid inhaling – if affected remove to fresh air and keep warm.
- Avoid prolonged contact as this can lead to dry skin.
- Avoid contact with eyes. If it occurs, wash well with water.

In the event of an accident

- Sweep or vacuum up, avoiding dust.

Storing

- Store in a cool dry place, keeping containers tightly sealed.

Handling

- Store in a cool dry place, keeping containers tightly sealed.

After-wax lotion

Hazards

- If used properly this product has no hazards.

First aid procedures

- If ingested, drink milk or water
- If it gets into the eyes, wash well with water; if irritation persists seek medical advice.

In the event of an accident

- If spillage occurs, clean up with an absorbent material, followed by washing with detergent and water to avoid a slippery floor.

Storing

- No special precautions considered necessary.

Handling

- No special precautions considered necessary.

Wax equipment cleaner

Hazards

- It is highly flammable and is hazardous.
- It should not be used in an enclosed space, as the fumes are highly noxious.

First aid procedures

- If the eyes are affected, irrigate immediately with copious quantities of cold water for at least five minutes. Obtain medical attention.
- Do not inhale, as this may cause dizziness. If this happens remove to fresh air.
- Avoid ingesting. If ingested, drink plenty of milk or water.
- Avoid prolonged contact with the skin. If irritation occurs seek medical advice.

Fire-fighting measures

- Contents are highly flammable.
- Evacuate the area and inform fire-fighters of the hazards.

In the event of an accident

- Clean contaminated area with lots of water, and add detergent, to avoid slippery floors.
- Do not absorb onto combustible material.

Storing

- Store in a cool place away from direct sunlight; large quantities should be stored in a fire-resistant store.

Benefits and effects of waxing

Type of wax	Benefits	Effects
Hot wax	As hot wax needs to be heated to a high temperature it is extremely effective on strong hair growth.	The solid wax turns into a liquid when heated and when applied to the skin, it coats the hairs, gripping them firmly. The wax is applied with a disposable spatula unit in a thick layer. A lip of the wax is then lifted to allow a firm hold to take the whole patch off.

Possible drawbacks

Only really suitable on longer hair growth – results not good if the hair is shorter.

Hot wax may cause a slight skin reaction, so not suitable for sensitive skin, or sensitive areas.

Application is a skill that needs a lot of practice to master.

As the wax needs to be kept at a constant working temperature it can be time-consuming if the wax keeps over-heating and therefore needs time to cool again.

The wax needs to be applied quite thickly, so it can be quite costly in materials.

Wax should not be applied over the same area twice, as the skin may burn.

Can be messy to apply so it is hard to keep the equipment clean.

These considerations need to be thought about when choosing equipment.

Type of wax	Benefits	Effects
Warm wax	More comfortable on sensitive skins than hot wax, and can be reapplied over the same area. Even short hairs can be successfully removed with warm wax. The equipment is easy to maintain and keep clean. Very little preparation is needed and application is easy and quick.	Warm wax is applied with a disposable spatula, in a very thin coating and a fabric or paper strip is applied over the top of the wax for easy removal – rather like a plaster coming off. The wax and hairs adhere to the strip. A single strip can be used over again until it reaches saturation point.

Possible drawbacks

There is some risk of infection, as loose skin cells may also be lost during waxing, leaving hair follicles open to infection.

As the wax is applied quite finely, it may not remove all of a strong growth, in one go.

Strips have to be used with warm wax, and may add to the cost of the treatment if not used economically.

Type of wax	Benefits	Effects
Cold wax	This treatment can be done at home for a top-up treatment, and is therefore convenient	Hairs are removed by an impregnated strip, with no heat.

Possible drawbacks

Not very economical if using on large areas as lots of strips will need to be purchased.

Not suitable on large areas of strong hair growth.

As it can be applied to oneself, there is more pain and discomfort than when a trained therapist does it.

For self-administration the angle of removal may not be correct for a swift, clean taking off, and that may be another reason for it to hurt.

Type of wax	Benefits	Effects
Roller wax	Very little possibility of cross-contamination from the rollers. Very quick, clean and easy to use. Very economical Safe – no possibility of spillage as the wax is contained within the cartridge.	Precise application of the wax can be achieved because there is a variety of roller head sizes, allowing more accuracy.

Possible drawbacks

Very few, except that the initial outlay may be high for purchase of the heaters and cartridges.

The units are specially made to fit each manufacturer's make of cartridge and therefore are not interchangeable if the type of wax proves to be unsuitable.

Suitability of hair removal products

Method	Eyebrows	Facial hair	Legs	Bikini line	Forearms
Warm wax	✓	✓	✓	✓	✓
Hot wax	✓ Depends on skin sensitivity	✓ Depends on skin sensitivity	✓	✓	✓
Sugaring	✓	✓	✓	✓	✓
Hair removal creams	✓ Care required	✓	✓	✓	✓
Plucking / tweezing	✓	✓	✓ Only for stray hairs after depilation	✓ Only for stray hairs after depilation	✓ Only for stray hairs after depilation

Method	Eyebrows	Facial hair	Legs	Bikini line	Forearms
Mechanical depilators	✗	✗	✓	✓	✓
Cutting / shaving	✗ Only to shorten brows	✓	✓	✓	✓
Bleaching	✗	✓	✓	✓	✓

Preparation for waxing treatments

Preparation is the key for the professional beauty therapist, regardless of the treatment being carried out. Good preparation sets the whole atmosphere of any treatment, creating a calm and efficient feel to the treatment. If preparation is not in place, the client will pick up that the therapist feels disorganised and rushed, and that can detract from the benefits of the treatment.

In the case of waxing, preparation is vital – most wax needs preheating so that the client is not kept waiting. All equipment and materials should be in place to avoid leaving the client alone, which is unprofessional, and does not make the client feel important or pampered.

Preparation of working area

Many salons have designated rooms or areas for waxing, and the room stays prepared only for waxing, with heaters and all necessary products never leaving the room. The golden rule here would be to leave the room fully prepared for the next therapist to use, which means replenishing anything that has run out, or is low, cleaning and being tidy during the actual treatment. It would be most off-putting for the new client to be lead into the waxing area only to find the remains of the previous client's treatment remaining.

The preparation of the working area should include the following.

- Protective covering for the couch, so that any spillage or residue is easily removed, and will not cause permanent damage.
- Where plastic sheeting is used, a paper couch roll should be placed over the top. This is good practice for hygiene as it prevents cross-infection, as the paper can be replaced easily, as well as providing client comfort.
- The couch should initially be placed in an upright position to allow the client to be comfortably seated, and then placed into the appropriate position for the area to be treated. A pillow covered with a towel, and protected with couch roll, should be used.
- Two waste bins are required, both with inner liners, placed behind or under the couch: one waste bin for wax waste – contaminated materials, which will be put into a designated bin for collection by a licensed removal firm for incineration; the other waste bin is for general waste.
- The chosen heating unit for the wax type to suit the client's needs and enough wax product for the area to be treated. Obviously a lip wax requires a small amount of product, whereas a full leg wax means the heater needs to be quite full. Remember that it may take a full half-hour to heat the wax to a working temperature, so that needs to be the first job of the day. (Many salons keep a heater on all day, in anticipation of clients dropping in, without appointments.)

Remember

Not all methods of hair removal are suitable for all clients. A full consultation will be needed to establish which method is suitable and agreeable to you both.

- Antiseptic cleaner for the skin, or the manufacturer's recommended skin cleanser.
- Talcum powder.
- Fabric or paper strips that are compatible with the manufacturer's requirements for the wax chosen.
- Disposable gloves, usually vinyl with talced lining for ease – refer to your professional body's guidelines for use.
- Disposable wooden spatulas or a suitable applicator – again refer to the professional body to fulfil their requirements (no spatula requirements for roller waxing, of course).
- Tissues, cotton wool and a jewellery bowl for the client.
- A pair of scissors and tweezers should be in a container soaking in suitable disinfectant to sterilise – the scissors may be required to trim the hair length prior to treatment, and the tweezers to remove the odd stray hair, which has escaped the wax.
- After-wax lotion or oil.
- Aftercare leaflets for the client to take away and refer to.

> ### In the salon
>
> Many salons have names for bikini styles of waxing – a 'Brazilian' is full and total hair removal; this is high maintenance and can be painful, with the client visiting the salon very regularly.
>
> A 'Californian' is not quite total removal, but a small line of pubic hair is left centrally in a vertical line. This allows for a narrow cut thong bikini to be worn. Some salons call this a Mohican.

The consultation

If the client is a regular to the salon, a record card will be on-going, with each treatment recorded on it along with the area treated and any reaction to treatment.

With a new client, a full consultation will be needed and a patch test carried out prior to treatment, to make sure the client does not have an allergic reaction to the wax. A treatment plan will be needed that is mutually agreeable to both client and therapist.

The treatment plan will depend on:

- hair growth – coarse, thick, thin, light, short, or long
- the area to be treated
- first or consecutive treatments
- skin type and sensitivity
- any reaction to any previous treatment
- success of the patch test
- any contra-indications present.

Warm wax and roller waxing operate at much lower temperatures than hot wax, so it may be that an alternative product is used, to prevent a reaction from occurring. Another patch test will be required using the different product, and if that proves satisfactory and the client is happy, then the treatment can go ahead.

> ### Reality Check!
>
> Accidents can, and do, happen. Advise the client not to wear her favourite expensive underwear when having a wax. Protect the client's clothing with towels and tissues to prevent them leaving with a sticky residue attached. Also, remember, if the client is having a bikini wax prior to her holiday, she should wear the swimsuit or bikini bottom for waxing to ensure that the line is the right shape for her. If not, an old pair of briefs with the same leg line will give the correct line.

> ### Reality Check!
>
> A patch test should be carried out on a clean, dry area of skin, usually on the forearm, as this is hair-free. Having heated the correct type of wax to be used for the client, test it on yourself for correct temperature, and then apply a small circle of wax to the client's forearm. Remove as for hair removal and note any immediate reaction on the skin.
>
> Put the details onto the client's record card and then ask her to monitor the result for the next 24–48 hours.

> ### Remember
>
> If a reaction is likely to occur, it will be noticeable as redness in the same shape as the patch, and may be itchy. This would indicate that either the wax type is not suitable for the client, or that waxing cannot take place at all.

Waxing and record of treatment client file copy

Client reference:

Initial consultation date:	Therapist:
First treatment:	Yes ☐ No ☐
Contra-indications checked:	Yes ☐ No ☐
Contra-indications noted: _____ None ☐	

Allergies:	Disorders:
Skin conditions:	Wax used:

Date and treatment no.	Area	Contra-action	Special notes Contra-indications or adaptations	Therapist	Patch test
1					
2					
3					
4					
5					
6					

NB After 6 treatments client requires new consultation and analysis

Leaflet given: Yes ☐

Aftercare – for a period of 24 hours:

- ◆ No sunbathing or sunbeds
- ◆ Avoid bathing in sea or swimming pool
- ◆ Do not take a *hot* bath or shower
- ◆ Do not use deodorant / anti-perspirant
- ◆ Avoid tight clothing
- ◆ Do not use perfumed products on the area
- ◆ No make-up or self-tanning preparations
- ◆ Do not keep touching or picking at the area

Waxing treatment record card

⚠ Contra-indications to waxing treatments

A contra-indication means that the treatment cannot be carried out, as the client is unsuitable for this particular treatment. (Refer back to Professional basics, page 25.) Or it may be that the area has to be protected, or avoided, e.g. a mole or skin tag is present.

The areas to be treated should be examined in good lighting to judge if any of the following conditions are present:

- skin diseases or disorders
- open skin, infection, inflammation or healing skin (scabs present)
- bruising

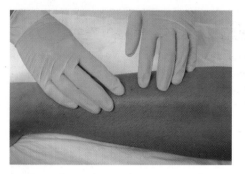

Look out for moles or skin tags, which may restrict the treatment in the area.

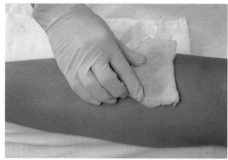

Cleanse the area with suitable product to ensure the area is clean and dry.

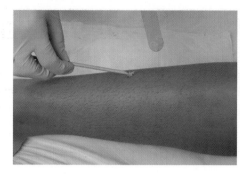

Cover the mole with petroleum jelly to prevent the wax adhering to it – this will ensure you do not cause any damage to the mole.

- very thin skin, or papery skin (diabetics have thin skin and do not heal very well, because of poor circulation)
- after any heat treatment – sauna steam bath, infra red
- after a sun bed or natural tanning – or if sunburn is present
- recent scar tissue
- moles, warts or any unidentified skin problems
- varicose veins or broken capillaries on the legs
- cold sores, eye infections, styes or colds if treating the face
- unidentified lumps, breast-feeding and mastitis if treating under the arm
- previous reactions to treatment
- excessive ingrown hairs from previous treatments
- prior to or during menstruation – the client may have a lower pain threshold at this time and the skin is more sensitive and may react unpredictably.

> **Remember**
>
> The golden rule is 'If in doubt – don't treat!'
>
> Always get a doctor's written approval, and keep it with the record card, along with the client's signature agreeing that the treatment can go ahead.
>
> Much better safe than sorry.

Remove unwanted hair to meet client requirements

7.3

In this element you will learn about:

- waxing
- sugaring.

Waxing

 ### Possible contra-actions

A contra-action is an unfavourable reaction of a client to a treatment.

Even when you have been faultless in hygiene, safety and product use, your client just may react unfavourably to the wax – even if she has had the same treatment for years. It could be a reaction caused by medication being taken, or it could be the influence of fluctuating hormones or it could just be an allergic reaction.

Possible contra-actions to waxing may occur immediately before, during or immediately after the treatment, or it could occur when the client gets home or back to work after the treatment. Whenever it occurs, you should act responsibly and make your client aware of what action to take.

> **Remember**
>
> There is usually a slight reaction to hair removal, and that is to be expected, but a strong reaction should not occur.

Contra-action	How to recognise it and what to do
Unfavourable skin reaction	This is recognised as redness or soreness in the area being treated. It could be caused by the wax being too hot on the skin, by an allergic reaction or by vigorous scraping of the spatula on the skin during application. Stop the treatment, apply a cold compress to the area, and apply and give aftercare cooling lotion for the client to continue applying.
Burning or blistering appearing	This is a burning sensation, caused by the wax being too hot. Before treatment the therapist should test the wax for temperature on herself, and apply a little to the area to be treated. Refer back to the individual waxes for first-aid recommendations
Swelling in the area	The area is tender and the skin has a puffy appearance. This is caused by the wax being too hot or by the strips being lifted off in an upward motion rather than back on themselves. Refer back to the individual waxes for first-aid recommendations. Give your client an aftercare leaflet to take away and refer to, so that any potential contra-action can be avoided and so that maximum benefit can be gained from the treatment.

Possible contra-actions with waxing

Aims of the treatment

During the consultation the therapist also needs to discuss the *realistic outcomes* of a waxing treatment.

Unrealistic aims of waxing	Realistic aims of waxing
Waxing is permanent hair removal .... False	Waxing lasts for 3–6 weeks depending on hair growth .... True
Waxing makes the hair growth weaken .... False	As the blood supply to the hairs are increased with waxing the hairs may grow back slightly more thick and coarse .... True
All the hairs grow back at the same time .... False	The hairs grow back spasmodically as the hair growth cycle for each follicle is different ...... True
Waxing lightens the hair colour .... False	Waxing does not change the hair colour .... True
The hairs grow back with sharp spiky feel to them ....False	Shaving and cutting blunts the ends of the hair, making them feel spiky, after waxing the hair grows back with its natural tapered end, feeling smooth to the touch .... True
Waxing does not hurt .... False	Waxing feels like a plaster being taken from the skin. Pain thresholds will vary and some clients will feel more than others.......................... True

Remember

It is important to be honest with your client, and that they know what to expect and what information is correct. Honesty between therapist and client is part of the ethical conduct expected to maintain the high professional standards for all beauty therapists.

Aftercare and homecare advice

It is important that you discuss homecare and aftercare with your client during the consultation, so that her skin reactions and contra-actions can be explained and understood. Give your client a leaflet to take away to refer to, as she may not take in all the information, especially if she finds the treatment painful.

Aftercare – for a period of 24 hours:

- ◆ No sunbathing or sunbeds
- ◆ Avoid bathing in sea or swimming pool
- ◆ Do not take a *hot* bath or shower
- ◆ Do not use deodorant / anti-perspirant
- ◆ Avoid tight clothing
- ◆ Do not use perfumed products on the area
- ◆ No make-up or self-tanning preparations
- ◆ Do not keep touching or picking at the area

Immediate aftercare

Your client should realise that the area waxed will be red and there may be some blood spots, especially where the hairs are strong, i.e. in the bikini area and under the arm. The after-wax cleanser should be applied to remove any sticky remains on the skin and then after-wax soothing lotion applied to help cool the skin and keep it moisturised.

Homecare

Your salon may like to devise a homecare card like the one here:

Health and safety for waxing

Health and safety information for the types of waxes used in a salon are described in the wax descriptions earlier in the unit. The potential hazards and first-aid required are tackled individually.

Please refer to the Professional basics section for all required legislation for all beauty treatments.

Here are the general precautions to be included in your safe practice of waxing:

General precautions

- Do not have any naked flame near waxing preparations or equipment as the ingredients make them very inflammable.
- Do not have heating units near anything flammable, in case the thermostat breaks and the wax ignites, e.g. curtains.
- Do not have the heater on a glass-topped trolley, in case the glass breaks and molten wax spills everywhere.
- Do a thorough consultation, check for contra-indications and patch test prior to treating the client.
- Firmly stretch and support the skin in fleshy areas to avoid bruising, especially in the bikini and underarm areas.
- Be aware of your own professional body guidelines regarding insurance cover and the use of gloves and protective clothing.
- Thorough moisturising after waxing can help to avoid the problems of ingrown hairs, which is when the hair grows back under the skin, causing infection, always a problem with continual waxing.
- When hot waxing never allow the wax to become too cool on the skin, as it will be too brittle to remove effectively, and may cause the client a great deal of discomfort.

Homecare card

You may also experience dry skin. After the 24-hour period you may remove the dead skin cells by slight friction, and then apply a cream.

Ingrown hairs

You may experience this condition when the hairs begin to grow. They grow underneath the skin. Sometimes friction with an abrasive mitt will release them, but if it doesn't, the skin needs to be broken with a sterile needle and hair released.

The hair must not be pulled out.

Waxing homecare card

- With hot wax always test on yourself and do a small patch test on the client to test for temperature and avoid giving a burn.
- With organic wax do not allow too much of a build up on the muslin strip, as this can cause undue lifting of the skin during removal.
- With organic wax it is important to keep the angle of pull on the muslin strip horizontal to the skin's surface, as the hairs can break off at the skin's surface and bruising can occur in fleshy areas.
- A thin layer of wax is more effective than a thick build-up of wax on a strip, as a barrier is created between the wax and the hairs.
- For maximum comfort and minimum embarrassment do not be afraid of giving the client lots of towels to protect her modesty, especially with a bikini wax.
- Lots of comfort protection will make the client feel a lot more secure and means that the therapist can manoeuvre her into good positions for easy and effective removal. Ensure that the waxing area has adequate ventilation, especially with hot wax, which can give off fumes when first heated.

Remember

Follow all electrical precautions, i.e. no trailing leads to fall over, regular equipment maintenance checks for efficient and safe working of machines, follow manufacturer's instructions, follow health and safety guidelines.

General checklist before applying wax – warm and hot

Check the following list before applying wax.

Has the following been carried out?

1 Is the working area fully prepared and the wax pre-heated?

2 Are you fully prepared with protective clothing and gloves?

3 Have all safety and hygienic precautions been observed?

4 Are the manufacturer's instructions being adhered to?

5 Has a full consultation been carried out?

6 Can the treatment proceed with no contra-indications present?

7 Has a patch test for sensitivity been carried out before the treatment?

8 Has the client had a full explanation of the treatment and knows what to expect?

9 Has the client been fully informed with regard to aftercare and homecare?

10 Has a record card been filled out for the client, or the existing one updated?

11 Has the area for waxing been examined in a good light and the best method of waxing decided and agreed between therapist and client?

12 Has the area to be waxed been cleaned, is grease-free, talced, and has pre-wax lotion been applied?

If the answers to all of the above are yes, wax application can begin.

Warm wax application

Warm wax is applied in a thin film using a spatula in the direction of hair growth, with a firm press, without hurting the client.

The procedure is as follows.

1   Test the wax on yourself, on the inner wrist. Then, if the temperature is comfortable, test on the client on the area to be worked upon, in a small patch. If the client confirms that she is happy with the feel of it, commence.

2   Gather a manageable amount of wax onto the spatula, and keep the spatula twisting to avoid drips, wiping off any excess onto the edge of the heater. Hold a tissue in the free hand, underneath the spatula to ensure no dripping on the journey from heater to couch.

3   Transfer the wax onto the skin following the hair growth, holding the spatula at a 90° angle and spread a strip-sized width of wax onto the hairs. (As your skill levels increase through practice, you will be able to apply longer strips and remove them quickly.) Support the skin with the free hand.

4   Firmly press the fabric or paper strip and rub down several times to bond the wax to the hairs, in the direction of the hair growth. Leave a small flap free at the end of the strip with which to grip the strip for removal.

5   Gripping the strip firmly (use the flap) and stretching the skin slightly with the free hand, pull the strip away from the skin. You are aiming to pull the strip against the direction of hair growth, with the strip almost going back on itself – in one swift movement. Try not to lift upward, as this can cause skin damage. The swiftness of the hand really does make a difference to the pain the client will feel. Do not hesitate, or stop halfway through, as that is just prolonging the agony.

6   Apply a little pressure to the area with your hand to help reduce the tingling and pain, which occurs after strip removal.

7   Work in a logical sequence all over the whole are to be treated. Take care not to miss any hairs, but avoid overlapping the strips, as this will make the skin in that area sore.

8   The strip will last for several removals before it becomes too laden with wax to pick up any more hairs. When that stage is reached, fold the wax strip in on itself so that the clean side is on the outside, and place it in the bin, with liner, designated for contaminated waste. Use a fresh strip for the next removal, and continue.

9   On inspection after the waxing is complete, if any stubborn, stray hairs still remain, they should be tweezed out with a sterile pair of tweezers. With warm wax it may be possible to reapply a strip over an area with lots of hairs remaining, as there is little skin reaction at low temperatures. This not advisable with the higher temperature of hot wax.

10 You can now apply afterwax lotion liberally and advise the client on aftercare.

11 Finally, you can clear up. This stage is just as important as the rest of the treatment, as cross-infection can occur through the contaminated waste. Dispose of used spatulas, wax strips (unless the strips are to be used again), gloves and couch roll in the appropriate bags. Clean the equipment with the recommended manufacturer's cleaner and clean the plastic couch covering. Wash hands and begin with next client.

Remember

Check with your own professional body as to the use of spatulas. Most state that once the spatula has come in contact with the skin it has become contaminated and should be thrown away and a new one used for the next application.

In the salon

Some manufacturers make strips for use with water soluble wax, and if the correct washing instructions are followed the fabric strips are boiled and re-used.

Area	Time
Eyebrows	10 minutes
Facial (lip and chin)	15 minutes
Full leg	45 minutes
Half leg	20–30 minutes
Underarm	15 minutes
Bikini	l5 minutes
Forearm (wrist to elbow)	20 minutes

Treatment time guide for warm wax

The information given in the table for treatment times is a guide only for information – the time it takes to complete a treatment wax will depend upon the amount of hair growth, how strong the growth is, and how experienced the therapist is. In time, with experience, timings can greatly improve as the confidence and judgement of the therapist improves. However, it is important to remember to be cost-effective when waxing with both time and use of materials.

Remember

The abdomen is also suitable for warm wax hair removal, but it is not a range in NVQ level 2 and has not been included here. However, the same application techniques would apply.

Step-by-step wax application for legs – warm and hot

The lower leg is a simple area to treat as the hair growth can be seen easily. The hairs usually grow towards the ankle on the front of the leg, but may go slightly sideways on the calf. Hair growth may be coarse due to the client shaving and results are usually good as the hair growth in the area is strong. Moving the leg around slightly will allow access to the ankle hair, if the growth pattern is not straight down, and the client may ask for the toes to be waxed, too. The general steps below apply whether you are waxing the legs using warm wax (see below for procedure) or hot wax (see page 221 for procedure).

1 The client can be lying down, or sitting up for the front of the legs, to chat if she wants to, however remember, to put the couch back into a flat position before the client is turned over for treatment to the backs of the legs.

2 It is important that the client's clothing is protected, so provide a towel for cover, and be aware of protecting the client's modesty, if repositioning is required.

3 Cleanse the area; and prepare for waxing following usual sanitising procedure.

4 Start from the ankle and work up the leg systematically.

5 To keep the skin taut at the knee, ask the client to bend it.

6 Turn client over (lowering the couch!) and follow same routine with the back of the leg, with special attention given to the hair growth, which may be not straight down.

7 Do not apply wax to the back of the knee, there are usually no hairs present there

anyway, but if there are a few, then tweeze.

8   If completing a full leg wax continue up the thigh at the front and then turn the client over, again paying attention to the growth direction.

Step-by-step warm wax application for legs

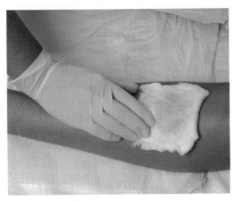

Clean the whole area to be waxed with a suitable antiseptic wipe or hibitane on damp cotton wool.

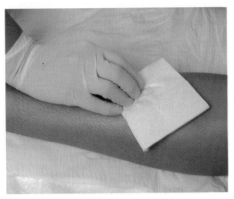

Blot the area with a tissue to ensure the skin is dry and grease free.

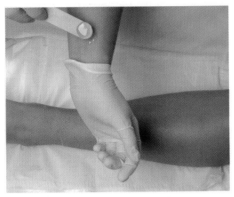

Test the wax on your inner arm to make certain you will not burn the client.

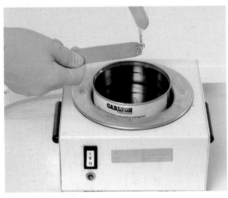

To avoid cross-infection drizzle the wax onto another spatula – it will also help you check that the consistency is workable.

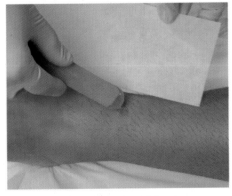

If temperature is acceptable to you, apply a small area onto the legs to check with the client that the temperature is tolerable for her.

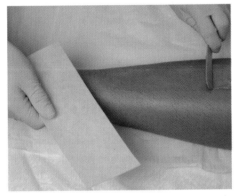

Following the hair growth, i.e. downward, apply a thin even strip of wax to the leg, approximately the width of the paper strip.

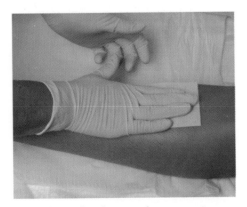

Press down firmly over the wax strip, to ensure all the hairs are fully attached to the strip.

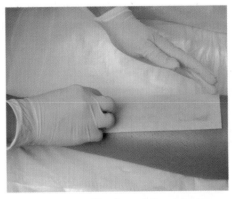

Peel back a small edge of the strip to hold onto.

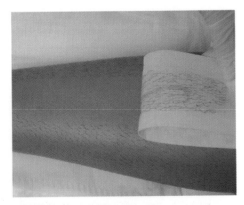

Holding the ankle, grip the wax strip edge and pull the strip off. It is almost a peeling back of the strip, but it must be quick, to minimise pain.

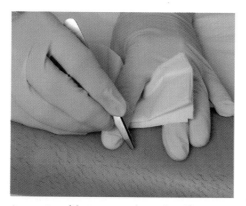

Any missed hairs, too short for the wax to pick, can be plucked out. Sterilise the tweezers first.

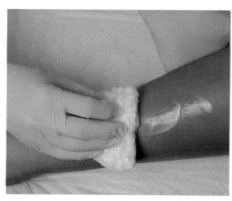

After-wax lotion will remove any wax residue.

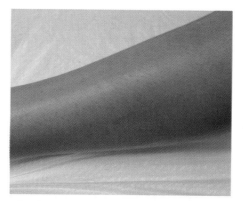

The finished result should be a moisturised, hair-free front of leg.

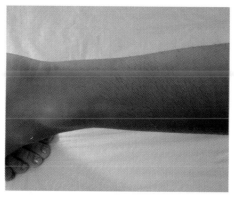

Ask the client to turn over – remember to ensure you put the back of the bed down first. Repeat the cleansing and blotting process.

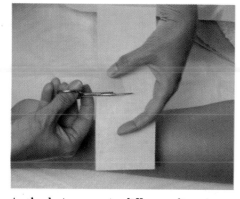

As the hairs grow in different directions, you will need to cut the wax strips into manageable sizes.

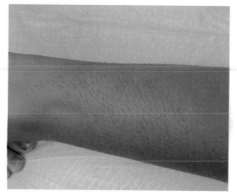

Check the direction of the hair growth, which may be diagonal as shown here. Remember to test the wax again – first on yourself and then on your client.

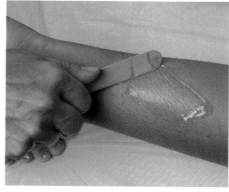

Apply a thin even strip of wax to the leg, following the hair growth, i.e. diagonally as shown here, and repeat the process as for front of leg.

NB Some awarding bodies only expect gloves to be worn if there is a danger of drawing bodily fluids, for example, underarm or bikini line. Therefore, it may be permissible to wax without gloves.

Step-by-step warm wax application for eyebrows

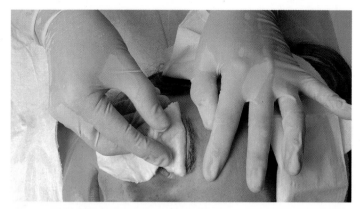

Cover the closed eye with a damp cotton wool round and cleanse the eyebrow area with suitable cleanser. Cut up some small pieces of paper or material strips

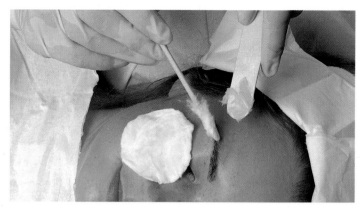

Decant petroleum jelly onto a spatula, using a covered orange stick; apply to hairs you do not want to remove. This barrier stops the wax sticking to the hairs.

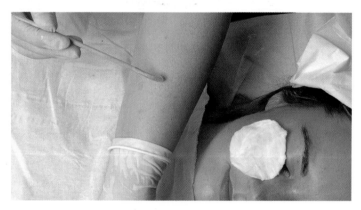

Remember to test the wax on your forearm, before applying to the client. You do not want to burn the delicate eye area.

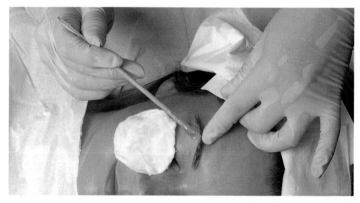

Apply a small amount of wax to the area under the eyebrow, working in the direction of the hair growth. Take care not to dribble wax onto the client's face.

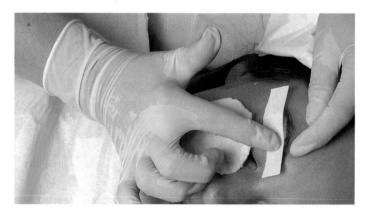

Using a small piece of wax strip, press onto the arch, under the eyebrow. Smooth over with your finger, to ensure all of the hairs are stuck to the strip.

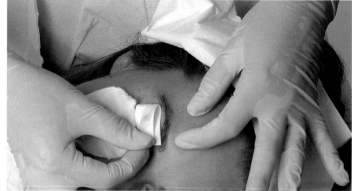

Stretch the eyebrow. Remove hairs against the hair growth i.e. working inwards towards nose. The movement needs to be quick to avoid pain, and it is like peeling back on the strip. Apply after-wax lotion.

Step-by-step warm wax application for the chin

1 Remove make-up and cleanse the area, following normal sanitising procedures.

2 If the hairs are very long, trim with scissors, but not too short for waxing.

3 Protect lower lip with a barrier cream in the lip area.

4 Apply the wax following the hair growth.

5 Stretch the area and remove with a small strip against the hair growth, keeping the skin as taut as possible. The client can help by jutting out the lower jaw and placing the tongue over the lower teeth.

6 Repeat until all hair is removed.

> **Remember**
>
> Do not press too hard on the jaw area, especially in the case of clients wearing dentures.

Step-by-step warm wax application for the bikini and thigh area

The following is the procedure for warm waxing.

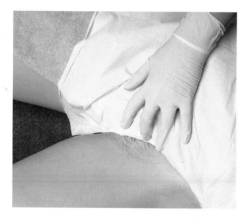

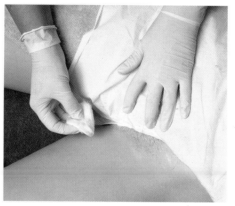

> **Remember**
>
> Make the client aware that as the hair in this area is strong terminal hair, there may be blood spotting, and that it is not unusual for this to occur. Cold compresses can be applied and careful aftercare and homecare must be adhered to.

Protect the edge of the client's underwear with couch roll. You can avoid embarrassment by asking the client to tuck the couch roll in.

Clean the area with suitable cleanser, leaving the skin clean, dry and grease free.

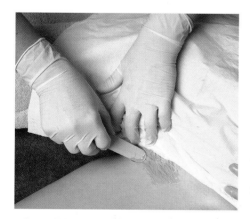

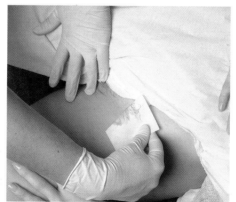

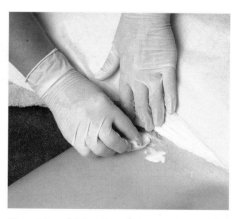

After testing temperature on yourself, apply the wax with the hair growth, in a firm pressing motion. Usually this is a downward direction towards the inner thigh.

Apply the wax strip and press onto the hairs. Ask the client to help stretch the skin, to minimise pain, and remove the wax strip against the direction of hair growth.

Should any blood spots appear, apply light pressure with a clean tissue and then wipe them away. Apply after wax-lotion.

Step-by-step warm wax application for forearms

1   The client can be semi-reclined, or if this is the only area of the body to be waxed the client could sit opposite the therapist across the couch.

2   If the client has just her sleeves rolled up, remember to protect the clothing.

3   Follow the usual pre-wax preparation and cleansing routine.

4   Wax is applied in the same way as on other parts of the body i.e. following hair growth.

5   The skin can be kept taut by grasping the underside of the skin for being worked upon.

6   Follow aftercare and homecare routines.

Step-by-step warm wax application for underarms

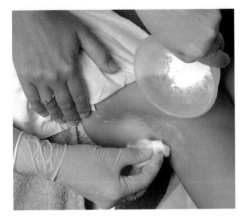

Protect the client's clothing with couch roll and cleanse the area. A light dusting of talcum powder will absorb any residue perspiration and make the hair stand out from the skin.

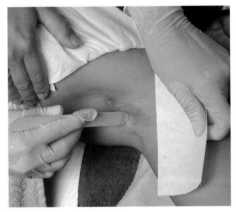

After testing on yourself, apply the wax, going with the hair growth. If hairs are diagonal then go in that direction.

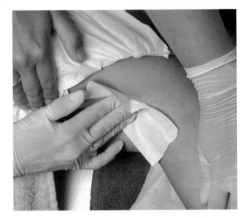

Firmly press the strip down to bond the hairs to it.

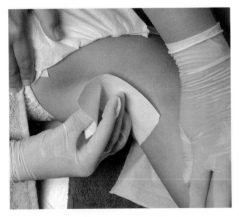

Stretch the armpit area and, if necessary, ask the client to help, with her free hand.

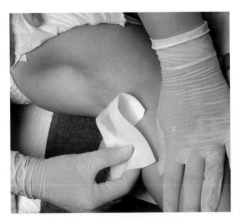

Grip the edge of the strip and quickly and firmly remove the strip against the direction of hair growth.

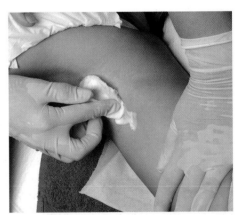

Should any blood spots appear, apply light pressure with a clean tissue and then wipe them away. Apply after-wax lotion.

Hot wax application

Hot wax application is a skill that needs more practice than warm waxing, but once they have been trained in its use, many beauty therapists prefer it to warm wax. As the temperature is higher, removal of strong coarse hairs is very effective and the technique gives a nice clean finish. Unlike warm wax, hot wax is applied as a thicker layer, which is built up by first going against the hair growth and then with the hair growth, until sufficient thickness for removal has been achieved.

The procedure is as follows.

1   Test the wax on yourself, on the inner wrist. Then, if the temperature is comfortable, test on the client on the area to be worked upon, in a small patch. If the client confirms that she is happy with the feel of it, commence.

2   Closely look at the hair growth in the area, as this affects both application and removal.

3   Gather a manageable amount of wax onto the spatula, and keep the spatula twisting to avoid drips, wiping off any excess onto the edge of the heater. Hold a tissue in the free hand, underneath the spatula, to ensure no dripping on the journey from heater to couch.

4   The wax should be the consistency of icing ready to go on a cake – spreadable but not too thick. Apply the wax, and build up several layers, working first against, and then with, the hair growth. Ensure that the edges are quite thick, too, as when the wax is removed, the edges may break off if too thinly applied.

5   Try not to make the strips too large, to avoid difficulty in removal, and two or three applications should give a covering of about 3 mm in thickness – avoid the temptation to apply too many layers, as the wax will just build up on itself, and not adhere to the hairs.

6   The trick is to be quick, and apply several patches in one go. As the first one is setting slightly, the second and third ones can be applied, but do not let any of them dry out totally on the skin, as they will become brittle and break off, like toffee slabs, and hurt the client when removed.

7   A thick lip on the edges of each patch will allow a firm grip to be taken, when removing.

8   As each strip starts to set slightly, press with the fingers; it should feel dry but still supple to the touch, and the lip can be flipped up.

9   Grip the lip you have created and with the other hand pull the skin slightly away from the wax patch, to minimise client discomfort. Be quick and firm, and swiftly remove the wax against the direction of hair growth.

10   Immediately soothe the area by applying pressure to the area. Quickly move onto the next patch as that will be setting.

11   Fold each wax strip in on itself, with the hairs inside, and dispose of into the lined bin, for disposal into the collectable waste bin.

12   Any small remains of wax can be picked up by pressing the larger patch over it and lifting it.

13   Work methodically all over the area to be waxed, in a pattern, so that all hairs are removed, but avoid overlapping and therefore over-waxing.

14 Any escapee hairs may be tweezed away, and the result should be clean and clear. The skin will be slightly pinker than with warm waxing, because of the higher temperature.

15 Aftercare and homecare can be given. A soothing after-wax lotion is applied, and a nice gesture is to provide the client with a small sample size aftercare lotion to take away and apply at home.

16 Clearing up can now take place, and is as important as the rest of the treatment, as cross-infection can occur through the contaminated waste. Dispose of used spatulas, wax, gloves and couch roll in the appropriate bags.

17 Clean the equipment with the manufacturer's recommended cleaner and clean the plastic couch covering. Wash hands and begin with next client.

Area	Time
Eyebrows	10–15 minutes
Facial (lip and chin)	10–15 minutes
Full leg	45–60 minutes
Half leg	20–30 minutes
Underarm	15 minutes
Bikini line	15–20 minutes
Forearm (wrist to elbow)	20 minutes

Treatment time guide for hot wax

Step-by-step hot wax application for legs

Before starting the procedure for waxing legs using hot wax, read the general section on waxing the legs on page 215.

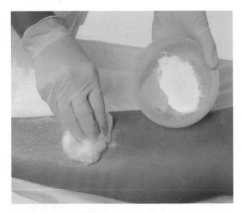

Cleanse the area with a suitable cleanser, to make sure that the skin is dry and grease free. Apply a light dusting of talcum powder – this will make the hairs stand up.

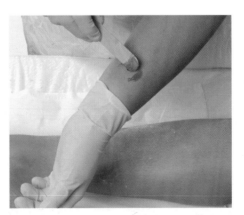

Test the hot wax on your forearm before applying any to the client.

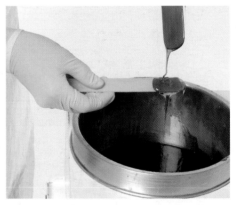

Decant a good amount of hot wax from the pot onto another spatula, to avoid contamination. The consistency of wax should be like soft treacle.

Remember

Some of the older wax heaters have a second tub to them. This was because the used wax was reheated and passed through a small filter, a bit like a sieve, and then reused. This is no longer acceptable practice and not hygienic. Ignore the second tub on the machine.

Remember

This treatment guide depends very much on the skill of the therapist. Hot wax needs to be nurtured up to the correct working temperature and consistency, and then used quickly. It may cool down, and start to solidify, in which case the heater needs turning up, and sometimes that causes the wax to get too hot. Time is then spent waiting for it to cool back down to a good consistency, and the client is kept waiting. Then the whole cycle starts again! This therefore has a big effect on treatment times, and that is why hot wax is considered to need more training and higher skill levels – it's a bit of an art form.

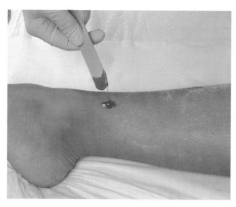

Test a small patch of wax on the client, to avoid burning the skin.

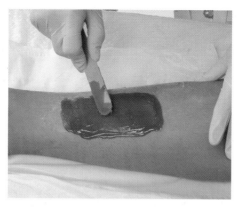

Working against the hair growth to begin with, apply the wax in a figure of eight shape. As you keep applying, you will build up a thick patch of wax.

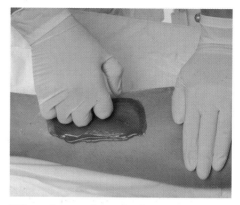

When the wax layer looks set, pressure from the knuckles will help bond the hot wax to the hairs. The wax takes on a matt finish as it cools.

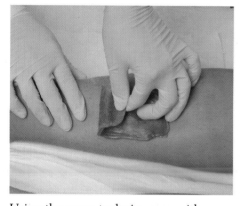

Using the same techniques as with a wax strip, flick a lip up, and gripping firmly, quickly remove the patch of wax – against the direction of hair growth.

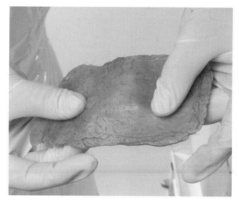

The hairs should be clearly visible, embedded in the wax strip you have removed.

Step-by-step hot wax application for eyebrows

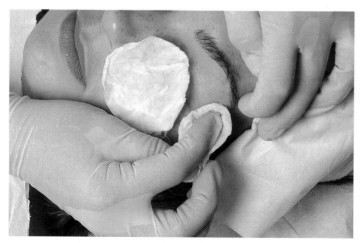

Cover the client's eye and protect the client's clothing from accidental spillage. Clean the area to be waxed.

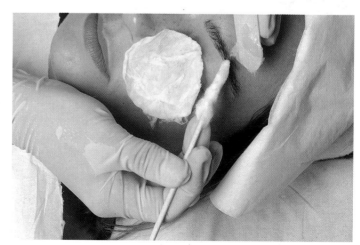

Decant petroleum jelly onto a spatula, using a covered orange stick; apply to hairs you do not want to remove. This barrier stops the wax sticking to the hairs.

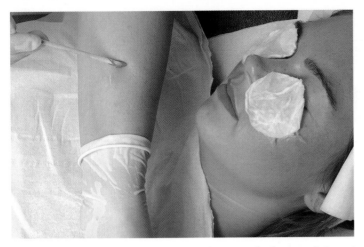

Remember to test the wax on your forearm, before applying to the client. You do not want to burn the delicate eye area.

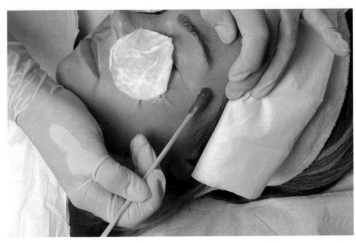

Patch test a small drop of wax near the eye, to test that the temperature is acceptable to the client.

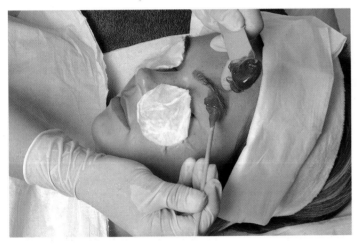

Apply a small amount of wax to the area under the eyebrow, working against the direction of hair growth. Take care not to dribble wax onto the client's face.

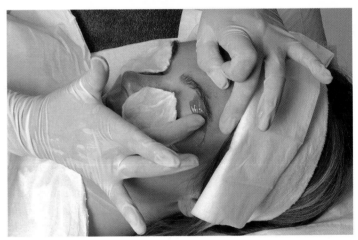

Press down on the wax, under the eyebrow. Smooth over with your finger, to ensure that the hairs have stuck to the wax.

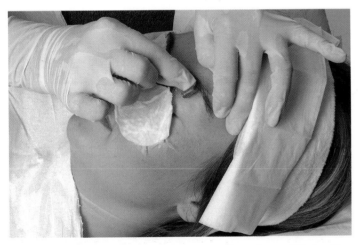

The wax takes on a matt finish as it cools and sets. Flick a lip up, grip firmly, and quickly remove – against the direction of hair growth. Apply after-wax lotion.

Step-by-step hot wax application for lip and chin

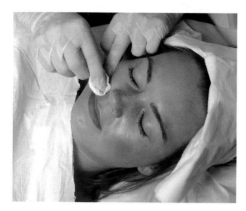

Cleanse the upper lip area. The skin should be clean and grease free. Blot if necessary.

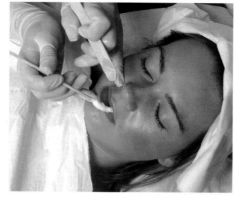

Decant petroleum jelly onto a spatula, using a covered orange stick, and cover the lip up to the lip line.

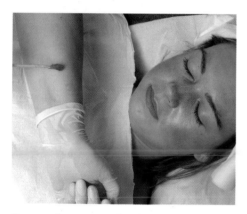

Remember to test the wax on your forearm, before applying to the client.

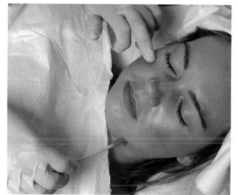

Patch test a small drop of wax near the area, to test the temperature is acceptable to the client.

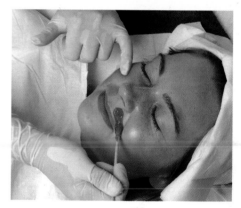

Build up a good layer of wax on upper lip. Ask the client to smile slightly to help stretch skin. Remove as for all hot wax application and apply after-wax lotion.

Step-by-step hot wax application for bikini and thigh area

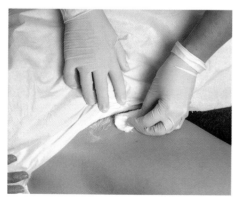

Protect client's underwear with couch roll. Clean the area with suitable cleanser, leaving the skin clean, dry and grease free.

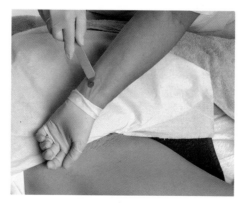

Test wax temperature on yourself on the inner wrist area.

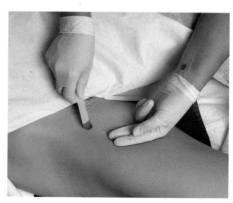

Test the wax on the client near the area to be treated to check the client's tolerance of the temperature. It may vary from yours.

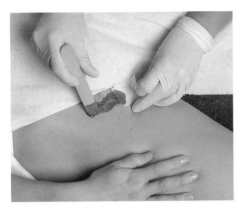

Ask the client to help stretch the skin, and begin to apply an even patch of wax. Use the figure-of-eight method of application.

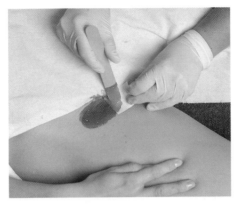

To help removal, you can create an edge to grip by working the wax over a small wax strip, cut to size.

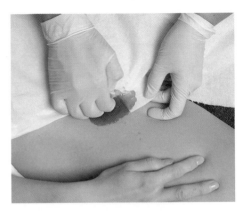

The wax takes on a matt finish as it cools and sets. Press to help the hairs bond to the wax.

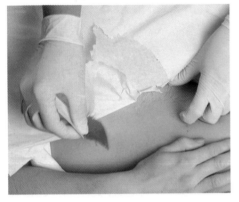

Grip the paper strip edge firmly, and quickly remove – against the direction of hair growth. Apply after-wax lotion.

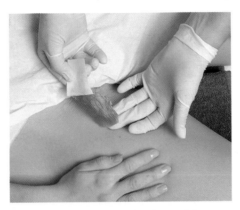

The hairs should be clearly visible, embedded in the wax strip you have removed.

Step-by-step hot wax application for the underarms

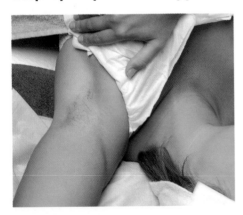

Protect the clothing with couch roll and stretch the underarm out as flat as possible.

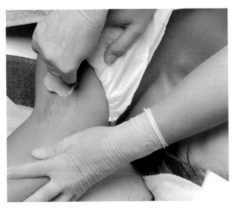

Cleanse the area, to make it clean, dry and grease free.

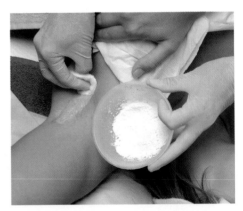

A light dusting of talcum powder can be applied to absorb any perspiration and make the hair stand out from the skin.

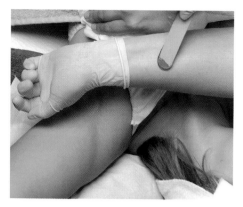

Test wax temperature on yourself, on the inner wrist, to avoid burning the client.

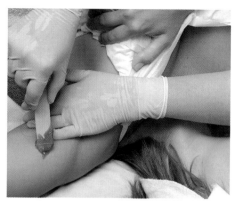

Patch test the wax near the area, for correct temperature. Remember that your client's tolerance may not be as high as yours.

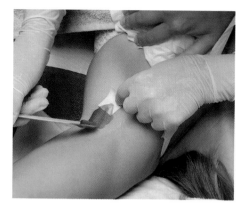

Using a small strip to help you grip, apply the wax. The direction of hair growth under the arms is sometimes circular and therefore the application may need to be circular too.

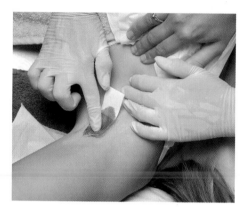

Build up a layer of wax and, using your fingers, press onto the hairs. The wax takes on a matt finish as it cools and sets, ready for removal.

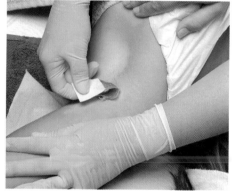

Stretch the area and, if necessary, ask the client to help, with her free hand. Grip the edge of the strip. Firmly remove the strip – against the direction of hair growth.

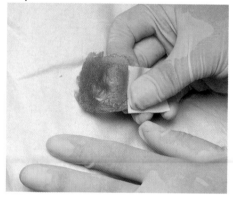

The removed hairs are clearly visible, embedded in the wax.

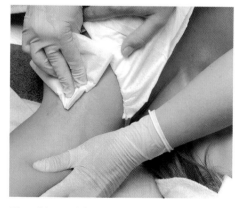

Should any blood spots appear, apply light pressure with a clean tissue and then wipe them away. Apply after-wax lotion.

Sugaring

What is it?

Sugaring is the removal of hairs using a paste. Many women prefer this method of hair removal, as they find it less painful than waxing.

What is the paste made of?

Sugar paste is made up of sugar and water, citric acid (lemon juice) and oil, with other natural ingredients. Most manufacturers of sugar paste will not reveal the actual proportions of the ingredients in their secret recipes, so it does have to be purchased by a sugaring wholesaler. It can be used either as a paste or as strip sugar.

What are the hazards?

Sugar paste ingredients are completely natural and are no threat to health in this natural form. However, as the product needs to be heated for use, great care should be taken to avoid causing burns.

What do you do in the event of an accident?

In the case of burns, flood the area immediately with cold water for a minimum of ten minutes. Twenty minutes are needed for burns to the eyes. Cover with a sterile dressing and seek medical aid. If ingested – seek medical advice.

To avoid accidents only a person who has been fully trained in the art of sugaring should use sugar paste.

How do you handle / store it?

Most suppliers use firm plastic tubs for their products, which can be heated in the tub, just as warm wax is. Store in a cool dry place, and keep containers airtight to avoid the product degenerating. The normal shelf life is about 12 months, but if looked after, it may last up to two years. The main reason for product deterioration is continual over-heating.

Types of treatment paste

Soft paste

Soft paste often needs no adjusting, especially if the weather or the practitioners' hands are warm. If the paste becomes wet and sticky, hard paste can be added to absorb moisture. If the paste becomes hard, add steam or water to adjust. Soft paste is ideal for using with strips.

Soft sugar paste

Super soft paste needs less time to heat and is ideal for use by practitioners with cool hands. It may need no adjusting, especially if the weather or the practitioners' hands are warm. If the paste becomes wet and sticky, hard paste can be added to absorb moisture. If the paste becomes hard, add steam or boiled water to adjust. Super soft paste is also ideal for use with strips.

Hard paste

Hard paste is darker in colour and takes longer to heat. It is ideal for use by practitioners with hot hands and in very hot weather. It often needs adjusting, especially if the weather or the practitioners' hands are cool. If the paste becomes hard, adjust with steam or boiled water. Firm paste is not recommended for use with strips.

Extra hard paste

Extra hard paste is the darkest in colour and takes longest to heat. It needs adjusting within a few minutes of use and so is not recommended for use with strips. This paste is mainly used abroad in hot humid climates.

Benefits and effects of sugaring

As the product is made up of natural ingredients and the working temperature of the paste is low, it is very effective on a more sensitive skin, and on some skins that would react unfavourably to waxing and would therefore be contra-indicated. Clients do say that it feels less painful than warm waxing. Sugar paste is water soluble, so is less inclined to stick to everything, and very easy to wipe off the skin and other surfaces. Very short hairs can be removed, as the paste grips the hairs and not the skin, so there is no need to wait for re-growth, as there is with waxing. Sugaring is very successful on facial hair, as the hairs are pulled out cleanly, and the soft vellus hair is left intact, whilst the coarser hairs are removed – this leaves the face with a natural look to it.

Strip sugaring

Strip sugaring is applied in the same way as warm waxing, and has all the benefits and effects of sugaring, as well as the advantage of being able to be heated in a microwave. Those in mobile businesses favour its use.

Care must be taken when heating in a microwave as the centre of the tub is very much hotter than the outside and there is a risk of burning.

Pre-care for sugaring

Sugaring sticks best to the hairs when there is no grease on the skin, and when the hairs are of a good length to grip.

If the client is booking a sugaring treatment, and she is a regular client, she can be gently reminded of the following; if she is a new client, these considerations need to be discussed, for maximum results.

> For 24–48 hours before treatment there must be:
>
> ✗ **No** body lotion applied to area.
> ✗ **No** bubble baths.
> ✗ **No** body or baby oil.
>
> And at least three days before treatment:
>
> ✗ **No** shaving of the hairs.

It will be too late to explain these to the client, once she is in the salon expecting to be treated.

The receptionists should also be aware of the expected pre-care for sugaring, so that if a new client makes an enquiry about sugaring, she can be primed before the salon visit. The last thing a salon wants is an angry or disappointed customer.

Remember

Most sugaring wholesalers will supply the complete kit for strip sugaring and there are lots of complementary accessories available, should the therapist wish to purchase them. It is advisable to carry out a little research, and shop around for the best purchases, for both value for money and reliability of aftercare service. Comparing prices and wholesalers will give good indications as to which manufacturer to go for.

Step-by-step sugaring depilation

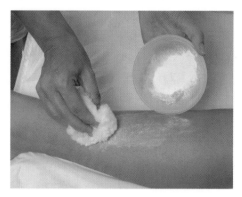

Cleanse the area, so that it is clean, dry and grease free. A light dusting of talcum powder can be applied to the area.

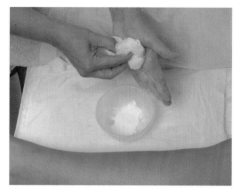

Apply talcum powder to your palms to ensure they remain free from grease and perspiration.

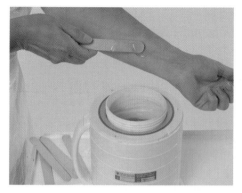

Test sugar paste temperature on yourself, on the inner wrist, to avoid burning the client.

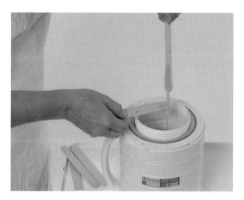

Decant a small amount of sugar paste from the pot onto another spatula, to avoid contamination. The consistency of the paste should be like soft treacle.

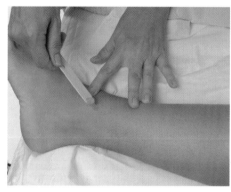

Test this small patch of paste on the client, to avoid burning the skin.

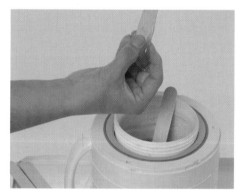

Draw off some of the paste onto your fingertips. (Cool hands are best for this.)

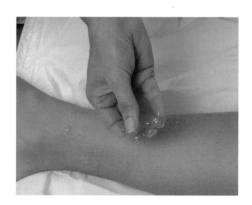

Using a circular wrist and hand motion, begin to work the paste between the fingers.

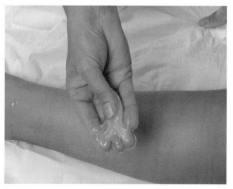

The paste begins to cool and become more treacle-like in consistency. It is now ready to use.

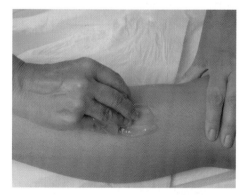

Firmly spread the paste onto the hairs, keeping the skin taut in the area.

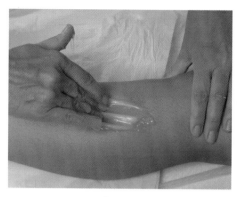

Drag and spread outwards, pressing as you go.

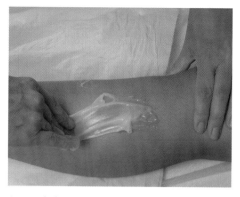

Spread the paste in the direction of hair growth.

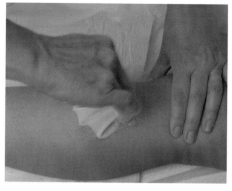

Begin flicking the edge of the paste inwards towards the centre of your patch, just as in waxing, but without leaving the skin.

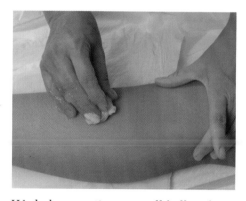

Work the paste into a small ball and remove.

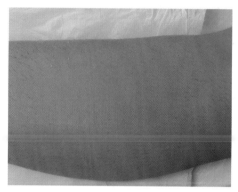

The successful result should be a hair-free, clean area, with no remaining paste on the leg.

Items required

- sufficient sugar and heating unit to pre-heat to temperature
- paper and plastic sheeting to protect couch and surrounding area
- paper to protect client's clothing
- antiseptic lotion – cleans and degreases skin
- talcum powder – dries skin and lifts hair
- cotton wool – for application of products
- spatulas
- tissues
- scissors – to cut long hairs or strips (in autoclave)
- tweezers - removal of stubborn hairs (in autoclave)
- soothing lotion
- barrier cream
- orange stick
- two bins and bin liner
- disposable gloves and protective apron
- pillow
- after-sugaring lotion
- cleanser
- towels
- strips – muslin, fibre
- jewellery bowl.

Preparation of couch

- Plastic sheeting covering base of couch, disposed of after use.
- Paper tissue over top of sheeting where client will be laid.
- Couch in an upright position with pillow, towel and tissue for hygiene.

Preparation of trolley

- Wipe over whole area with antiseptic lotion.
- Place wax heater at top of trolley and position away from client, with no trailing wires.
- Make sure all products required are on the trolley and to hand. This promotes a professional image and saves time.

Preparation of client

- Check for contra-indications to prevent any harm to client and operator.
- Examine area and note which way the hairs are growing for speed and efficiency when applying the paste.
- Explain treatment – to relax client and prepare her for the feeling.
- Remove lower garments, skirt, trousers, etc., for leg sugaring. Place a modesty towel over lap with protective paper tissue.
- Underarm sugaring – remove client's upper garments. Place a modesty towel around upper chest, with protective tissue.
- Bikini sugaring – remove lower garments, ask client to place a folded tissue each side of her briefs.
- Facial sugaring – cover client's upper half with a towel and paper tissues.
- Wipe the area to be treated with antiseptic, or cleanser and toner if working on face, to remove dirt and grease – enabling wax to adhere to skin and hair.
- Position the client in a comfortable position for the area to be treated.
- Make sure all the surrounding area is protected with paper towel.
- Apply a fine dusting of talc to the area where you will be lifting the hairs away from the skin; this dries and lifts hairs so that the sugar can get a firm hold on the hairs and remove them successfully.

Areas to sugar

There are many areas which can be treated:

- eyebrows
- chin
- face
- upper lip
- toes
- underarm
- abdomen
- bikini line
- legs.

The areas to be treated must be agreed with the client prior to treatment. This requires discretion from you. Allow your client to tell you the areas she requires treatment for, as you may have a different opinion.

Consultation

Before starting treatment it is necessary to discuss certain points with your client. These points should be noted on a card, called a record card, and kept in a safe place for future reference (refer to the Professional basics section).

Hygiene and sterilisation

During treatment two of the main rules are:

- Wear disposable gloves.
- Dispose of sugar paste after use and do not reuse it.

This is to avoid the possibility of spread of any infections and HIV.

Contra-indications

- Varicose veins / ulcers – waxing would aggravate condition.
- Defective circulation i.e. diabetes – the client would be easily bruised and damaged.
- Skin diseases – cross-infection.
- Cuts, abrasions, recent scar tissue – could worsen a problem and cross-infect.
- Stings or sepsis – cross-infection or client discomfort.
- Warts or hairy moles – protect with barrier cream.
- Hyper-sensitive skin (due to wind or sunburn) – client discomfort.
- High blood pressure – circulation problems.
- Areas of discomfort to client – bruises.
- Recent haemorrhage or operation.

Remember

The golden rule is: if you are unsure of a problem, request a physician's approval.

Other health and safety precautions are as follows.

- As wax is very desquamating, serum may be excreted from the skin, along with small amounts of blood deposits. Students are strongly advised not to touch such areas and to advise the client to have the affected area treated.
- Cotton wool, tissues, spatulas, wax should disposed of be in a sealed dustbin liner and placed in the main bin.
- Use autoclave – to sterilise tweezers, scissors.
- Use antiseptic lotion – to sanitise the area of the body to be treated, the treatment area, the trolley and equipment.
- During hot wax treatment, scrape residue wax onto large spatula – not onto the sides of machine.
- Please refer to health and safety for information on legislation and by-laws.

⚠ Safety precautions

- Certain rules must be followed to ensure client and operator safety.
- During sugaring, have folded tissues in one hand to catch drips, to prevent them dropping onto client.
- Check the machine, wires, plugs etc.
- Do not rest the machine on glass (on the trolley).
- Do not heat the wax near inflammable materials.
- Do not over-heat the paste.
- Always test the temperature in relation to the client's tolerance.
- Protect the client's clothing.
- Do not re-apply immediately after removing a strip.
- Explain procedure thoroughly and warn client of possible skin reaction.
- Explain after-care procedure.
- Ensure all equipment is clean and sterile.
- Do not leave heating paste unattended.
- Do not heat paste too near client.
- Check contra-indications.
- The therapist should be familiar with machine, e.g. what temperature the wax should melt at and work with.
- Barrier cream applied to moles and birthmarks.
- Make sure you avoid area behind knee.
- All heaters must comply with British Safety Standards.

Testing paste temperature

Once the therapist has tested the paste, test a small amount on the client to check tolerance and also to prepare her for the feeling. This is usually done on the inner ankle.

Application of sugaring

1 Take up a manageable amount of paste, and if it needs it adjust the consistency with a few drops of water, and mould it to make it elastic enough to use.

2 With the spreading technique, massage the paste onto the area with fingers and thumb. The skin will need to be stretched and supported, as when applying wax.

3 Make sure the edges are thickly enough applied to make a lip for easy removal.

4 Remove the paste with a firm flicking motion – without hurting the client.

5 Work over the whole area to be treated in a methodical sequence, so that all hairs are removed.

> **Remember**
>
> The reason for the test is to prevent any burning or discomfort to the client. The paste must also be tested on the therapist during treatment to make sure the temperature hasn't altered.

> **Contra-actions**
>
> If a treatment is applied and the area reacts by:
>
> - swelling
> - blistering
> - becoming sore.
>
> *You must stop sugaring*
>
> A *normal* reaction to sugaring is:
>
> - slight heat builds up in area being treated
> - blotchy red patches
> - some itchiness.
>
> These reactions must only be mild, any other reaction would prevent treatment from either being carried out in the first place or from being continued.

6   Using the antiseptic wipes and soothing lotion that is compatible with the product used, wipe over the area.

7   Provide aftercare and homecare advice.

Top and bottom lip

1   Work from corner of mouth, towards centre of lip in small strips.

2   Ask client to open her mouth or twist to opposite side, before applying paste against hair growth.

3   Place hand on top of area to soothe.

4   Move to other side of couch and repeat on the opposite side.

5   Always support with thumb and index finger.

6   Second application may be necessary to strip the hair growth.

7   Some manufacturers recommend that diluted witch hazel be applied after treatment to soothe.

Chin and jaw line

1   Use strips if the hair is long; if too long, trim with scissors.

2   Treat as for top lip, using wider strips, working first against and then with the hair growth.

3   If the hair is strong, apply worked paste and remove by strip.

4   Ask client to support by lifting her neck and using thumb and index finger to pull skin taut. (Cover a maximum of three times.)

Neck

1   Work by hand, unless hair is particularly strong.

2   Work first against the growth and then with the growth.

3   Witch hazel may be applied after sugaring to prevent the skin from drying.

Underarms

1   Look at direction of hair growth and check support for maximum effect, asking client to help.

2   Work elbow to breast; apply paste against hair growth with side of index finger. If using strips to remove paste, the direction of application may need to be varied. When using strip sugar, wear disposable gloves.

3   Take a strip and press firmly, leaving room at the ends to flick; always check beneath and hold away from this point with your fingernails and flick forwards.

4   Always flick long and low, not forgetting to place hand on skin after treatment.

5   Then work breast to elbow if necessary, to remove remaining hairs, still with client supporting breast.

6   Treat other side in the same way.

7   Dry area and remove any remaining hairs with tweezers and pad.

8   Apply after-sugaring lotion, using gentle massage techniques.

9   Give aftercare advice.

Step-by-step sugaring for lip and chin

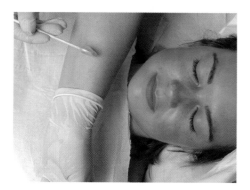

Prepare the client by covering the clothes, and clean the area to be sugared. Patch test the paste on yourself for correct temperature.

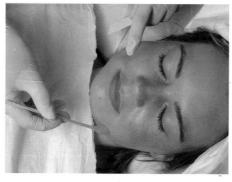

Test the paste on the client prior to application – remember her temperature tolerance may be different to yours.

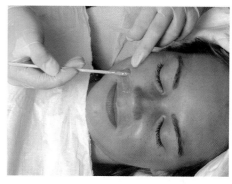

Work from the outer edge of the upper lips inwards.

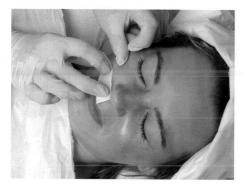

Use a small length of paper or fabric wax strip to help grip the hairs. Press down to bond the hairs to the strip.

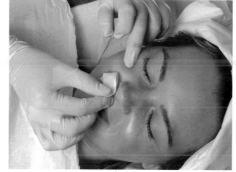

Using the same removal technique as for waxing the upper lip, quickly remove the strip – avoiding contact with the nose.

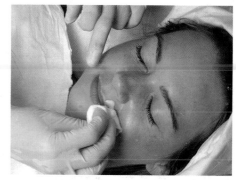

Carry out the same procedure on the other side of the upper lip, and apply after-sugar lotion.

Step-by-step sugaring for the underarms

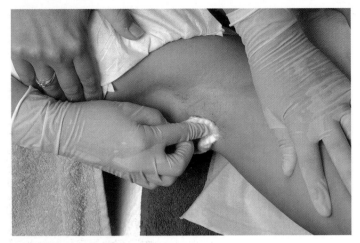

As with the procedure for warm wax application on the underarm, protect the clothing, cleanse the area and make sure the skin is dry and grease free.

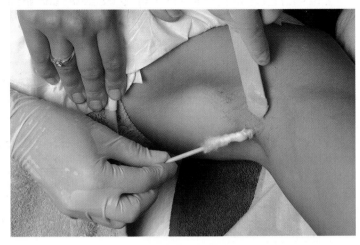

Look for skin tags or moles in the armpit and, should you find one, cover with petroleum jelly to avoid causing any damage.

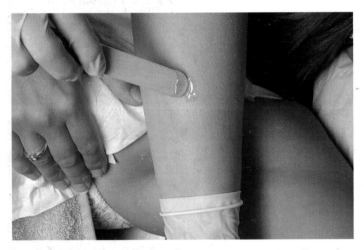

Test the paste on yourself.

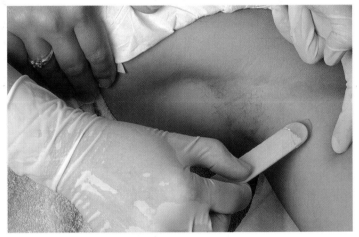

Apply a test patch on the client and remove in the same way as for warm wax, following the direction of hair growth. Pluck any stray hairs out and apply after-sugar lotion.

Eyebrows

As for warm waxing.

Lower legs

1 Prepare as for other sugaring areas. The client may wish to have feet and toes included in the treatment.

2 Treat ankles in small flicks in both directions.

3 Treat knees first against and then with the hair line, then from side of knee and then from opposite side of couch. Ask client to place leg flat and treat side of knee asking for client's assistance, treating first against then towards hair growth.

Remember

Sugaring, like hot waxing, is a skill that develops over many hours of practice. All skills that include a certain amount of dexterity take time – after all, could anyone learn to play the piano in a day? Practice makes perfect and treatment times will improve with experience!

4   Treat in rows from ankle to knee, first against and then with hair growth. Always start with the backs of the legs, with ankle flexed and short flicks.

5   Aftercare and homecare as usual.

Aftercare and homecare

Once you have finished an area you must soothe it with a lotion before commencing another area. This can be done with soothing after-sugar lotion or cream spread over area with cotton wool.

The client should also follow guidelines of care after treatment at the salon. These are for a period of 24 hours.

- Do not take a hot bath or shower.
- Do not expose skin to the sun or use sunbeds.
- Do not use perfumed products on area – e.g. body lotion, deodorant, make-up, perfume.
- Avoid wearing tight clothes or clothes that cause friction.
- Avoid bathing in sea or swimming pool.
- Avoid touching area where possible.
- Do not apply antiseptic or similar product to area.
- Treat ingrown hairs with a scratch mitt.

It is quite normal to experience slight soreness and redness for up to 24 hours following treatment. This redness is called an erythema and can be treated by after-wax lotions at home or soothing substances such as calamine lotions. The client may also experience dry skin. After the 24-hour period she may remove the dead skin cells using slight friction, then apply a cream.

Ingrown hairs

The client may experience this condition when the hairs begin to grow again. They grow underneath the skin. Sometimes friction with an abrasive mitt will release them, but if it doesn't the skin needs to be broken with a sterile needle and the hair released. *The hair must not be pulled out.*

Possible depilation problems

It can be very frustrating to find that the 'perfect' treatment isn't perfect after all, and that some stubborn hairs remain.

Here are a few possible reasons for this.

- The hairs were just too short – even for sugaring.
- The application was too thickly applied to grip the hairs.
- The hot wax was too thick to contract around the hairs.
- The wax / sugar was applied in the wrong direction.
- The wax / sugar was removed too slowly.
- The skin was not pulled taut and the hairs were caught in the skin folds.
- There was grease on the skin.

The simple answer is practice, practice, practice!

Waxing / sugaring

Preparation – you, your working area and the client.

⬇

Two waste bins with liners.

⬇

Choose wax / sugar most suitable for client / area. Heat it up – an hour before appointment.

⬇

On the trolley:
- antiseptic cleaner
- talc
- fabric / paper strips
- disposable gloves
- wooden spatulas
- tissues and cotton wool
- jewellery bowl
- scissors and tweezers
- after-treatment lotion
- record card.

⬇

Consultation, with record card. Fully explain treatment.

⬇

Wash hands.

⬇

Test on self and patch test on client.

⬇

Area to be clean and grease free. Commence treatment.

⬇

Wash hands.

⬇

Aftercare / homecare.

⬇

Dispose of used spatulas, etc. Clean working area.

⬇

Wash hands.

⬇

Start again with next client.

Lighten hair using bleaching techniques

7.4

In this element you will learn about:

- bleach
- bleaching hair – how it works
- application of bleaching
- other methods of hair removal.

Bleaching

What is it?

Bleach comes in a ready mixed cream form, or as a dry powder that needs activating by mixing with liquid hydrogen peroxide.

What is it made of?

Most bleach-based products are made up of hydroquinone. A compound of ammonium and mercury can also be used. Check with individual manufacturers regarding proportions of chemicals. Domestic bleaches used in cleaning obviously have a higher proportion of active ingredients than those preparations used on the skin. They have sodium hypochlorite in a water base for disinfecting.

What are the hazards?

Mercury is classed as a poison and hydroquinone requires great care when handled as it can cause skin irritation. Bleach can also cause respiratory inflammation in its dry powder form.

What are the first-aid measures?

Eye contact Rinse eyes immediately with plenty of water and seek medical advice.

Skin contact Wash contaminated skin and if irritation persists seek medical advice.

Inhalation If dry powder is inhaled, remove to fresh air. If coughing, choking, or breathlessness continues for longer than 10–15 minutes seek medical advice.

Ingestion Seek medical advice immediately.

What do you do in the event of an accident?

Use water to dilute and mop up spillage. Do not dispose of dry powder – wash it down the drain with plenty of water.

How do you handle bleach?

Use only in a well-ventilated area and always use protective gloves. Avoid inhalation of the dry powder and contact with eyes. Do not use on damaged or sensitive skins.

How do you store bleach?

Store in a cool, dry place away from direct sunlight and other sources of heat. Reseal container after use.

Bleaching hair – how it works

Bleaching has a lightening effect on the hair, i.e. it removes or lifts the colour, without penetrating the skin. This makes the hair less visible, but the hair's true colour will be visible as re-growth begins to appear.

Bleaching is a good alternative to offer a client who wants to make a small area of superfluous hair, e.g. on the face, less visible without having it depilated. As it does not interfere with the follicle of the hair, it is also ideal for clients going through epilation – other methods of hair removal will distort the follicle and make permanent removal more difficult.

Bleach affects the cortex of the hair. The bleach contains ammonia and hydrogen peroxide, which swell out the hair to open the protective outer covering, the cuticle, and enter into the hair shaft to destroy the pigment in the cortex. The bleaching agents then mix with the hydrogen peroxide and oxygen is released. The oxygen that enters the cortex, oxidizes the melanin to oxymelanin, which bleaches out the colour.

> ### Remember
>
> It is not acceptable to use any old bleach that is in the cupboard. The only types right for the skin are the ones prepared for salon use, or the retail products sold in chemists.

Contra-indications to bleaching

In a good light, cleanse the area to be bleached and look for:

- ✗ open or broken skin
- ✗ the presence of infection or disease
- ✗ moles or warts
- ✗ recent sunburn
- ✗ recent scar tissue
- ✗ healing skin, i.e. scabs
- ✗ swelling or unrecognised inflammation
- ✗ signs of heat treatment / sunbed
- ✗ eye infections, styes etc
- ✗ loss of pigment already present in the skin
- ✗ over-pigmentation of the skin colour of the area
- ✗ failure of the patch test.

> ### Remember
>
> Because of the strong nature of the ingredients within bleach, always use a patch test prior to treatment for the client's well-being and the therapist's protection.

The patch test is similar to an eyelash tint patch test.

Cleanse an area in the elbow and apply a small amount of the mixed bleach product. Leave for five minutes, or as long as the manufacturer's instructions for treatment states, and remove with damp cotton wool. Over the next 24 hours the client must check for any adverse reaction to the bleach and report back, before the treatment can be carried out

It is likely that a reaction will occur almost immediately, if there is one. A burning or stinging sensation with redness and itchiness are common. Remove immediately and place cool compress to the area.

Safety precautions for bleaching

Refer to the COSHH regulations for first-aid and safety. Also refer to the Professional basics section for legal responsibilities under HASWA (page 33).

> ### Remember
>
> - Always follow the manufacturer's instructions for mixing and application.
> - Never apply bleach after a hot bath or shower as the pores are open and bleach will enter the skin and cause irritation.
> - Ensure the client's clothing is protected – the bleach will also make fabric lose its colour.
> - When bleaching the eyebrows, do not allow any mixture to fall into the eye.
> - Always wear protective gloves.
> - Never leave the client while the bleaching process is taking place.
> - Never mix products from different manufacturers as the stability of different ones may not be compatible.
> - Never exceed the processing time and do not guess – use a clock.

Step-by-step bleaching for the forearms

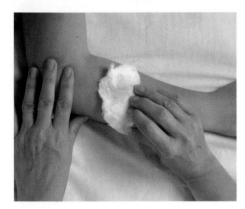

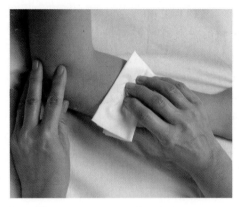

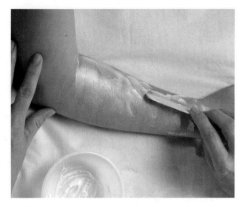

Cleanse the area well, checking for contra-indications, broken skin or signs of infection. Never treat unless a patch test has been completed 24 hours before.

Providing no contra-indications are present, blot the skin with a tissue to keep the skin clean, dry and grease free.

Follow manufacturer's instructions for mixing the bleach and apply all over the forearm in light strokes. Leave for recommended time and wipe off with damp cotton wool.

Step-by-step bleaching for the upper lip

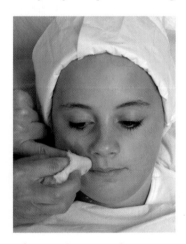

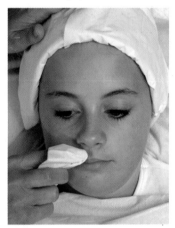

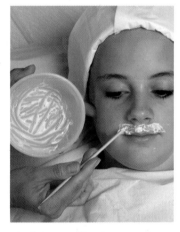

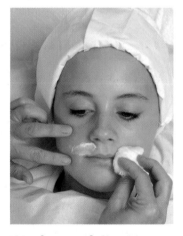

Cleanse the upper lip.

Blot with a tissue to dry the skin.

Apply a small amount of paste all over, avoiding going too far into the nostrils – it may make the client inhale.

Wait for manufacturer's development time, and remove with damp cotton wool. Give aftercare and homecare advice to the client.

Aftercare for bleaching

- Do not apply make-up for 4–6 hours.
- Do not expose skin to sun or use a sunbed for 24 hours.
- Do not touch the area.
- Do not re-bleach within 24–48 hours.
- Avoid highly perfumed products for 24 hours.

Need to know

Other methods of hair removal

Hair-removing creams

These creams include chemicals to break down the hair structure. The chemical is calcium thioglycollate, which attacks the hair keratin layer. The hair dissolves and can be scraped or washed away. Most over-the-counter preparations have a full list of instructions for use, and timings may vary. This type of product is not always suitable for young or sensitive skins and a reaction can occur. The re-growth is soft and with a tapered end, so the hair does not feel spiky and sharp.

Cutting / clipping

Scissors are used to trim the hair, and they can be used in between treatments, as using them does not distort the follicle. Scissors can be used to shorten long 'whiskers' but they are not ideal for achieving a smooth finish. They are not a long-term solution to superfluous hair.

Shaving

Shaving is the chosen option for many women who wish to avoid the pain of waxing. It can produce clean results, provided care is taken, a clean razor used, and a suitable lubricant on the skin is applied. Many of the large razor companies have recognised how big the female market is, and designed razors, creams, shaving foams and after-shaving preparations in feminine colours and with attractive smells.

However, the ends of the hair are chopped at skin level and are very blunt, so the re-growth is spiky and gives stubble.

Shaving the face or arms becomes quite a chore as you have to keep doing it, and if the hair growth is dark and thick, it could become a twice-weekly job.

Plucking

Plucking of the eyebrows involves taking hairs out individually so it really is not suitable for large areas of hair removal. The hair is pulled out of its follicle, and if the hair is taken out at the right stage of growth, re-growth can take some time. The hair eventually grows back with its natural tapered end, so does not feel spiky to the touch. Care must be taken to avoid infection. The tweezers should be clean and disinfected, and the skin cleaned and wiped with antiseptic. Avoid applying make-up straight away, as the follicle is open and there is a risk of infection.

Threading

Threading is similar to plucking and practised mostly in Asian communities, and sometimes in the Mediterranean. A piece of cotton is entwined around the fingers and twisted over the hairs. The hair gets caught up in the thread and is plucked out of its follicle. This is quite a skill and practice makes perfect.

Abrasives

An abrasive glove or pumice stone is rubbed over the skin and the hair is broken off at the skin's surface. There are many over-the-counter preparations that have this effect, and they come in glove or mitt form and are sold as 'a sensible alternative to waxing and shaving'. They tend to resemble fine sandpaper. For best results the skin must be dry, and the glove is rotated in a gentle circular fashion.

Remember

When using abrasives, do rub gently, do rub in circular motions, don't rub up and down.

The fine powder that appears is an accumulation of skin exfoliation. This means skin cells are shed. This makes the product ideal on dry rough skin, provided soothing body moisturising creams are applied after use.

How to be cost effective

What being cost effective means:

Cost = the price paid or required for acquiring, producing, or maintaining something. This is measured in time, money or energy.

Effective = capable of producing a result, or equipped and prepared for action.

So, in terms of hair removing, how does this apply?

Imagine you own your own business and you have to pay for everything: equipment, overheads, stock and wages.

How can a therapist be economical?

Only use the amount of product needed. Do not use a heavy application of wax – it does not give the best results.

Don't be wasteful with disposable items. Couch roll can be split in half, cotton wool pads split and you can use smaller tissues, rather than the 'man sized' ones.

Plan your time. Remember time is money. If the treatment times are not planned carefully through the day, there may be gaps between clients, say 15 minutes between each. This adds up to an extra hour at the end of the day – which could have been put to good use, either with vital chores, or another client.

Be organised and prepared – extra time preparing the working area not only gives a professional appearance, it is also very time-saving.

Don't engage in false economy. Paying out to have equipment maintained and repaired makes good financial sense. If the equipment starts failing, and the therapist is unable to offer some treatments because of it then revenue may be lost. Bad advertising through word of mouth is definitely not being cost-effective.

In the beginning invest in some good labour-saving equipment – for example, borrowing an old twin tub to wash all the towels may look like cutting costs, but an industrial one will be more effective, with no maintenance and costly bills.

Work out overhead costs on a realistic basis, and try and gear your prices to that figure. Work out the days and hours working – remember, you do not work 24 hours a day.

Be wary of both consultation and aftercare times: some clients love to chat, and whilst the therapist wants to give a quality treatment, time can slip away and that is expensive. Leaflets are always a good time-saving trick, and the client can take them away to refer to.

It is a good idea to do some research and find out what sort of prices the competition is offering for waxing / sugaring treatments. This way prices can be adjusted to be about the same, not too expensive so that custom is lost, but not too cheap so that clients think there is a catch.

Remember

A patch test would be advisable for people with a sensitive skin.

Remember

Remember to keep practising, and the skills will develop with experience. Be patient while learning and it will pay off.

Do some of your own research – find out what manufacturers can offer in terms of equipment, products and prices, and visit trade shows for a preview of all future developments.

Your questions answered

Why must we advise clients to avoid using grease-containing products on areas 24 hours prior to a sugaring treatment?
Because the grease forms a barrier and prevents the sugar fully adhering to the hairs, preventing a clean hair removal.

What action would you take if the sugar became soft?
You would need to add hard paste to the soft paste to achieve a workable consistency.

How often should sugar or wax be tested for temperature?
Throughout the treatment, especially when changing to a different area of the body, to prevent burning the skin.

What homecare advice would you recommend to a client with erythema?
Apply a soothing lotion, i.e. calamine. If the erythema persists accompanied by swelling, consult a GP.

How do industry codes of practice and by-laws affect treatment in the salon?
One must adhere to the codes of practice and the legislation, which requires:
- couch roll on bed
- decanting of sugar from one spatula to the other, to prevent cross-infection
- gloves to be worn when sugaring in certain instances, i.e. the bikini area
- follow the cut-out system of splitting couch roll and washing hands prior and after treatment
- full consultation done before treatment commences
- where appropriate, a doctor's letter may be required.

What advice would you give a client with dry skin conditions?
- The use of body lotions on a daily basis.
- Using suitable bath products, i.e. oil-based.
- Exfoliation with loofah or body scrub.

Test your knowledge

Choose the correct answer to each of the questions below.

1   *Waxing is a:*
    a permanent method of hair removal
    b temporary method of hair removal
    c long-lasting method of hair removal
    d short-term method of hair removal.

2   *Hot wax is most suitable for use on:*
    a strong hair growth
    b weak hair growth
    c bent follicles.

3   *Hair removal creams are:*
    a suitable for all skin types
    b not suitable for all skin types
    c a painless method of hair removal
    d a permanent method of removal.

4   Warm wax is:
     a   most suitable for all areas
     b   easy to apply
     c   not easy to apply
     d   a temporary method of removal.

5   Hot wax works best at a temperature of:
     a   48–68 °C
     b   20–30 °C
     c   60–80 °C
     d   15–20 °C.

6   Warm wax works best at a temperature of:
     a   48–68 °C
     b   40–43 °C
     c   60–80 °C
     d   15–20 °C.

7   The main ingredients used in hair removal wax are:
     a   resins and beeswax
     b   starch and flour
     c   sugar and water
     d   crystals and polish.

8   Pre-wax lotion must be used to:
     a   dry up the skin
     b   cleanse the area
     c   make the area smell nice
     d   make the hairs stand on end.

9   Talc is used to:
     a   make the skin smell nice
     b   provide a coating for the wax to stick to
     c   make the hairs stand away from the skin
     d   make the skin white.

10   After-wax lotion helps:
     a   soothe the skin
     b   stop the area going pink
     c   makes the skin smell nice
     d   helps calm the client down.

11   A patch test must always be carried out, to:
     a   try out the heat of the wax on the client
     b   see if the client is suitable for treatment (i.e. no reaction occurs)
     c   let the client know it hurts
     d   give the client a bald patch on her arm.

12   After-care is important, because:
     a   it prevents the client from irritating the area after the treatment
     b   it stops you from being sued for poor treatment
     c   it's just part of the job
     d   it stops the client from picking at the area.

Enhance the appearance of eyebrows and lashes

Unit 8

This unit focuses on ways to enhance the appearance of eyebrows and lashes by carrying out a range of treatments. The unit will cover the following areas.

8.1 Assess clients and prepare treatment plans.
8.2 Prepare the work area for eyebrows and eyelash treatments.
8.3 Shape the eyebrows to meet client requirements.
8.4 Tint eyebrows and eyelashes to meet client requirements.
8.5 Apply artificial eyelashes to meet client requirements.

Each of the elements in this unit can be either combined or carried out independently to meet the requirements of the client. If you are completing an assessment on tinting you will need to complete elements 8.1, 8.2 and 8.4 for example.

Some therapists view this section as 'small treatments', but it should not be undervalued. Clients can instantly see an improvement with an eyebrow shape, eyelash tint or eyelash perm. Eye treatments can be easily slotted into other treatments, e.g. added into the facial, whilst the tint is processing. Remember to include these 'extras' into the cost, as lots of small treatments soon mount up.

Assess clients and prepare treatment plans

8.1

In this element you will learn about:	
• the contra-indications to treatment	• measuring the eyebrows to decide
• the client's requirements	length.

As with all treatments, you will need to carry out a consultation, to check for any contra-indications that may prevent the treatment taking place and to discuss the client's requirements. These contra-indications apply to all eye treatments.

Contra-indications to treatment

- **Conjunctivitis** – This is a nasty eye condition. The eyelids are red and sore, with itching. Mainly caused by bacteria present. It can be irritated by a virus or an allergy.
- **Stye** – This is a small boil at the base of the eyelash follicle. It is raised, sore and red, there may be considerable swelling in the area.
- **Blepharitis** – An infection of the lid causing inflammation of the eye, which will look red and sore. Depending on the severity of the condition, it may be better to avoid eye make-up application altogether, and focus attention on the mouth, with a pretty lipstick shade.
- **Viral infections** – This could include a cold.
- **Bruising** to the area.

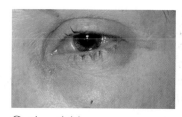

Conjunctivitis

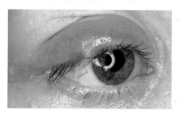

Stye

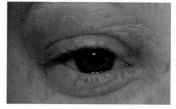

Eczema

Other conditions include:

- **Hyper-sensitivity** – If a client has hypersensitive eyes it is very important to use hyposensitive products when cleansing the eyes and ensure a patch test is carried out before the products are used.
- **Active eczema or psoriasis** – the area should not be treated, especially if the skin is open or weeping, when it is vulnerable to infection and the condition can be spread.
- **Common cold** – easily recognised: runny or blocked nose, dry skin around the nose, sneezing, watery eyes, headache.
- **Hay fever text** – an irritation of the nasal membrane resulting in watery eyes, runny nose and sneezing.
- **Watery eyes** – an irritating condition, in which the eye area becomes moist, causing make-up application to be difficult.
- **Recent operations** – a general rule of thumb is to wait six months before treating an area with scar tissue. However, if it is a minor operation, and you have your client's and her GP's approval, go ahead, but avoid the area itself.
- **Bruising to eye** – easy to recognise, a bruise shows as blue / black and yellow skin colouring. Do not treat a bruised eye.

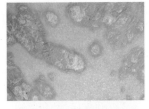

Psoriasis

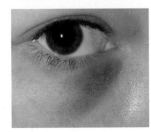

Bruising to the eye

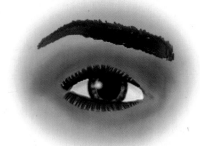

Remember

It is very easy to cross-infect the eyes, so care must be taken at all times. When carrying out any treatment on the eyes ensure that you use a fresh piece of cotton wool, cotton bud, or make sure your tweezers are sterile when transferring from one eye to the next.

The client's requirements

Shaping the eyebrow

Eyebrow shaping is the removal of superfluous hair to enhance the shape of the natural brow. Superfluous hair is the term used if hair growth is normal but the client feels it is unattractive. When shaping the eyebrows you need to plan the treatment carefully, because once removed the eyebrows *cannot* be stuck back on. So, discuss the needs with your client before commencing the treatment. You may have very different ideas.

Important tools for shaping are a mirror and an eyebrow brush.

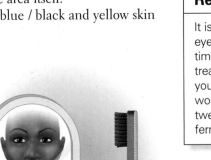

Mirror   An eyebrow brush

Facts about eyebrows

Every natural eyebrow is different in shape, hair type and colour.

As well as this, to achieve the most flattering effect, you need to consider both facial and eye types.

Most hairs on the brows are terminal hairs. The terminal hairs of the brows, unlike other terminal hairs, are usually short in length but are still there for protection. The reason we have hairs on the brows and surrounding the eyes is to stop debris entering the eyes and to keep germs out. The hairs are also there to protect the eyes from excessive light damage.

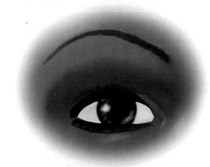

Eyebrows differ in shape, hair type and colour

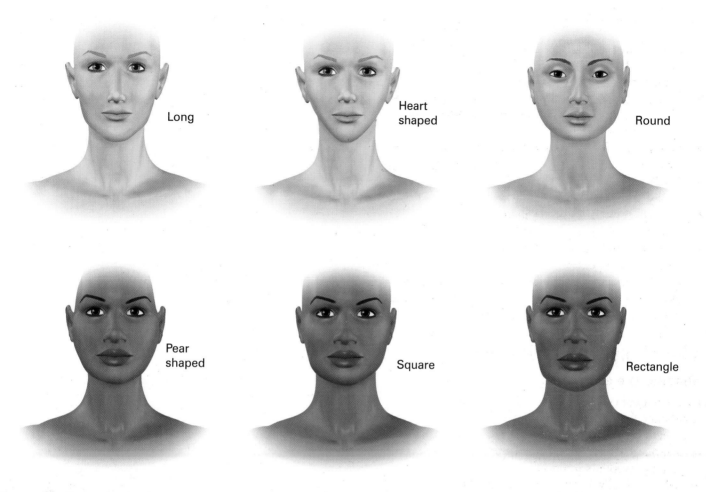

Face types influence brow shape

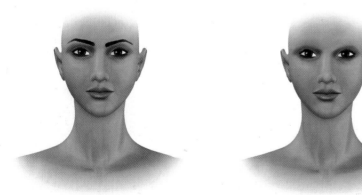

Brows give the face definition

It is suggested that the normal eyebrow should look like the wings of a bird in flight: thicker at the inner corner of the eye tapering to an arch and narrowing at the end of the brow. As the eyebrows frame the face, they should be in balance with the rest of the facial features.

The following indicate the effect of shapes.

Angular shape

This shape can define a round face. Enhance this shape with shading and contouring of the eye make-up for elegance.

Rounded shape

Suitable for clients with large eyes or a wide forehead, a rounded shape can enhance the client's eyes. The eyebrow line should follow the frontal bone and be shaped to a taper.

Arched shape

Sometimes referred to as 'sweeping', this shape is very flattering on most clients. It gives width and expression to the eye. It opens the eye and can help to balance a prominent nose or a large mouth. An arched shape can also be used to detract from a high forehead.

Low arched shape

This shape works well for a client with a low or small forehead by giving the illusion of more length. It is sometimes referred to as a straight shape.

Wide-set eyes

If a client has wide-set eyes, extend the eyebrow to inside the corner of the eye.

Other factors that may influence the shape of the brows are:

- The natural shape of the brows. If the client has been shaping her own brows, it may be necessary to let them grow for a short time before shaping them professionally; in the meantime, stray hairs can be removed to keep them neat.
- Client age. More mature clients might have some coarse hairs, which can be long, white and discoloured. These can be removed, provided that doing so does not alter the brow line or leave bald patches. Ideally, the brow should be of medium thickness. Too thick, and it can give an older appearance. Thin eyebrows give a severe appearance.
- Fashion trends. Each season sees new fashion trends, which have an effect on eyebrow shapes and eye make-up. This should also be considered before shaping the brows.

Other approaches which may be suitable for the client

- Semi-permanent make-up. This should be applied only by professionals in this technique. Pigment is applied to add colour to the brows, for example to disguise a bald area.
- Hair transplants. These are already available in the USA for clients with sparse brows.
- False individual eyebrow hairs. These are applied in the same way as individual eye lashes and are not permanent.

Measuring the eyebrows to decide the length

Once you have carried out your consultation and discussed the requirements with the client, you need to measure the length of the brows. Here are some points to help you when deciding the correct length and shape for your client.

- Place an orange stick in a straight line from the side of the nose to the inner corner of the eye. This is where the eyebrow should begin.
- Place an orange stick from the side of the nose to the outer corner of the eye. This is where the eyebrow should end.

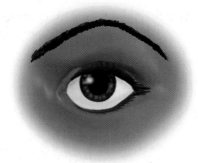

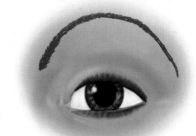

Rounded shape

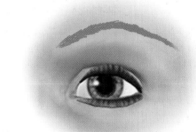

Arched shape

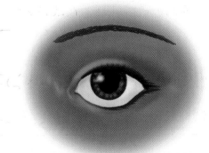

Low arched shape

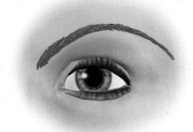

Wide-set eyes

- Ask the client to look straight ahead. Hold the stick vertically so that it runs through the lateral edge of the eyes. This is where the highest point of the arch should be.
- Hold the stick horizontally and it should more or less connect the beginning and end of the eyebrow.

These are useful guidelines. With practice you will learn to train your eye.

> ### Check it out
>
> Look at different photographs of famous people. Do their brows suit their face shape? Also look at your own brows. What do you think about them? Be honest.

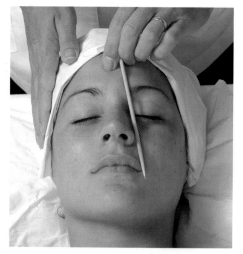

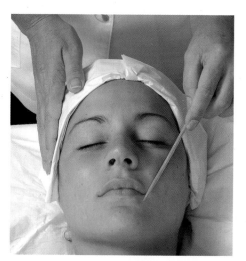

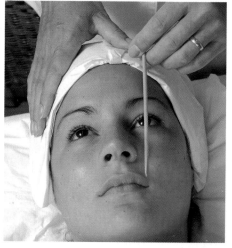

Line up an orange stick with the corner of the mouth and edge of nose: the beginning of the eyebrow should start where the orange stick rests on the skin

Line up orange stick with the edge of the mouth and outer corner of eye: the end of the eyebrow should be where the orange stick rests on the skin

The arch of the eyebrow should match the middle of the pupil. This is your shape guideline; any stray hairs outside this shape can be plucked out

> ### In the salon
>
> A client comes to you with thick bushy eyebrows and wants them thinned out unrealistically.
>
> How would you deal with this?

> ### Remember
>
> You can only work with the eyebrow's natural shape, so you may need to discourage your client from expecting unrealistic outcomes.

Prepare the work area for eyebrows and eyelash treatments

8.2

> ### In this element you will learn about:
>
> - equipment required for eyebrow shaping
> - preparation of the client.

Equipment required for eyebrow shaping

- Tweezers (rounded, slanted, pointed)
- Damp cotton wool
- Orange stick
- Antiseptic solution

> ### Remember
>
> Good lighting or a magnification lamp may be useful for clients with fair brows.

- Aftercare solution
- Disposable gloves (please refer to your professional body for guidance)
- Tissues
- Bin and bin liner
- Sterilising dish
- Mirror
- Eyebrow brush.

Tweezers

There are two types of tweezers used for eyebrow shaping.

Automatic tweezers

These are designed to remove the bulk of excess hair. They have a spring-loaded action (see the photograph of automatic tweezers in use on page 251).

Manual

These are used to remove stray hairs and accentuate the shape of the brow. Various ends are available – slanted ends are generally considered to be the best for eyebrow shaping.

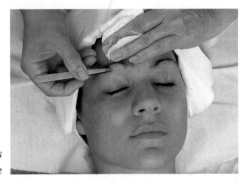

Manual tweezers in use

Preparation of the client

- Carry out a consultation – checking for contra-indications.
- Secure client's hair with headband or turban.
- Place towel or tissue or cape over the client's chest.
- Position client comfortably; couch or chair should be slightly elevated.
- Remove all accessories, e.g. earrings. Clients who wear contact lenses may find treatment more comfortable if they remove them prior to treatment.

> **Remember**
>
> It is important that all tweezers are ready for use, and they should be sterilised between clients, either in an autoclave or by soaking in a sterilising solution. It is important that this is carried out, as blood and tissue fluids could be drawn during the treatment, and these could cause contamination. Any tissue fluid drawn should be disposed of, in accordance with health and safety regulations, to prevent contamination.

> **Remember**
>
> Be sure to clarify the shape required with the client before commencing any treatment. If the client is nervous, explain the procedure and reassure her as you progress. Details of shape, thickness, texture and required shape should all be added to the client record card.

Shape the eyebrows to meet the client requirements

8.3

> **In this element you will learn about:**
>
> - procedure for eyebrow shaping
> - trouble-shooting eyebrow problems.
> - aftercare

Step-by-step eyebrow shaping

1 Remove all traces of make-up and clean the area with an appropriate cleanser. Wipe with sanitising solution and prepare the area.

2 Inspect the treatment area to assess the amount of work required. Measure shape and consult the client. A magnifying lamp can be used to give maximum visibility.

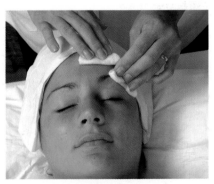

Placing hot cotton wool pads on the brow opens the pores (Step 4)

3 Brush the brows into shape before you begin.

4 Open pores – it is often suggested that before you begin shaping, you should place warm, damp cotton wool pads over the area. This relaxes hair follicles and softens the eyebrow tissue, making hair removal easier.

5 To remove hairs, gently stretch the skin between your fingers and pluck out the hairs in the direction in which they grow. Begin by removing the stray hairs between the eyes. Hairs below the natural brow shape can then be tackled. The few odd hairs that grow unevenly above the brow may also be removed, provided they do not form part of the main eyebrow growth.
   If there are any tough, spiky or white hairs these can sometimes be removed without spoiling the overall shape.

6 Consult the client as you work, ensure she has a hand mirror and consults with you as you proceed.

7 Place the removed hairs on a tissue placed at the side of the client, or held wrapped around your fingers.

8 Periodically soothe the client's brow with antiseptic, as this helps to remove any stray hairs.

9 When all the shaping is complete, place a dampened cotton wool soaked in witch-hazel over the area to soothe, cool and remove excess erythema.

10 Give aftercare advice and book the client's next appointment.

If blood or tissue fluid is accidentally drawn during the treatment, the following steps should be taken.

1 Apply pressure to the area with clean cotton wool soaked in sanitising solution

2 Do not panic, keep calm, and explain to the client so she is aware of the problem.

3 Apply soothing solution to the area.

4 Dispose of waste carefully in accordance with health and safety regulations and local by-laws.

An eyebrow re-shape may take up to half an hour and an eyebrow tidy up to 15 minutes. In all cases it would depend on the density of the hairs, shape required, hair growth and the client requirements. Clients who visit the salon regularly often have an eyebrow tidy as an integral part of their treatment plan. On average an eyebrow tidy would be carried out every 4–6 weeks.

Aftercare

Clients should be given the following aftercare advice when they have had an eyebrow shape or tidy.

- Cooling mild antiseptic products, e.g. witch hazel, should be applied.
- No make-up should be applied to the area for 12 hours, as the follicles are open and infection may occur.
- Stray re-growth hairs can be removed at intervals to prolong the effect.

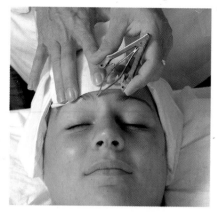

Using spring-loaded automatic tweezers makes plucking very quick and virtually painless (Step 5)

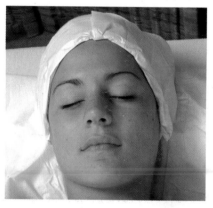

The finished look should be clean and tidy and opens up the whole face.

Remember

A nervous client may require eye pads or be advised to keep eyes shut. Heavy brows should be gradually reduced over two or three visits to minimise discomfort and allow client to become accustomed to her new image.

Contra-actions

These usually take the form of erythema to the area, but in some cases blood spots occur and sometimes swelling. As a therapist you should try to reduce the swelling before the client leaves the salon, by applying a soothing antiseptic. In extreme cases, a cold compress or ice should be applied. All contra-actions should be recorded on the client record card.

Trouble-shooting eyebrow problems

Bare sparse brows

Fill in with pencil, using short strokes in the direction of the hair growth, and blend with a brow brush. Ensure that the pencil is sharpened as you move from one eye to the other, to prevent cross-infection

Stray hairs

Remove any stray hairs with tweezers.

Thin brows

Instead of a pencil, try a shade of powder that matches the brow colour. Apply with a stiff brush, following the natural line, and ensure that you blend in well to prevent the line looking harsh. This will create the illusion of doubling the thickness.

Wild stubborn brows

Long unruly hairs should be trimmed. Hold the brows straight with a brow comb and trim to the required length. To help the hairs to lie flat, either use a little hair gel or a small amount of hairspray on a comb. Never spray directly onto the face.

Eyebrow shaping

Ensure all equipment is sterilised and accessible

Carry out consultation

Check for contra-indications

Discuss client requirements

Remove contact lenses if necessary

Cleanse area

Measure brows

Pre-warm area

Shape as required

Soothe area with suitable solution

Give aftercare

Show client finished result

Record details of treatment on client card

Tint eyebrows and eyelashes to meet client requirements

8.4

In this element you will learn about:

- eyebrow and eyelash tinting
- how colour works
- choosing a tint
- equipment for tinting
- preparing the client for tinting and lashes and brows
- applying the lash tint
- applying the eyebrow tint
- assessing the results
- aftercare.

Eyelash and eyebrow tinting

The benefits of tinting

- Eyebrows help to emphasise facial expression and eyelashes frame the eyes.
- Tinting may be carried out on clients with light-coloured brows and lashes to define their appearance.
- Brows and lashes can be tinted to complement hair colour.
- Tinting can mean that coloured mascara need not be applied, which is good for those who are allergic to it, or in the summer months when mascara is likely to smudge if it is very hot.
- Eyebrows help to emphasise facial expression and eyelashes frame the eyes. Tinting may be carried out on clients with light-coloured hair.
- Tinting is also ideal for clients who wear glasses or contact lenses.

Patch test for eyelash and eyebrow tinting

The skin around the eyes is very sensitive to chemicals and is liable to become irritated. It is therefore an important safety precaution to carry out a skin test on the client. This should be carried out every six months, even on a regular client, as you may have changed products or the client may have become sensitised to the product and suffer an allergic reaction.

The patch test should be carried out at least 24 hours prior to the treatment taking place.

Method

- Cleanse the area of the skin to be tested (behind the ear or the crook of the arm).
- Mix the same make and colour of tint to be used with manufacturer's recommended quantity of 10% volume peroxide
- Apply the tint to the area selected with a brush, about the size of a ten pence coin.
- Allow to dry.
- Ensure the client is aware that the tint should be left on the skin for 24 hours. If no reaction occurs then wash off.
- If a reaction occurs, the tint should be removed immediately with water and a soothing lotion applied to the area.
- A reaction will be recognised by itching, red-hot inflamed area. This should be treated with a soothing substance.

Precautions for lash and brow tinting

- Discuss the client's requirements with her.
- Ensure all equipment is clean and sterilised.
- Ensure that all eye make up is removed with a non-oily product.
- Check for contra-indications.
- Remove contact lenses.
- Apply barrier cream to the skin around the eyes only and not to the hair to be tinted, as the tint will not act. The barrier cream is used to prevent the tint spreading beyond the area being treated.
- Ensure the client keeps eyes closed at all times when the tint is on the eyes. As a therapist you are responsible for giving your client full instructions. This is vital, especially when treating nervous clients.
- Do not leave the client while the tint is processing.
- Complete details of the tint on the record card.
- Ensure that the eyebrows are tinted prior to shaping, to avoid tint seeping into the follicles, resulting in a reaction.

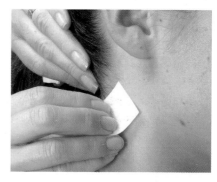

Patch test: cleansing the area first

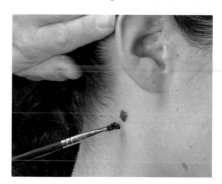

Patch test: applying the product

Remember

Always note the date and the results of patch tests on client record cards.

Remember

The details on the client record card should include:

- date of patch test
- products used
- development time of the treatment
- areas treated
- contra-actions
- aftercare.

253

How colour works

- The selected dye and hydrogen peroxide are mixed together to produce a chemical reaction. When first applied to the hair, they enter the middle of the hair as small particles, but, because of the chemical reaction, they swell. This swelling prevents the colour from coming out when washed and so becomes permanent. This process is known as oxidation. The colour of the natural hair changes and this will remain until the hair grows or falls out.
- Never mix the ingredients until you are ready to use them. Oxidisation starts to occur and the tint starts to work as soon as it is mixed, so the product will not be able to enter the hair properly, resulting in poor colour.
- Replace caps on the tint and hydrogen peroxide, as they will oxidise and again the result will be unsuccessful.

Choosing a tint

The skin around the eye is very thin and sensitive, therefore dyes designed for lash and brow tinting have been specially formulated to avoid any eye or tissue reactions. The application of any other type of dye or any hydrogen peroxide solution stronger than 10% dilution should not be used in this area. It is dangerous and may even cause blindness.

The products used for eyelash and brow tinting are usually available as creams or gels in basic colours of black, blue, brown and grey. These colours are mixed to form variations in tone, i.e. blue / black provides a darker colour.

The choice is a matter of personal preference and depends on:

- the client's overall skin type and hair colouring
- the type of eye-make-up usually worn
- the age of the client.

As clients grow more mature, they lose a lot of natural colour from hair and eyes. Brown or grey tints are preferable to black for producing a softer, more natural effect. This is an example of when you need to be aware of the fact that the client's expectations may not be realistic. The client's expectations may be a very dark unnatural finish or longer eyelashes. It is therefore your responsibility to explain to the client that certain expectations cannot or should not be achieved, due to suitability. It is important to provide the client with sufficient professional advice and emphasise that lash and brow treatments are designed to enhance the natural features.

This applies to shaping and lash extensions too. Expectations are realistic when they can be achieved with success and when the treatment is suitable for the client. The effect of tinting depends on the natural colour of the hair, e.g. blonde hair colour develops rapidly, i.e. 5 minutes. Red hair is more resistant and development will take longer, i.e. 10 minutes.

Preparing the client for tinting lashes and brows

- Help the client into a comfortable, semi-reclined position and protect hair and clothing.
- Clean and tone the area to ensure that all grease and make-up is removed from lashes and brows. If grease is left on the skin, a barrier will be created and the tint will not take properly.

Tinting

You will need:

- tinting equipment
- protective headband and towel
- couch roll to protect the work area
- small non-metallic bowl for mixing tint (a metal one would react with the hydrogen peroxide)
- lined container for waste
- sterile spatula
- sterile applicator or tipped orange stick
- clean water in the event of eye irrigation
- hand mirror
- client record card
- materials
- damp cotton wool and tissues
- eye shields made from cotton wool or paper shields
- selection of coloured tints
- hydrogen peroxide (usual 10% volume, but always check manufacturer's instructions)
- eye make-up remover (non-oily)
- cleanser
- toner
- barrier cream.

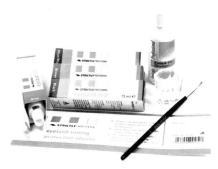

Tinting equipment

- Protect the skin and above the eyes with a barrier cream. Take care not to get any barrier product on the lashes or brows that require tinting.

Barrier cream

This prevents the tint from staining the skin and spoiling the effect of the treatment. It will also prevent the tint from penetrating the hair if it touches it.

Use a tipped orange stick or cotton bud to apply the barrier cream to the skin above the eyes.

When applying the cream below the eyes, either:

- stroke it directly onto the skin and position the eye shields on top, close to the base of the lashes,

or,

- coat the underneath surface of the shields with barrier cream and slide them into position.

Applying the tint

Precautions should be taken to ensure that neither the tint nor the applicator penetrates the eye. There should not be any problems provided:

- the eye is well supported by gently holding the area
- the tint is carefully applied
- the lashes are not overloaded with tint
- the client's eyes are kept still.

Step-by-step eyelash tinting

1 Once the client has been correctly positioned and the make-up removed mix the correct colour of tint according to the manufacturer's instructions. A guide is a 5mm length of tint with 2 – 3 drops of hydrogen peroxide, mixed in a tinting bowl with a disposable brush or orange stick to a smooth paste.

2 Remember, before applying the tint a barrier cream should have been applied to prevent staining.

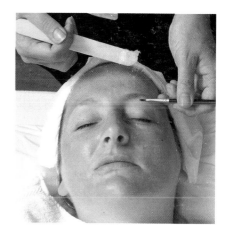

Decant barrier cream onto a spatula and paint onto the skin surrounding the eyebrow to prevent accidental staining

Remember

Make sure you do not ask the client to look up into an overhead light because this will over-sensitise the eyes and make them water!

Check it out

Check out the COSHH regulations referring to the products that you use for tinting.

3   Ask the client to look upwards and cover the lower lashes with tint (if the client has watery eyes the lower lashes can be covered with the upper lashes when the eyes are closed, but the result is often not so effective). (See photo.)

4   Ask the client to close the eyes and apply the tint to the upper lashes. (See photo.)

5   Gently lift the skin to the eyebrows, so the tint can be applied right down to the base of the lashes and include shorter hairs which grow near the inside corner of the eyes.

6   If the client complains of discomfort or the eyes begin to water, remove the tint immediately using damp cotton wool pads, and irrigate the eye.

7   Note the time and allow for the tint to work according to the manufacturer's instructions. The colour should be checked at intervals and the tint reapplied if necessary. As a guide allow 5–10 minutes, depending on the colour characteristics of the client.

Removal of eyelash tint

1   Place a pad of damp cotton wool on each eye. Hold the eye shield and pad of cotton wool together at the base and swiftly remove, enclosing any excess tint.

2   Remove any remaining tint with slightly damp cotton wool, using a gentle downward motion, and remove excess with a cotton bud. (See photo.)

3   When both eyes have been cleaned, ask the client to carefully open the eyes.

4   Support the eye and work quickly on the lower lashes with damp cotton wool and a cotton bud.

5   Stand in front of the client to check that all the tint has been removed.

6   Finally, wipe the area over with damp cotton wool to remove traces of the barrier cream.

7   Offer a hand mirror to view the final results.

8   Inform the client of possible contra-actions and aftercare. If irritation occurs, apply a damp cotton wool compress to the area.

9   Enter details onto the client's record card. This should include the colour selected and the processing time for the tint, and any contra-actions and other information relevant to the treatment.

The process of eyelash tinting should take about 20 minutes.

Step-by-step eyebrow tint

This can be performed after lash tinting, prior to shaping. Many salons and therapists perform this treatment while the lash tint is processing, to ensure they are cost-effective with their time. If shaping is carried out first, the tint will seep into the open pores causing irritation.

1   Prepare the skin and brows the same way as for treating the lashes. Apply barrier cream around the eyebrows taking care to avoid the hairs.

2   Apply the tint against the hair growth using an orange stick or a fine brush, working gradually from the outer and underneath hairs towards the centre.

3   After one minute, remove a little tint from the inner corners of the eyebrow and check how the colour is developing. Apply more tint and repeat colour checks at one-minute

Eyelash tinting

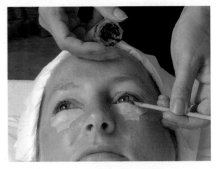

After placing shields under the eyes, begin to apply tint to lower lashes, made up to manufacturer's instructions (Step 3)

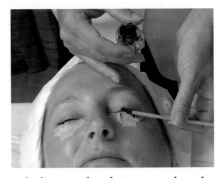

Ask client to close her eyes, and apply tint to the top lashes. Cover the eyes (Step 4)

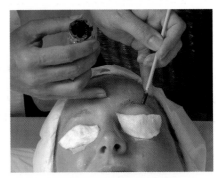

While the lash tint is developing, you can tint the eyebrows if required

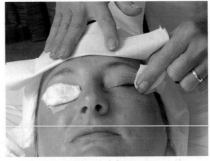

When processing time has elapsed, remove all traces of the tint (Step 2 – Removal)

intervals until the desired effect has been achieved. The developing time for tinting brows is much shorter than for lashes, usually between one and three minutes. Always refer to manufacturer's instructions for product guidance. Care must be taken to prevent the brows from becoming too dark as this can create an unattractive harsh effect.

4   Remove tint with clean, damp cotton wool.

5   Wipe over the area to remove all traces of barrier cream.

6   Discuss the final effect, possible contra-action and aftercare with the client.

7   Enter details of the treatment on the client record card.

The process of eyebrow tinting should take approximately 15 minutes.

How to irrigate the eye

If tint accidentally enters the eye, do not panic; the client may be feeling discomfort and a slight burning sensation. Calm the client and explain the procedure you are going to follow.

1   Tilt the client's head slightly to one side. Carefully trickle some tepid water into the corner of the eye and allow the eye to be rinsed of the foreign body.

2   Hold some tissue or a small kidney dish to collect the excess water.

3   Apply a damp cotton wool compress to cool and soothe the eye.

It is not acceptable to use an eyebath because of the risk of cross-infection.

Possible causes of eye irritation:

- very sensitive eyes
- too much or incorrect strength of hydrogen peroxide
- something in the eye
- inadvertently poking the eye.

Assessing the results

- A successful tinting treatment produces the required colour changes to the lashes and brows without staining the skin.
- Even the shortest eyelashes should be coloured from the base.
- Blonde roots after the eyelash tint shows that not enough care was taken. The skin fold of the eyelid was probably not lifted away from the base of the hairs when applying tint.
- The tint will not have covered the brows successfully if:
  – there was grease or make-up on the hairs
  – old tint was used
  – the hydrogen peroxide had lost strength
  – the tint and peroxide were incorrectly mixed
  – the tint was removed too soon.

Aftercare

- As with all treatments, the client should be advised against touching or rubbing the areas immediately after the treatment.
- If redness or irritation occurs, apply a damp cotton wool compress.
- The client should be aware that the effects will last approximately 4–6 weeks as the hairs grow out. Strong sunlight will make the results fade *faster*.

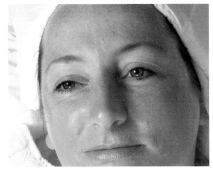

The finished eyelash tint defines the lashes and enhances the eyes

Tinting

> Ensure all the equipment is hygienic and close to hand.

> Carry out a consultation (ensure a patch test has been carried out). Check for contra-indications.

> Remove contact lenses, if required.

> If shaping is to be carried out always tint first and shape after.

> Cleanse area with non-oily product.

> Apply barrier cream and pre-formed shapes if tinting lashes.

> Mix tint and apply (never pre-mix the tint). Note processing time on client record card.

> Remove tint after the required processing time.

> Show client results. Give aftercare advice.

> Record details on client record card.

Apply artificial eyelashes to meet client requirements

8.5

In this element you will learn about:

- false eyelashes
- semi-permanent individual lashes
- equipment for individual and strip lashes
- preparation of the client
- strip lashes.

False eyelashes

False lashes are designed to enhance and emphasise the eyes by giving the natural lashes a fuller and more defined appearance. They come in the form of individual lashes or strip lashes.

Using false lashes can have the following benefits.

- They are a good option for a client who is allergic to mascara and eyelash tint.
- They can be convenient for someone who is going on holiday.
- They make the natural lashes appear longer and thicker.
- They add definition to the eye area.
- They can enhance a photographic make-up.
- They can enhance an evening or fantasy make-up.
- They can complete a corrective make-up.

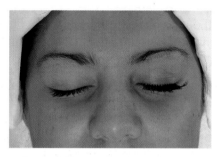

False eyelashes

Effects

- **Deep set eyes** Fine pointed upper and lower lashes will give added definition to the eye.
- **Round eyes** Individual lashes can be used to thicken the lash line from the centre of the eye outwards.
- **Small eyes** Individual lashes placed at the outer corner will make the eyes look larger.
- **Close set eyes** False lashes applied to the outer third of the eye will have the effect of widening the eye.

At the consultation stage it is important to establish what result the client is expecting to achieve. If their expectations are unrealistic, this should be explained to the client. Once a plan has been agreed, treatment can commence.

Factors to consider when choosing false eyelashes

- **Client's age** Artificial lashes create a very bold, dramatic effect, which can make an older client look harsh.
- **Client's natural lashes** Choose artificial lashes to complement the natural lash.
- **Occasion for wearing false eyelashes** This can determine whether individual or strip lashes are more appropriate, e.g. individual for corrective, strip for fantasy make-up.
- **Maintenance of lashes** Strip lashes are easily maintained as no special product is needed for removal, and they can be reused. In the case of individual lashes, maintenance may be required to replace lashes due to natural hair loss. Solvent product is required to remove lashes.

- **Time for lash application** Strip lashes add 10 minutes to a make-up time. Individual lashes take 20–30 minutes, depending how many are applied.
- **Further appointments** Strip lashes need to be applied daily. Individual lashes need three to six weeks for maintenance and to replace lashes lost naturally.

Semi-permanent individual lashes

This type of lash is also known as an eyelash extension. One advantage is that it can be placed on top of the client's own lashes individually. They can therefore be placed independently to create different effects: they can be used sparingly on the outside of the eye to improve the client's eye shape, or placed across the entire upper eye area for a fuller effect.

The lashes are usually available in black or brown and come in four lengths: mini, short, medium and long. Individual lashes also come in single lashes or flared. The flared have two or more strips from one bulb.

Individual lashes may be worn for up to six weeks, and will be lost when the natural lash falls out. These can be replaced each week if the client requires. The client should be made aware of this as part of the aftercare. Individual lashes are usually made from synthetic threads of nylon although some of the more expensive lashes can be made of real hair. The lashes made of synthetic fibres hold a permanent curl for a longer time than natural hair. Whichever type is applied, they are fixed by using special adhesive which bonds the false eyelash to the natural lash. This is available in black or clear.

Patch test the adhesive

This test is required for individual and strip lashes.

Place a small amount of the adhesive in the crook of the elbow or behind the ear, at least 24 hours prior to the treatment. If a reaction, occurs i.e. swelling, irritation or inflammation, do not proceed with the treatment. It is important to remember that dates of all the tests should be recorded on the client record card.

Equipment for individual and strip lashes

You will need:

- basic trolley products – tissues, cotton wool, etc.
- oil-free eye make-up remover (if oil-based products are used the adhesive will not
- adhere to the lashes)
- magnifier lamp
- lash kit – containing a selection of lashes, adhesive and adhesive solvent
- tweezers and orange stick
- small scissors
- mirror
- small bowl of water to irrigate the eye if required – refer to lash and brow tinting for the procedure.

Remember

Always carry out a skin sensitivity test for the adhesive at least 24 hours prior to the application of lashes. As with tinting, this needs to be carried out every six months.

Remember

Glue can be an irritant, so always refer to manufacturer's instructions and COSHH regulations when using this product.

Check it out

Research the COSHH regulations for the adhesive you use.

Contra-indications

These are the same for all eye treatments, so remember to check. Also remember that it is very easy to cross-infect the eyes, so strict hygiene must be followed, e.g. use separate cotton wool, etc, for each eye.

Preparation of the client

- Full consultation checking for contra-indications and ensure a patch test has been carried out
- Discuss length, colour and type of lash and client expectations.
- Ensure the client has removed contact lenses, and jewellery that may get in the way.
- Place a hair band or turban around the hair.
- Cover client's clothing with a cape, towel or tissue.
- Seat client in a semi-reclined position in a good light or with access to a magnifier lamp.

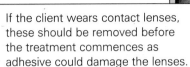

Remember

If the client wears contact lenses, these should be removed before the treatment commences as adhesive could damage the lenses.

Remember

Always refer to manufacturer's instructions when using and applying lashes, using solvents, and adhesives. If the client indicates irritation, remove the lashes at once and soothe with a suitable solution.

Step-by-step application of individual lashes

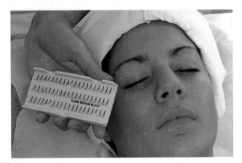

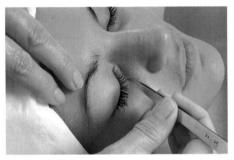

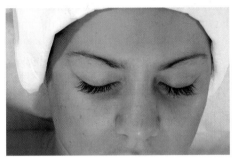

Cleanse the eye with oil-free cleanser. Select eyelash – choose a colour and length of lash nearest to the client's lashes for a natural look – and, using tweezers, dip the root into adhesive.

Place the lash with bulb at, or as near to as possible, the client's natural eyelash roots. Check as you go, with the client's eyes open, then closed, that the lashes follow the natural curve of the eyelid. Apply shorter lashes around the inner and outer eye, and longer ones around the centre of the eye.

Comb through, when the glue is dry, to blend in with the natural eyelashes. Apply eye make-up. The finished result should enhance, but not look too obvious.

Maintenance and care of individual lashes

- As extensions are designed to be worn for some weeks, the adhesive used with them is quite strong. It is therefore acceptable to apply eye make-up in the normal way.
- Removal of eye make-up must be oil free, as oil will dislodge the lashes.
- The lashes should be touched as little as possible.
- Mascara will clog the lashes and is difficult to remove.
- After initial application of lashes the client should wait several hours before showering.
- Avoid rubbing eyes, as this will loosen the lashes.
- Avoid extremes of temperature, e.g. sauna.
- You should use the solvent specially designed for the adhesive when removing the lashes. The solvent dissolves the adhesive so that no damage occurs to the natural lashes. A cotton bud soaked in the solvent should be gently rolled down the lashes, onto a tissue, until the lash detaches itself. Always refer to manufacturer's instructions when using solvents.

Contra-actions

Contra-actions to individual and strip lashes:

Eye irritation
- Always remember to do a patch test for the adhesive. If eyes start to water, blot with a tissue.
- Never place eyelashes underneath the natural lashes, irritation will occur.
- Products which are suitable for soothing eye irritation vary but commonly contain witch hazel, calamine and antiseptic.

Adhesive or solvent in the eye
- If either of these products accidentally enter the eye, irrigate immediately. If serious seek medical advice.
- Record all details on the client record card.

Strip lashes

As the name suggests, these synthetic fibres are attached onto a fine strip and secured onto the eyelid as near to the natural lashes as possible, with a special adhesive. This enables the lashes to be placed over the entire eye for a full appearance. Strip lashes are manufactured in many colours and shapes, and can include glitter effect and multi-coloured lashes, which can be used in fantasy or photographic make-up. Strip lashes not only add length but also add thickness and texture. When applying strip lashes the client should be advised that they are for short-term wear, unlike individual lashes, for a maximum of a day. As with individual lashes, they also come in a variety of lengths for a realistic appearance.

Step-by-step application of strip lashes

1   After discussion as to the style and colour of the lash that the client requires, trim to the correct length.

2   Complete the face make-up – foundation, blusher and eye shadow.

3   Seat the client in a semi-reclined position and work from above.

4   Apply a fine film of adhesive to the base of the false lash.

5   Using tweezers to hold the eyelash, place them gently onto the skin of the eyelid as close as possible to the client's lashes.

6   With firm careful pressure, use an orange stick to gently press the false lash into place from the tear duct outwards.

7   Come round to the front of the client and check fitting, keep client's eyes closed, wait for a few seconds before checking the results with the client.

8   Continue with the eye make-up, applying eyeliner to give a professional finish. Mascara should be applied to both natural and false lashes to seal them. Use eyelash curlers if necessary.

Maintenance and care of strip lashes

Strip lashes should always be removed at the end of the day – sleeping in them will distort their shape. Their shape will also be distorted by rubbing the eyes as this will loosen the adhesive. To remove the lashes, support the side of the eye and gently pull the lashes from the outer corner to the inner eye.

Clean strip lashes in the following way.

- **Human hair** Clean with manufacturer's recommended cleaner or 70% alcohol.
- **Synthetic lashes** Place in warm, soapy water for a few minutes. Rinse in tepid water.
- **Re-curling lashes** After cleaning, lashes should be rolled and secured around a barrel-shaped object, such as a pencil. Keep the base of the lash straight so the whole lash length curls around the object. Once recurled, store in the original container for further use.

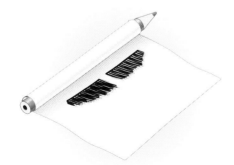

A simple way to restore the shape of strip lashes

> **Remember**
>
> When trimming the lashes, do not cut straight across; rather, cut on a taper to avoid a blunt appearance.

> **Remember**
>
> Always follow manufacturer's instructions for the use of adhesives and solvents. If irritation, swelling or stinging occurs, remove immediately and soothe with a suitable solution. Refer to COSHH regulations.

Eyelash perming

This treatment is a semi-permanent way of curling the upper lashes and the result will last from 4–6 weeks; as the old hairs are lost and replaced with new hairs the curl diminishes. The use of perming solutions, although chemically based, is far less damaging than regular use of eyelash curlers.

Eyelash perming is recommended:

- to emphasise the eyelashes, making the eye look larger and to give more definition
- for clients who wear contact lenses or glasses
- for mature clients with sagging eyelids
- for clients who do not wish to wear mascara
- for holidays or for sports women
- for clients living or working in hot environments
- for clients who have short straight lashes
- for special occasions.

There is a variety of eyelash perming products available and most companies offer training sessions. It is always important to follow the manufacturer's instructions when using any product, but special care should be taken when working with chemicals around the sensitive eye area. Refer to COSHH regulations.

How perming works on the eyelashes

When perming, the lashes are curled and stretched over small rods and curled into shape by the use of a chemical product. Today, most of the products are referred to as cold wave gels or lotions. This term is used to distinguish these products from heat perms, which require heat to activate the chemical process. This would be unsuitable for the delicate eye area.

The gel breaks down the structure of the hair, and once broken, the hair can then take on the shape of the curling rod. When this curl has taken place, a second gel is applied to fix the eyelash into the new shape. This gel is often referred to as a neutraliser or oxidising agent.

Consultation

It is important with all treatments to carry out a thorough consultation and to establish what a client requires from the treatment. The same contra-indication checks apply to perming as for other eye treatments. It is vital that no skin infections or open wounds are present, as a chemical is being applied to the skin. Ensure that no reaction has occurred to the products patch-tested. A reaction would show itself as itching, redness and swelling. Treat with a suitable product.

Preparation of the client

- Ensure the client is in a semi-reclined position.
- Remove jewellery.
- Remove contact lenses, if required.
- Secure hair away from the face.
- Protect the client's clothing.
- Ensure all products and basic trolley equipment are close to hand. Use non-oily eye make-up remover, to remove any make-up.
- Have a bowl of water ready to irrigate the eye if required.

Remember

The products to be tested are adhesive perm solution and neutraliser and they should be tested, as with tinting and lash application, in the crook of the client's elbow or behind the client's ear.

False eyelashes

Ensure all materials are to hand and are hygienic.

Consultation and ensure an adhesive patch test has been carried out.

Contra-indication check.

Discuss client requirements (it may be worth taking into consideration the type of event the lashes are being worn to, as this will determine the type most suitable).

Cleanse area using non-oily product.

Apply lashes.

If lashes require cutting, remember to cut so that they are tapered to avoid an unrealistic appearance.

Show client the finished look.

Give aftercare advice.

Fill out record card. If individual lashes are used remember to include details of the lash number and where they were placed on the eye so that the effect can be recreated.

Step-by-step eyelash perming

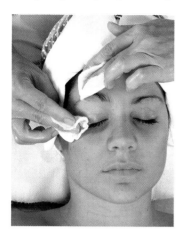

A full consultation follows a patch test, which should have been done 24 hours previously. Thoroughly cleanse the eye and lashes, removing all traces of make-up.

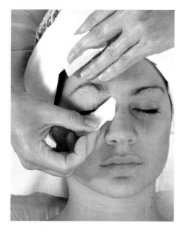

Blot the eyes to ensure they are grease free and dry. A non-oily remover should be used so as to avoid any grease forming a barrier (a witch-hazel-based remover is often used).

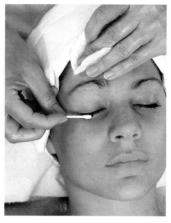

Use a cotton bud to thoroughly check the lashes are clean and dry.

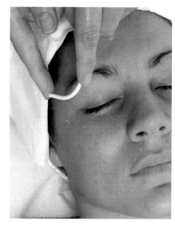

Choose a suitable-sized rod, depending on the lashes and the curl required.

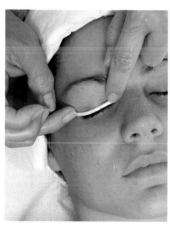

Apply a small amount of adhesive to the main body of the rod. Check that no lashes are caught underneath. Bend and shape the rod to sit tightly in the eye shape.

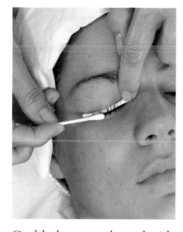

Curl lashes over the rod with no bends or kinks. Use a cotton tip to apply solution to the lashes. Follow manufacturer's instructions for development and neutralising times.

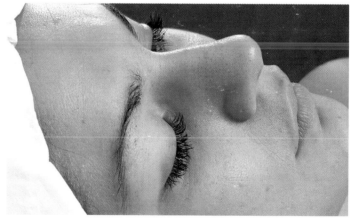

The finished result should be curly but natural looking, with not too tight a curl. Tinting can be carried out during this procedure, but check recommended instructions before attempting it.

Problems with eyelash perming

Problem	Possible cause	Solution
Too curled	Rod too small	Re-perm larger rod, half time
No result	Too large a rod	Re-perm
	Insufficient processing	
	Incorrect neutralising	
	Oil barrier on lashes	
Uneven curl	Incorrect positioning of rod	Re-position rod
	Uneven application of lotion/gel	
	Not curling all the lashes over the rod	
Buckled or hooked ends	Failure to wrap hair correctly around the rod	Trim off ends

Product safety data

Eye make-up remover

Description

- The product is prepared from mild cleaning agents in a cosmetic base.

Ingredients

- All ingredients are commonly used in cosmetic products and meet accepted standards of purity.

Hazards

- This product is considered to be non-hazardous under normal conditions of use.

Flammability

- Non-inflammable.

First aid procedures

- Ingestion: drink milk or water.
- Skin contact: N/A.
- Eye contact: Wash well with water; if irritation persists, seek medical advice.

Spillage

- Clean using absorbent material, followed by washing with detergent and water to avoid slippery floors.

Handling and storage

- No special precautions considered necessary.

Eyelash tint

Description

- Oil / water-emulsion (cream).

Ingredients

- Water/ cetearyl alcohol/ PEG-sorbitan lanolate/ sodium cetearyl sulfate/ diaminotoluene/ aminophenols / dyest. CI 77499 and / or 77007 / no preservatives.

Hazards

- This product is considered to be non-hazardous on its own but it becomes a hazard when mixed with hydrogen peroxide.

Flammability

- Non-inflammable.

First aid procedures

- Ingestion: drink a lot of water, seek medical attention.
- Skin contact: remove with water; if irritation occurs, seek medical attention.
- Eye contact: Avoid by careful observation of the instructions for use; if contact occurs, rinse immediately with warm water.

Spillage

- Clean area immediately to prevent staining.

Handling

- Always wear gloves and avoid contact with skin and eyes.

Storage

- At least three years, when kept under normal stocking conditions.

Eyelash tinting peroxide

Description

- The product is a mixture of oxidising agents, wetting agents, Ph adjusters, fragrance and water.
- Contents: Hydrogen peroxide.

Ingredients

- All ingredients are commonly used in cosmetic products and meet accepted standards of purity.

Hazards

- The product is considered hazardous if precautions are ignored.

Flammability

- Non-inflammable, but note comments under fire.

First aid procedures

- Ingestion: Seek medical attention immediately.
- Skin contact: Avoid and always wear rubber gloves when using this product; if skin contact occurs, wash well with soap and water; if irritation persists, seek medical attention.
- Eye contact: Avoid, wash well with water and seek medical attention.

Spillage

- Clean area with plenty of water and dispose down drain; do not absorb into combustible material.

Handling and storage

- Always wear gloves and avoid contact with skin.
- Storage: Store in a cool place away from direct sunlight; store in the original container only and keep closures tightly sealed. Contamination of solutions containing hydrogen peroxide can result in instability with liberation of heat and oxygen.

- Fire: Hydrogen peroxide may react with other chemicals to form explosive mixtures; combustion may occur if hydrogen peroxide is allowed to dry on paper, wood, hair etc.

Eyelash tint stain remover

Description

- This product is a mixture of ethanol and fragrance oils in solution.

Ingredients

- All ingredients are commonly used in cosmetic products and meet accepted standards of purity.

Hazards

- The product is considered hazardous unless normal safety precautions are followed.

Flammability

- Flammable. Ethanol content: 50% w/w.

First aid procedures

- Ingestion: avoid, drink plenty of milk or water.
- Inhalation: Avoid, may cause dizziness, remove to fresh air.
- Skin contact: Avoid prolonged contact with skin; if irritation persists, seek medical attention.

Spillage

- Clean contaminated area with plenty of water, wash with detergent and water to avoid slippery floors; do not absorb onto combustible material.

Handling and storage

- Storage: Store in a cool place away from direct sunlight; large quantities should be stored in fire-resistant store.
- Fire: Contents are flammable; evacuate areas known to contain products and inform fire-fighters of their presence.

Your questions answered

Why is it important to carry out a patch test?
To ensure that the client is not allergic to any of the products used in the treatment. This should be done prior to the first tint or application of lashes.

Why should a patch test be carried out every 6 months even on a regular client?
To ensure the client has not become sensitive to the product causing irritation. As a salon you may have changed products.

Do I have to pre-warm the area prior to shaping?
You do not have to pre-warm the area, but this procedure does help to minimise discomfort as the heat opens the hair follicles – making removal easier and less painful for the client.

Why is it important to use a non-oily eye make-up remover prior to treatment?
Oil-based products will form a barrier over the lashes, making the application of tint or false lashes non-effective. Tint will not take properly, and the lashes will not stick correctly.

Why should a barrier cream be applied prior to tinting lashes and brows?
This barrier cream prevents tint seeping onto the surrounding skin causing unsightly staining of the area.

Test your knowledge

1　How would you recognise blepharitis?

2　How would you minimise discomfort when shaping the brows?

3　What facial features would you use to aid measuring the shape of brows?

4　Name two types of eyebrow tweezers.

5　Why is it important to patch test before carrying out a tint?

6　How often should you carry out a patch test for tint/adhesive/perm products?

7　Why is it important to mix the tint just before you use it, and not in advance?

8　How long do you leave a tint on the brows for?

9　Why should you tint before carrying out a shape on the client?

10　What are false lashes made of?

11   How should you trim false lashes?

12   How are individual lashes applied?

13   Name the solutions required when perming lashes.

14   State three reasons why a client may require permed lashes.

Improve the appearance and condition of nails and adjacent skin

Unit 9

This unit focuses on the treatment of nails and adjacent skin on feet and hands.

It covers the following elements:

9.1 Assess clients and prepare a treatment plan for manicure and pedicure treatments
9.2 Prepare the work area and client for manicure and pedicure treatments
9.3 Improve the appearance of nails and skin using manicure and pedicure techniques
9.4 Improve the condition of nails and adjacent skin.

The practices of improving the appearance and condition of the nails and adjacent skin are known as manicure and pedicure. A **manicure** is the care of hands and fingernails. This is a popular treatment in salons as smooth skin, well-shaped and varnished nails are vital to promote a well-groomed appearance. Regular professional attention will help prevent minor nail damage, e.g. hangnails, split and brittle nails. This treatment is becoming increasingly popular with men who have regular treatments as part of their professional lives.

A **pedicure** is the professional treatment of feet and nails. This treatment greatly enhances the appearance of feet and toenails, which are often a neglected part of the body. Professional attention to the nails and surrounding skin encourages nail growth, keeps cuticles pushed back and can prevent minor skin conditions, e.g. corns and ingrowing toenails.

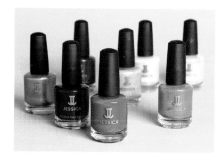

Nail polish

Assess clients and prepare a treatment plan for manicure and pedicure treatments

9.1

In this element you will learn about:	
• preparation of the working area	• nail shapes
• consultation	• contra-indications to manicure and
• treatment timings	pedicure.

Preparation is the key to being a professional beauty therapist, regardless of the treatment being carried out.

Preparation of the working area

Many salons have a designated working area for manicure / pedicure treatments, sometimes in the reception area, but wherever you carry out your treatment you should ensure all materials, equipment and products are within easy reach. The area required for manicure and pedicure varies greatly, with more versatility in manicure than in pedicure.

Manicure	Pedicure
Client across a couch	Sitting only – can be combined with a manicure
Sitting across a table	
At a manicure station	
In a hair salon while having hair done	
Client lying on a beauty couch while having a facial	

Working areas for manicures and pedicures

Consultation

Whichever method you use to carry out your treatment, you need to be prepared. Have all the equipment, materials and products you will need to hand and also keep with you a client record card to ensure a professional treatment. The consultation should cover the following points:

- contra-indications
- skin and nail conditions (treatable)
- occasion (e.g. wedding)
- products used
- contra-actions

- varnish used
- homecare advice
- sales
- next appointment / recommendations
- therapist's name.

Treatment timings

When you perform your first manicure or pedicure treatments, they may take you some time. Once experienced, you should be able to perform treatments within a commercially acceptable time. It is important at the consultation stage, and when booking, to allocate enough time for the treatment. Always confirm the amount of time with the client – he or she may only have a lunch hour for their treatment. Here are some commercially acceptable times for these treatments:

Treatment	Timings
Manicure without polish	25–30 minutes
Manicure with polish	35–40 minutes
File and re-polish	10 minutes
Pedicure without polish	40–45 minutes
Pedicure with polish	50–55 minutes
Pedicure soak, file and re-polish	15 minutes
Manicure and pedicure without polish	1 hour
Manicure and pedicure with polish	1 hour 15 minutes

Standard times for manicure / pedicure treatments

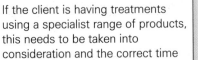

Remember

If the client is having treatments using a specialist range of products, this needs to be taken into consideration and the correct time allowed, and agreed with the client.

If the client requires treatment to improve both the condition and appearance of nails and the surrounding skin, the initial appearance at the consultation should identify that regular treatments are necessary, e.g. weekly over a six-week period, followed by a maintenance treatment every 4–6 weeks.

How you decide on the appropriate timing and type of treatment must be mutually agreed with the client. The same treatment plan will not be suitable for all clients because of individual needs, such as:

- work commitments
- home life
- leisure activities
- money available
- time available.

Nail shapes

At the consultation stage it is also important to consider the shape that would most suit your client: discuss this with the client. You will need to consider his/her working environment. Nail shapes should usually conform to the shape of the fingers for a more realistic and natural appearance. The following are shapes to be considered.

Square

This shape is usually most suitable for manual workers or clients who do a lot of work with fingertips, e.g. typists, pianists.

Round

This is a good shape for clients who require a short neat style. It decreases the likelihood of breakage or injury. It is suitable for clients with large square hands.

Oval

This shape can appear to lengthen the fingers for a more elegant appearance. It is usually suitable for small hands.

Pointed

This shape is liable to breakage due to the exaggeration of the shape. It is therefore most suitable for special occasions.

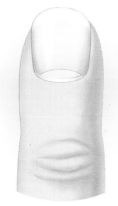

Square

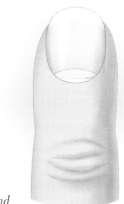

Round

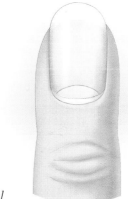

Oval

In the salon

Helen comes into the salon for a manicure and polish. She has badly bitten nails, but she insists that her nails look good enough for a special evening out.

What approach would you take?

What would you actually do?

Contra-indications to manicure and pedicure

It is important to establish at the consultation stage if contra-indications are present. A contra-indication means that the treatment cannot be carried out, as the client is unsuitable for this particular treatment, or that the treatment needs to be adapted. If an area with a contra-indication is treated, there is a risk of contamination and cross-infection occurring.

The area to be treated should be examined in good light to judge if any of the following conditions are present. Details should be recorded on the client record

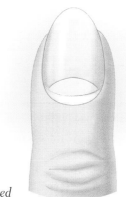

Pointed

card. Here are the most common contra-indications that are found and associated with manicure and pedicure treatments. The term Onychosis is used to describe any nail disease.

Fungal infections

Fungal infections spread very rapidly and often thrive in damp areas, and can appear soft and spongy. Fungal infections should not be treated.

Onychomycosis (pronounced on-i-ko-my-ko-sis) or ringworm

This is a fungal infection caused by the tinea unguim fungus, otherwise known as ringworm. The infection invades beneath the free edge, spreading into the nail bed and then attacking the nail plate. The nail plate becomes brittle, rough and opaque, and separation starts to occur due to the build-up of scales between the nail bed and nail plate. This can also make the nail plate appear very thick. Yellow discoloration may also be present.

Ringworm of the hands is a highly contagious disease caused by a fungus (tinea unguim).The symptoms are papular, red lesions, which occur in patches or rings over the hands. Itching may be slight to severe.

Athlete's foot (ringworm of the foot) – in acute conditions deep, itchy, colourless blisters can appear. These can appear singly, in groups, and sometimes on only one foot. They spread over the sole and between the toes, perhaps involving the nail fold and infecting the nail. When the blisters rupture they become red and ooze. The lesions dry as they heal. Fungus infection of the feet is likely to become chronic. Both the prevention of infection and beneficial treatment are accomplished by keeping the skin cool, dry and clean.

Bacterial infections

This type of infection is usually characterised by swelling, tenderness and redness in the area. Bacterial infection is a contra-indication to treatment.

Paronychia (pronounced par-on-ik-ee-ah)

This is a bacterial infection of the nail fold, the two types of bacteria generally responsible being staphylococci and streptococci. In paronychia, the nail fold is damaged either from a bad manicure, or by the hands being constantly immersed in water and harsh detergents. The symptoms are erythema, swelling and tenderness around the nail fold. There may be signs of slight shrinkage of the nail plate, which is separated from the nail bed. If the condition is not treated then the symptoms are accompanied by pus formation under the nail fold. After this, other types of bacteria set in, turning the nail plate a dark brown or black colour. Eventually, if the condition is not treated, a fungal infection known as candida takes over. Candida is the worst form of paronychia and is hard to destroy. The more common form of paronychia is very often found amongst dental and nursing staff. **Paronychia should not be manicured**.

Whitlows

This is a small abscess at the side or base of nail. The skin around the nail becomes soft and open to infection by herpes simplex virus or by bacteria, usually through a prick with a dirty pin or other sharp object. **Nails with this condition cannot be manicured**.

Onychia (pronounced on-ik-ee-ah)

This is the inflammation of the nail matrix, accompanied by pus formation. Improper sanitisation of nail implements and bacterial infections may cause this disease. **Nails with this condition cannot be manicured**.

Check it out

When you watch the television, look at the hands of the celebrities and people in the news. Look at the shape of their nails. Do they follow the guidelines for nail shapes listed above? Could you make any adjustments or other recommendations?

Remember

Ringworm is a highly contagious disease and must not be manicured. If in doubt refer client to a G.P.

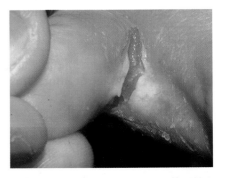

Athlete's foot (ringworm of the foot)

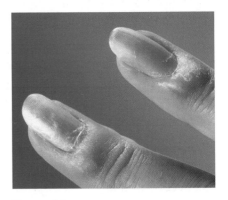

Paronychia

Viral infections

These infections are very common and treatment can be adapted by using a waterproof dressing and avoiding the area. However, viral infections are highly contagious if touched.

Verruca vulgaris (common warts)

These are small and highly contagious. They are caused by a viral infection. They are rough and hard and can be darkish in colour or natural skin tone. They are found either singly or in groups and appear around the nail fold area. They create pressure above the matrix, which can lead to deformities appearing in the growing nail plate (dystrophy). Warts should be left alone or untouched since they tend to disappear of their own accord, as suddenly as they appear. **Cannot be manicured unless covered**.

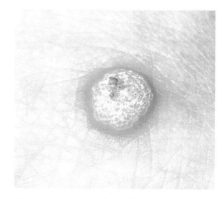

Verruca vulgaris (warts)

Verruca plantaris (verruca of the foot)

This condition belongs to the same family as the common wart, but instead of being raised on the surface of the skin, verrucas tend to grow inwards, so until they get fairly large the client can be unaware of having a verruca. They are often caught in swimming pool areas and are highly contagious. The skin's surface can be smooth and the appearance can be like a circular piece of hard skin with a black dot/s in the centre.

Now you know what to look for, refer to your GP for advice on treating these conditions.

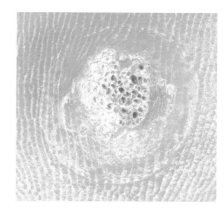

Verruca plantaris (verruca of foot)

Other contra-indications to manicure and pedicure

Onycholysis (pronounced on-ik-oh-lie-sis) or nail separation

This is a disorder where the nail separates from the nail bed (usually only part of and not the whole nail). It results from a build-up of debris found in the moist warm space between the digits, which attracts bacteria and fungal organisms, and in severe cases turns the nail plate a dark green or black colour. The infected nail plate grows faster than those that are uninfected. In feet, onycholysis occurs through wearing a tight-pinching shoe, poor general circulation and lack of attention to foot care. Non-infectious nails can be manicured or pedicured as long there is no fungal or bacterial infection. **Severe separation should not be treated**.

Onychogryposis (or ingrowing nails)

This may affect either the fingers or toes. In this condition, the nail grows into the sides of the flesh and may cause infection. Filing the nails too much in the corners or over vigorous cutting is often responsible for ingrowing nails.

Other nail conditions

There are also other conditions that may require an amendment in treatment but are not necessarily a reason for stopping treatment.

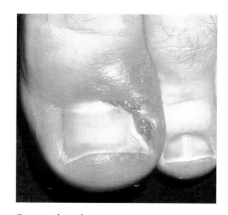

Paronychia due to ingrowing toenails

Split nails, brittle nails

Normally the result of abuse with drying agents, like those found in harsh detergents, cleaners, paint-strippers and film-developing fluids. Cotton-lined rubber gloves are good protection. Since the nail begins forming at almost the last finger joint, sometimes injury to the finger or diseases like arthritis can result in split nails. If accompanied by an overall dryness of skin and hair, split nails could indicate poor circulation.

Treatment will increase the circulation, bringing more nutrients and oxygen to help with cell regeneration. Hydrate the nail plate and surrounding skin with hot oil or paraffin wax. The use of a cuticle cream or oil for home use will be effective between treatments. **Manicure should be given.**

Blue nails

Usually a sign of bad circulation of blood or a heart condition. Manicures and pedicures may be given and massage usually helps circulation.

Beau's line

This is a disorder caused by an acute illness. As a result, the matrix temporarily stops producing new cells for the duration of the illness and, when it once again begins to reproduce, the period of the illness is clearly marked by a definite furrow or series of furrows. This grows forward and eventually disappears as it is cut away as part of the free edge.

This disorder is non-infectious and can therefore be manicured.

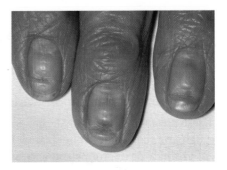

Beau's line

Nail / finger biting

This is a nervous habit whereby the individual is prompted to bite and chew the free edge of the nail plate right down to expose the bulging nail bed below. The individual may also chew at the hardened cuticle and nail wall, causing a multitude of hangnails.

Should be regularly manicured. Massage and buffing will help to increase circulation and therefore stimulate growth. The use of special preparations to discourage nail biting may be recommended.

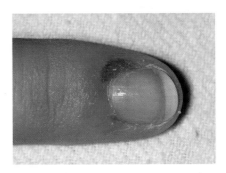

Finger biting

Hangnail

This is a condition whereby the cuticle around the nail plate splits leaving loose, flaky pieces of dry skin. It is caused by extreme dryness of the cuticle and from not keeping the cuticle free from the nail plate, so that it is stretched forward as the nail plate grows and eventually snaps leaving hangnails.

Splinter haemorrhages.

These appear as tiny streaks of blood under the nail plate, usually near the tip. Like nail separation, splinter haemorrhages can result from a traumatic blow to the nail. Sometimes, however, these red streaks can indicate a liver disease or possibly trichinosis (from improperly cooked pork).

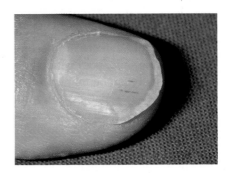

Splinter haemorrhages

Overgrown cuticles

This is caused by excessive cuticle growth that adheres to the base of the nail plate. Suggest that your client has a manicure or that she gently pushes the cuticle back with a soft towel after bathing and apply cuticle cream as often as possible. If the cuticles are very dry, a hot oil or paraffin wax manicure will help hydrate the area.

Pits and grooves

Linked to both dermatological disease and systematic irregularities. However, many people who complain about pits and grooves in their nails have no apparent systematic diseases. It is very common and sometimes an inexplicable phenomenon, which can be dismissed with gentle buffing.

Flaking and breaking nails

This is a very common complaint, and can be due to lack of vitamin A and B2, general ill-health, incorrect filing, excessive use of enamel remover, or excessive use of solvents and harsh detergents. Use of a nail strengthener may help this condition if applied regularly. It is also advisable to keep the nails fairly short to prevent the nails breaking.

Bruised nails

This occurs when the nail receives a heavy blow. This shows as a dark purple patch on the nail and will grow out with the nail. In severe cases the nail may detach itself from the nail base. Unless there is damage to the matrix, a new nail will grow normally to replace it.

Severely bruised nails should not be treated.

Eggshell nails

These are recognised by the nail plate being noticeably thin, white and much more flexible than in normal nails. The nail plate separates from the nail bed and curves at the free edge. This disorder may be caused by chronic illness or may be of systemic or nervous origin.

Corrugations (or wavy ridges)

These are caused by uneven growth of nails, usually the result of illness or injury. When giving a manicure to a client with corrugations, buff to minimise ridges and use a ridge filler when painting for a smoother finish.

Furrows (depressions)

In the nails these may either run lengthwise or across the nail. These are usually the result of an illness or an injury to the nail cells, in or near the matrix. The nails are fragile, so care must be taken.

Leuconychia (pronounced loo-ko-nick-ee-aah) or white spots

These appear frequently in the nails but do not indicate disease. They may be caused by injury to the base of the nail or they might be air bubbles. As the nail continues to grow, these white spots eventually disappear. This is a very common disorder.

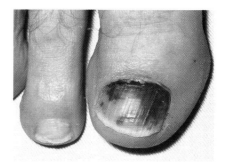

Bruised nails

Check it out
Have a really good look at your own fingernails and toenails. Can you identify any of the conditions mentioned?

Prepare the work area and client for manicure and pedicure treatments

In this element you will learn about:

- equipment required
- products required.

Equipment

To ensure that no cross-infection or contamination occurs, the manicurist must make sure everything is clean. Some pieces of equipment are only designed for single use. Therefore, the cost of these items should be reflected when setting prices for manicure and pedicure treatments.

Emery board

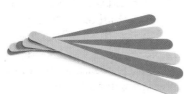

This has two sides, a coarse side for shortening nails and a fine side, which is used for shaping and bevelling. These cannot be cleaned, and should be used once only and disposed of, or given to the client.

Orange stick

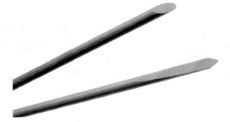

The two ends of the orange stick each have different purposes. The pointed side is used to apply cuticle cream and buffing cream. The other side, when tipped with cotton wool, can be used to clean under the free edge, remove excess enamel and ease back cuticle. When tipped with cotton wool this should be disposed of after each use. If not tipped they are for single use only.

Cuticle knife

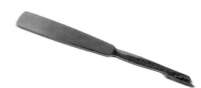

This is used to mould back the cuticle and remove any excess attached to the nail plate.

Cuticle nipper

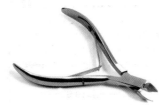

Used to remove hangnails and dead skin around the cuticle.

Nail scissors

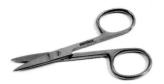

Used to cut nails.

Toenail clippers

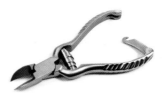

Used to cut and shorten nails prior to filing.

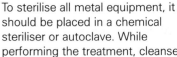

Remember

To sterilise all metal equipment, it should be placed in a chemical steriliser or autoclave. While performing the treatment, cleanse with a suitable sanitising solution.

Nail buffer

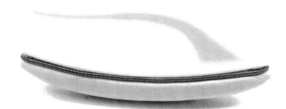

A pad covered with chamois leather and with a handle. Used in conjunction with buffing paste. Buffing adds sheen, stimulates circulation and growth at the matrix. Useful in male manicure or when nail varnish is not going to be applied. To clean wipe with a suitable cleansing solution.

3-way buffer

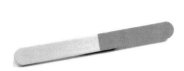

This is used to smooth the nail and to remove any longitudinal and horizontal lines. Wipe between use with a suitable cleansing solution.

Nail brush

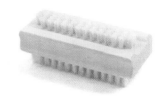

To brush the nails and clean them effectively, it's also used to clean the therapist's nails. Wash in hot soapy water or sterilise in a chemical solution.

Hoof stick

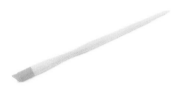

Usually plastic, may be wooden, with a rubber end to ease back cuticle. Pointed, and may be tipped with cotton wool to clean under free edge. When using from nail to nail, clean with a steriliser. On completion of treatment, sterilise in a cold sterilising solution.

Hard skin rasp/file/grater

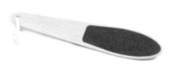

To be used after the feet have been soaked and can be used in conjunction with hard skin remover. Use on areas of hard skin in a rubbing action with light pressure. Wash after use in hot soapy water and remove debris, sterilise in chemical solution.

Pumice stone

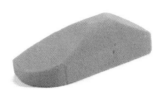

As with hard skin rasp.

Manicure bowl

This contains warm soapy water and sometimes a few drops of oil or a soaking solution. This softens the cuticle ready for pushing back. To clean, wash in hot soapy water and dry thoroughly.

Some chemical solutions may dissolve the glue that attaches the rasp element or bristles in this equipment.

Towels

A new clean towel for each client. It is useful to protect it with couch roll. Remember to have a separate towel for your personal use.

Couch roll

Dispose of all pieces after use.

> ⚠ **Remember**
>
> All metal equipment should be regularly checked, e.g. hinges and springs on scissors and clippers. Also check that cutting surfaces are smooth and sharp. Once sterilised all equipment should be stored hygienically, to prevent contamination occurring.

Tissues / cotton wool

Use a different tissue or piece of cotton wool for each hand / foot.

Spatulas

Break wooden spatulas after use. Wipe clean plastic or metal spatulas with a suitable cleansing solution when using between different products. Sterilise in chemical solution after use.

Products required

The following products are required for manicure and pedicure treatments:

- cuticle cream
- buffing paste
- hard skin remover
- massage medium
- talcum powder

- nail varnish / enamel
- base and top coats
- nail hardeners
- nail strengtheners.

For all these products use the cut-out system, or use pump action dispensers. When using pump dispensers, do not allow the spout to come into contact with the client's hands or feet. Chemicals contained within varnishes will prevent infection spreading, but to avoid any infection use the client's own product or sell the product to the client.

Improve the appearance of nails and skin using manicure and pedicure techniques

9.3

In this element you will learn about:

- products used in manicure and pedicure treatments
- suggested manicure procedure
- nail painting
- suggested pedicure routine
- French manicure
- massage.

Products used in manicure and pedicure treatments

Nail enamel / varnish remover

A solvent used to dissolve nail enamel. It is usually a mixture of acetone, glycerol and perfume. Acetone can have a drying effect on nails and surrounding skin.

Nail enamel / varnish thinners

A solvent used to thin down thick nail varnish / enamel, usually ethyl acetate. Nail enamel / varnish remover should not be used for this purpose due to the oil content contained in the remover. This may cause the varnish to discolour or separate.

Cuticle cream / oil

An emollient (softening, soothing) agent applied to cuticle to make it pliable. Cream contains soft white paraffin, mineral oils and some also contain lanolin. Oils contain a mixture of almond and jojoba and mineral oils.

Cuticle remover

A liquid or cream designed to dissolve and break down the cuticle to make removal easier. This contains potassium hydroxide (which is caustic), water and glycerol. As it is caustic, cuticle remover should be rinsed off the nails and skin directly after use. This product can be used as a nail bleach.

Nail hardeners

Used to strengthen fragile nails. It is a liquid which is painted on and allowed to soak into the nail plate. It acts as a binder to harden the nail.

Nail strengtheners

A mixture of powder acrylic and liquid plastic is painted on. Once set will reinforce the nail but still be flexible. This product is often combined in a base coat.

Rough skin remover

A cream or lotion containing abrasive particles, oils, emollients, perfume and water. Used to soften skin and aid removal of hard skin.

Buffing paste

An abrasive paste used in conjunction with a chamois buffer to smooth out ridges on nail plate. The abrasive elements in the paste may be a mixture of the following - kaolin, chalk, silica or talc.

Hand cream / massage cream

A cream that provides lubrication for massage and softens skin. It contains emollient, glycerol, lanolin, water, emulsifiers, colour and perfume.

Hand lotion

Contains the same elements as hand cream but has a higher water content. It is therefore less sticky than cream.

Nail enamels and varnishes, base coat and top coat

These products all have the same basic contents:

- a film firming plastic e.g. nitrocelluose
- a plastic resin e.g. aryl sufonamicide
- a gloss e.g. formaldehyde
- a plasticiser e.g. castor oil for flexibility
- solvents to dissolve other substances causing the nail enamel to dry e.g. ethyl acetate.

Coloured enamel / varnish

Colour is given by the addition of pigments, and a pearlised effect is made by adding, for example, bismuth oxychloride (for a metallic shine).

Base coat

Applied before colour, to prevent staining of the nail plate and to give a smooth surface for the coloured varnish to stick to.

Top coat

Applied after colour, to give extra durability against knocks and wear for cream colours. Pearlised varnishes/enamels already have these additives to give this durability.

Nail bleach

Cuticle remover may act as a mild bleach, but 20% hydrogen peroxide will be most effective on stains, e.g. dyes and nicotine.

Nail white pencils

Used on the underside of the free edge when coloured varnish is not used. Use moistened.

Nail repair kit

Used for splits or tears in nails – comprises of fibrous tissue and liquid adhesive.

Quick dry spray

Used for splits or tears in nails, comprised of fibrous tissue and liquid adhesive. Contains solvents that evaporate and speed up the drying process.

Step-by-step manicure

If you do specialised manicures and pedicures at your salon using a particular brand of products, you will probably go on a course which shows you how to use their products and gives an order for the procedure that should be followed. You therefore need to adapt your treatments at all times according to the manufacturer's instructions. However, whichever products you use, the basic principles for manicure and pedicure are the same.

Before starting the treatment, always carry out the following steps.

- Ensure equipment is sterile and all materials and products are easily accessible.
- Complete your consultation form, check for contra-indications on client and discuss the needs of the client.
- Remove all the client's jewellery, including watches, so that a thorough treatment can be carried out. Keep in a safe place.

> **Remember**
>
> Many of the products used in manicure and pedicure treatments are covered by COSHH regulations. Always refer to manufacturer's instructions prior to use.

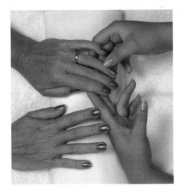

During the consultation discuss your client's needs, preferred shape of nails, and type of polish required. Providing there are no contra-indications present you are ready to begin.

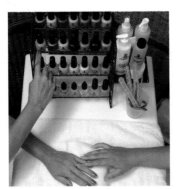

As your nail bar has all equipment and stock ready to begin treatment, ask the client to pick her choice of varnish – dark, plain, frosted or French manicure.

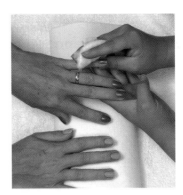

Remove the old varnish and check the nails for ridges and possible problems as you go.

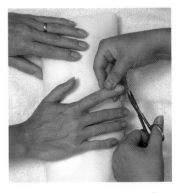

Cut the nails into shape if required, using sterilised scissors. Nail clippings need to be caught in a tissue and disposed of.

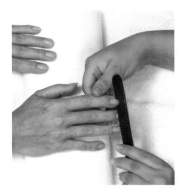

File the nails using an emery board working outside in, one way, one side then the other – avoid using a 'sawing' action. (There are different thicknesses of emery board.)

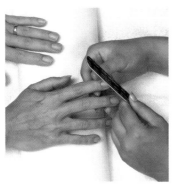

Bevelling seals the free edge layers to prevent water loss and mechanical damage.

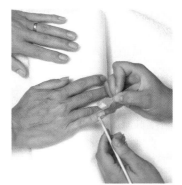

Using an orange stick, decant and apply cuticle cream around the cuticles.

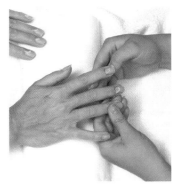

Gently massage the cream into the cuticles.

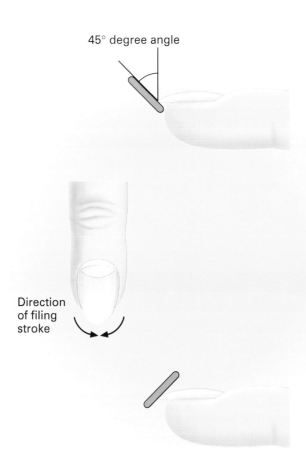

45° degree angle

Direction of filing stroke

Bevelling seals the free edge layers to prevent water loss and damage

Remember

Do not use a sawing action as this can cause the layers of the nail plate to split and separate.

Remember

The nail is made of three separate layers. 'Bevelling' holds the layers together and prevents splitting if the edge is traumatised.

Remember

There are some commercially prepared soaking preparations on the market, along with manicure bowls, to prevent spillage.

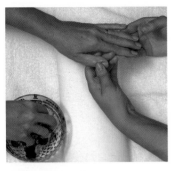

Soak the hands in warm water (tested by you first) to absorb the cuticle cream and to soften them.

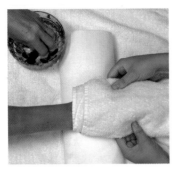

Remove one hand at a time and dry the hands thoroughly.

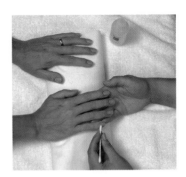

Apply cuticle remover with a cotton wool bud. It is caustic, so take care to apply sparingly and not onto the surrounding skin. Refer to COSHH regulations and manufacturer's instructions.

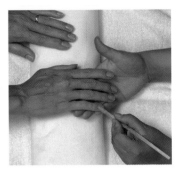

Using a hoof stick, flat to the nail plate, gently push the cuticle back, using circular motions.

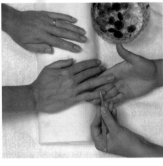

Depending upon the amount of work to be done on the cuticle, you may need to use the cuticle knife to ease the excess away from the nail plate.

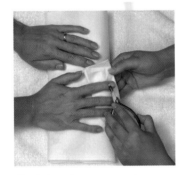

Cuticle nippers may be used to trim off the excess cuticle; use a tissue to dispose of the waste.

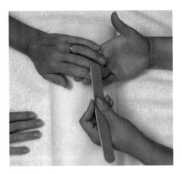

Bevel again, to give a smooth finish to the free edge.

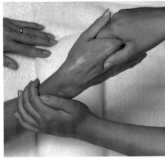

Using a suitable medium, begin your hand massage with light effleurage movements. Support the hand and effleurage right up to the elbow.

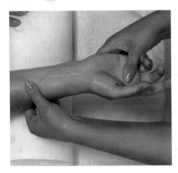

Circular thumb frictions get rid of tension in the flexors and extensors of the forearm.

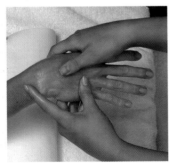

Do circular frictions over the back of the hand.

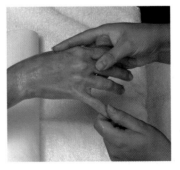

Support the hand and do gentle circular manipulations to each finger – this will free tension in the knuckles. Do not pull on the finger or make the circles too big.

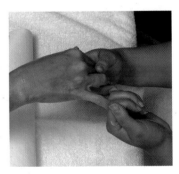

Grip the client's finger between your bent first and middle fingers and pull and twist gently down the length of the finger.

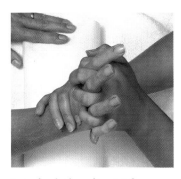

Interlock the clients' fingers with your own, and supporting the forearm, gently manipulate the wrist. First backwards . . .

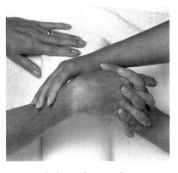

. . . and then forwards, to loosen the wrist and get rid of tension.

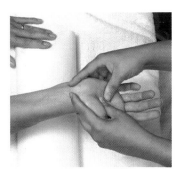

Apply circular thumb frictions to the palm. Stretch the palm out slightly.

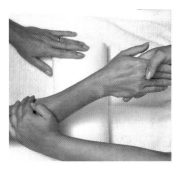

Finish your massage with effleurage up to the elbow.

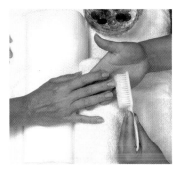

With warm soapy water, gently wash the nails with a soft brush to remove any grease from the massage medium.

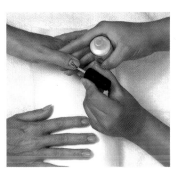

Apply a suitable base coat. Some nail systems have joint strengtheners or corrective properties within the base coat.

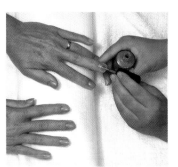

Apply the varnish of the client's choice, with clean strokes, without flooding the cuticle area.

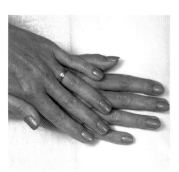

Top coat will give a professional finish and the results should look good for some time.

Pedicure

Before starting the treatment, carry out the following steps.

- Check for contra-indications, specifically: athlete's foot, bunions, corns, verrucas, ingrowing toenails and nail disease.
- Client should be seated comfortably with modesty towel over lap, and legs to knee exposed, to allow full pedicure with massage treatment.
- Therapist should have all materials to hand, be in a comfortable position with towel and single paper tissue roll on lap. Paper tissue to be replaced constantly through treatment to prevent cross-infection.

NB The client's feet may be pre-washed prior to commencement of treatment.

> ⚠️ **Remember**
>
> Diabetes may not be considered a contra-indication to manicure and pedicure but in some cases diabetes can cause limited sensation in the feet due to poor circulation. If this is the case GP approval is required. In the case of varicose veins: avoid massage – doctor's approval may be necessary.

Step-by-step pedicure

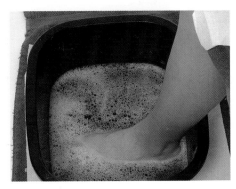

After a full consultation, remove the nail enamel and soak the feet to soften and refresh them.

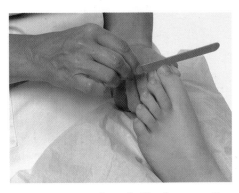

Using an emery board, file the toenails straight across – avoid any shaping, as it could cause ingrowing nails.

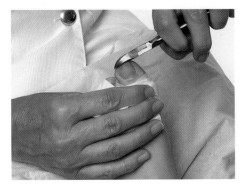

If the toenails are very long, use the clippers to get rid of the free edge, before filing.

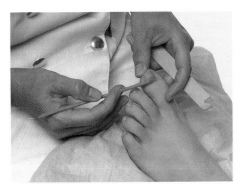

Apply cuticle cream and massage into the cuticle.

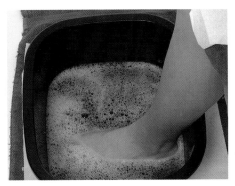

Soak the first foot in clean warm water, and repeat with second foot.

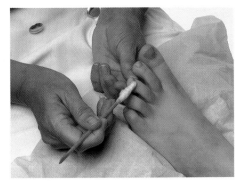

Apply cuticle remover with a cotton wool bud. It is caustic, so be careful only to apply sparingly and not onto the surrounding skin.

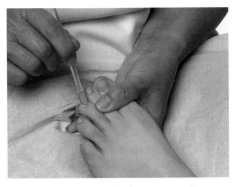

Using a hoof stick, flat to the nail plate, gently push the cuticle back, using circular motions.

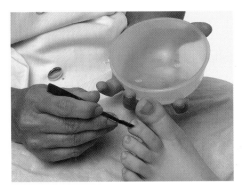

Depending upon the amount of work to be done on the cuticle, you may need to use the cuticle knife to ease the excess away from the nail plate.

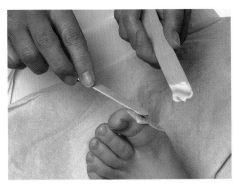

Rough skin remover may be applied to the areas that need attention, most commonly the ball of the foot, the heel and the side of the big toe.

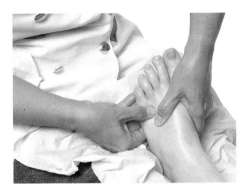

Apply massage medium and begin with effleurage to the whole foot, and follow with thumb frictions to the upper foot.

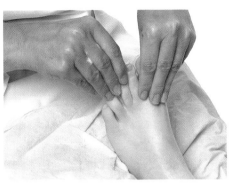

Follow the massage routine, as for manicure (see pages 282–283) – toe manipulations are really relaxing.

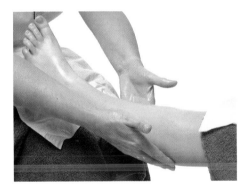

Finish with effleurage over the whole foot and lower leg.

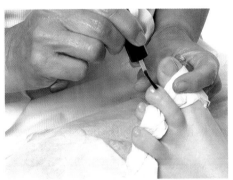

Paint toenails with client's choice of colour, using a base coat and top coat for extra durability. Remember to give the varnish plenty of time to dry, before the client puts her shoes back on.

Remember

Do not file nails to shape into the nail groove – keep free edge straight (square) or slightly rounded, to avoid problems with ingrowing nails.

Check it out

Do a small survey by asking how your friends and members of your family file their nails.

Are they filing correctly?

Nail painting

When painting nails, it is important to remember the following points.

- Try not to use more than four strokes per nail.
- Hold nail enamel in non-working palm of hand and use finger to support nail being painted.
- Always allow coats to dry before re-applying, this prevents smudging and streaking.
- When painting large wide nails, leave a thin unvarnished line at each side of the nail to produce a slimming effect.
- Avoid flooding the cuticles with nail varnish, as this has a drying effect on the skin.
- Tidy up any flaws with a cotton wool bud soaked in varnish remover.

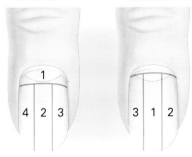

Method 1   Method 2

This is the better method for wide nails

In the salon

Jane has ridges on the nail plate and feels they are more noticeable when painted.

What recommendations could you make?

What colour varnish would you advise the client to wear?

Can you give any homecare advice?

Selection of colour

When selecting a coloured enamel it may help your client if you remember these few rules.

- Very bright colours draw attention to hands or feet.
- Dark colours make nails look smaller.
- Small hands or feet usually suit a light colour.
- Oval-shaped nails suit most colours.
- Orange, peach or beige tones emphasise the bluish tinges to the skin often seen in clients with poor circulation.
- Pearlised nails reflect the light and will emphasise any flaws in the nails.
- Coloured enamel is not suitable for very short / bitten nails, or hands and nails that are in poor condition.

Drying nail enamel

Nail enamel will dry quite well on its own, but on occasions it may be necessary to speed the process up. The application of either a top coat dryer or quick dry spray can be used. Nail drying preparations do not completely dry the varnish but form a barrier over the surface to prevent smudging. Always refer to manufacturer's instructions and be aware of COSHH regulations when using these products.

French manicure

This is a popular way of varnishing fingernails that gives a natural look. Kits that are sold usually contain white and flesh coloured enamels. Always refer to manufacturer's instructions for application. A suggested method of application follows.

1 Apply base coat.
2 Apply white enamel to free edge only. Allow to dry.
3 Apply flesh-coloured varnish to entire nail.
4 Apply a top coat.

Massage

Hand / foot and arm / leg massage (to elbow or knee) is included in manicure and pedicure treatments.

Massage helps to:

- moisturise skin
- aid desquamation (shedding of skin cells)
- improve poor nail conditions
- stimulate blood supply aiding cell regeneration
- relax tired muscles
- aid with the removal of waste products from the tissues
- aid client relaxation.

Types of massage movements

Effleurage

Effleurage movements are used for:

- introducing medium to area
- introducing hands to area
- helping relaxation with long flowing moves
- small amount of pressure with the fingers and palms of hands
- soothing nerve endings.

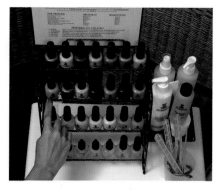

Helping your client select a nail polish colour

Check it out

Investigate a range of salon products that you can buy for manicure and pedicures and a range of products that you can purchase in a local store.

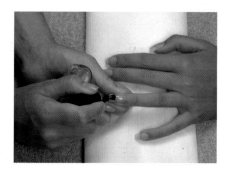

French manicures are very popular and are often chosen by brides

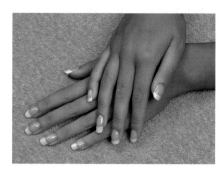

The finished results give a healthy, natural look

Petrissage

Petrissage movements are used for:

- increasing the blood flow feeding the muscular tissue and feeding cells
- desquemating cells from the surface of the skin
- increased removal of waste
- stimulating tissues, using deeper, more localised kneading or friction movements.

Tapotement

Tapotement movements are used for:

- breaking down areas of tension and nodules and adipose tissue
- a range of movements, such as hacking and cupping where hands work briskly to stimulate the area.

This type of movement needs adaptation depending on the area being treated and tissue density, e.g. not over a bony area.

Step-by-step arm massage

1 With effleurage movement, apply oil or cream.

2 With your left hand, effleurage the side of arm 3 times from out to in.

3 With your right hand, effleurage the other side of arm 3 times in to out.

4 Carry out thumb rotaries up the arm in 4 lines (2 at front and 2 at back).

5 Petrissage side of arm with your left hand out and in, and repeat on the other side from in to out 3 times.

6 Thumb-flicks in between the metacarpals 2 times between digits.

7 Rotaries in between metacarpals 2 times between every digit.

8 Thumb-flicks again, in between the metacarpals 2 times between digit.

9 Rotaries to phalange joints, traction 2 times, full mobilisation – 3 in one direction (in towards your client), then repeat in the opposite direction away from your client.

10 Effleurage whole hand once.

11 Rotaries on carpals, traction of hand 2 times.

12 Full mobilisation of carpals, 3 times in one direction (in towards client).

13 Knead the palm with your thumbs.

14 Effleurage arm alternatively 6 times and finish with pressure on the fingers.

Manicure / pedicure

Ensure all equipment is to hand and sterilised

⇓

Consultation to establish client requirements (discussion of occupation to help with suitable nail shape)

⇓

Selection of nail colour

⇓

File/cut if required

⇓

Cuticle work

⇓

Application of specialist product according to manufacturer's instructions if required

⇓

Massage

⇓

Buff

⇓

Paint

⇓

Homecare / aftercare advice

⇓

Record details on record card to include shape and varnish colour.

Improve the condition of nails and adjacent skin

9.4

In this element you will learn about:

- specialist treatments.

Specialist treatments

In some cases, the condition of a client's hands or feet might mean that a standard manicure or pedicure is not enough, and so a specialist treatment would be recommended. These treatments include abrasive products for hard skin and electrically heated mittens for intensive moisturising. It is vital when using these products that you follow manufacturer's instructions. You may need to attend specialist training courses to use some of the products.

Product	What it does	Benefits
Abrasives and exfoliants	These products contain abrasive particles, which help remove (desquamate) excess skin. This type of product is especially useful for pedicure treatments	Softens and removes hard skin while conditioning. For best results, feet should be soaked prior to application. A massage product should be applied to the area after use, to help replace lost moisture, making the skin feel soft and smooth.
Thermal masks	These products are usually wax- or oil-based, and they are applied to a well-moisturised area in a heated liquid form. The treated area is usually wrapped in either foil or cling film to maintain heat. The mask is usually left on for 15 minutes, but you should always check the manufacturer's instructions. An example of a thermal mask is paraffin wax.	Intensive re-hydration and softening of skin and nail plate. Ideal for dry skin conditions. Increases circulation, promoting healthier growth. Decreases joint stiffness. Relaxes aching muscles. Increases absorption of moisturising products.

Specialist treatment products

Step-by-step paraffin wax treatment

This can be used for both manicure and pedicure treatments. It is applied after the cuticle work and before the massage.

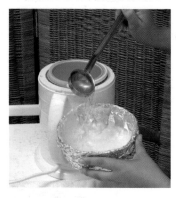

Prepare your working area and decant the melted paraffin wax into a bowl lined with tin foil.

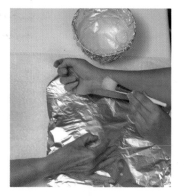

Test on self, prior to application on the client, over a sheet of tin foil, with a towel underneath it.

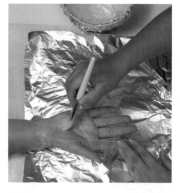

If the temperature is suitable, paint on a good even coating of the wax, working quickly before the wax sets, turning the hand to paint both sides.

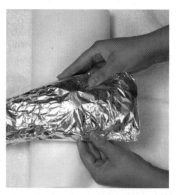

Wrap the hand in the tin foil, to retain the heat.

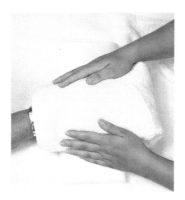

Wrap both hands in the towels and allow the heat to soothe and soften.

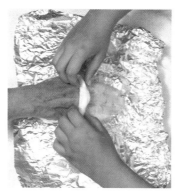

The wax cools and hardens, which makes removal easy – just peel it off. Any paraffin wax left in the bowl can be give to the client to use as a home treatment.

Warm oil treatment

This treatment is useful when treating dry hands / feet, cuticles and flaky nails.

The oil used should always be vegetable-based, for example:

- sweet almond oil
- olive oil
- cocoa oil.

Step-by-step warm oil treatment

1 Warm oil, either by immersing a suitable container in hot water or by using an infra-red lamp.

2 Proceed with treatment – do not apply cuticle massage oil at this stage. Soak fingers or toes in warmed oil for 5 minutes.

3 Massage in oil and wipe off any excess with a tissue.

4 Continue with routine.

NB It is not necessary to carry out a massage with this treatment.

Thermal mittens and booties

These are electrically heated items of equipment that are used on the same principle as thermal masks, with the added advantage of:

- maintaining heat more effectively
- easy and less messy to use
- more cost-effective over a period of time, as no special product required.

Step-by-step thermal treatments

1 Apply a moisturising product to the area.

2 Apply cling film to improve the re-hydration process.

3 Place hands / feet in mittens / booties for 10–15 minutes.

4 After that time continue with cuticle work and the rest of the treatment.

Contra-indications ⚠

- Skin infections
- Varicose veins
- Nail diseases
- Hypersensitivity.

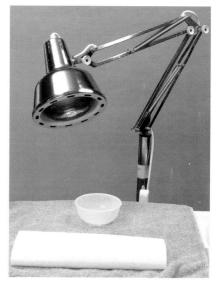

Preheat the oil in a plastic bowl

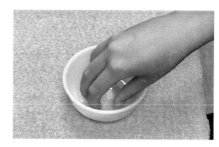

Soak the cuticles to help soften, and massage

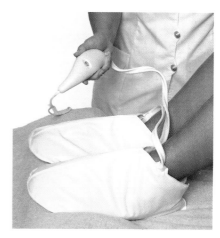

Thermal booties

These treatments are highly effective and clients feel pampered and relaxed. Specialist treatments usually take 1–2 hours, but frequency depends on severity or condition.

There are a number of professional nail companies that produce a wide range of specialist products designed for salon and home use, and often specialist training is required before salons introduce these products. Always follow the manufacturer's instructions for use to obtain the best results.

In the salon

Helema comes into the salon with dry hands and overgrown cuticles.

What intensive treatment could you carry out for these conditions?

What homecare advice could you give?

Homecare and aftercare

To ensure that your client gains maximum benefit from the treatment, you need to give aftercare and homecare advice that is both practical and achievable. Wherever possible it is advisable to show the client how to use the product. Many of the items and products listed are sold through salons. It is worth remembering that many therapists work on commission, so good product knowledge could earn you extra money.

To protect the client's hands and nails from damage, it should be suggested that suitable gloves or a special barrier cream is used when completing tasks involving any dirty work, or other work involving the use of water and or chemicals. Examples of these types of work include:

- gardening
- washing up
- hairdressing
- car maintenance.

The client should also be advised:

- not to bite their nails or surrounding skin and to keep an emery board available to deal with ragged free edges to their nails, so that the temptation to bite is removed
- to use a moisturising hand cream or lotion regularly
- to avoid using their nails as tools (e.g. undoing screws, removing tight lids from containers and opening tightly sealed letters and parcels)
- to stop using a product immediately in the event of contra-actions occurring, such as a reaction to products in the form of extreme redness, rashes, irritation or swelling – advise the client to cool the area with cold water and visit his or her GP if treatment is required.

Products

With nail care of the feet and hands the retail products you may stock to sell to clients is an important income booster to a salon, and many therapists boost their salaries with commission from these sales. It is therefore important to have excellent knowledge of the products your salon retails, which could include the following.

Nail varnish remover

This is used to remove old varnish. Do not use too frequently, as it can have a drying effect on the nails and surrounding skin. Always wash hands after use.

Base coat, nail varnish, top coat

It is advisable to sell a selection of varnishes, and ensure your client realises the importance of wearing a base coat to prevent staining the nail plate.

Nail strengthener

Use these products according to manufacturer's instructions. This is often built into base coat varnishes, to improve the condition of the nails.

Cuticle cream

This product can be massaged around the cuticles daily to keep them soft and smooth. The massaging action will help stimulate the growth of the nail.

Emery boards

Recommend the fine side for shaping finger nails and the coarse side for hard nails and reducing the length of the nails. Show the client how to file correctly. Avoid sawing.

Buffers

These can be used to smooth out ridges and to give the nails a natural sheen. Show the client how to use them correctly, going from the base of the nail to the free edge. Buffing will stimulate growth, so this is can be an incentive for nail biters.

Foot care

Clients should be advised of the importance of ensuring that all footwear is well fitting, so that the feet are not restricted, which may result in damage, discomfort and foot problems.

Rough skin remover

This is a slightly abrasive product that is effective against hard skin. Massage onto affected areas firmly in circular movements for softer feet.

Foot powder

This is a deodorised powder that can be applied regularly to keep feet fresh and dry. This product is worth recommending to clients who suffer with odour problems, or have a tendency to have athlete's foot (this condition thrives in damp conditions).

COSHH regulations for manicure and pedicure preparations

The Control of Substances Hazardous to Health (COSHH) regulations control the safe use, disposal and storage of products.

Many of the preparations that are used in manicure and pedicure treatments are governed by these rules. Therefore, as a therapist, you have to know how to use these products correctly.

Cuticle remover

Description
- A solution of sodium hydroxide in water with other cosmetic ingredients.
- Contains sodium hydroxide.

Ingredients
- All ingredients are commonly used in cosmetic products and meet accepted standards of purity.

> **Remember**
>
> Matching lipsticks could also be sold to colour co-ordinate with the nail varnish.

> **Check it out**
>
> Find out the COSHH regulations for the products you use.

Hazards

- Considered to be hazardous if precautions are ignored.

Flammability

- Non-inflammable.

First aid procedures

- Ingestion: drink milk or water and seek medical attention.
- Inhalation: avoid. If prolonged inhalation occurs, remove to fresh air and keep warm.
- Skin contact: avoid. If prolonged contact occurs, wash well with water. If irritation persists, seek medical advice.
- Eye contact: avoid. If it occurs wash well with water for a minimum of 15 minutes and always seek medical help immediately from a qualified doctor or hospital.

Spillage

- Clean using liberal quantities of water.

Handling and storage

- Always wear gloves and avoid contact with skin and eyes.
- Store in a cool place away from direct sunlight. Keep closures tightly sealed.

Cuticle massage cream

Description

- An emulsion of oils, waxes, water and water-soluble ingredients, emulsifiers, fragrance and preservatives.

Ingredients

- All ingredients are commonly used in cosmetic preparations and meet acceptable standards of purity.

Hazards

- Considered to be non-hazardous under normal conditions of use.

Flammability

- Non-inflammable.

First aid procedures

- Ingestion: drink milk or water.
- Inhalation: N/A
- Skin contact: N/A
- Eye contact: wash well, if irritation persists, seek medical advice.

Spillage

- Clean using absorbent material, wash with detergent and water.

Handling and storage

- No special precautions are necessary.

Non-acetone nail polish remover

Description

- A mixture of organic solvents.

Ingredients

- All ingredients are commonly used in cosmetic products and meet accepted standards of purity.

Hazards

- The product is considered hazardous if precautions are ignored.

Flammability

- Inflammable.

First aid procedures

- Ingestion: drink milk or water and seek medical advice.
- Inhalation: avoid inhalation. If affected, remove to fresh air and keep warm.
- Skin contact: avoid. If prolonged contact occurs, wash well with water. If irritation persists, seek medical advice.
- Eye contact: wash well with water for a minimum of 15 minutes. If irritation persists seek medical advice.

Spillage

- Clean using liberal quantities of water.

Handling and storage

- Avoid contact with skin and eyes.
- Store in a cool place away from direct sunlight. Keep tightly sealed and store in a fire-resistant cupboard.
- Fire: advise fire service of storage quantities.

Acetone

Description

- Dimethyl ketone or 2-propanone.

Ingredients

- This product is commonly used in cosmetic products and meets accepted standards of purity.

Hazards

- Considered to be hazardous unless normal safety procedures are followed.

Flammability

- Flammable.
- Flash point 17.2 = Highly flammable.

First aid procedures

- Ingestion: drink plenty of milk or water.
- Inhalation: may cause dizziness, remove to fresh air.
- Skin contact: avoid prolonged contact with the skin. If irritation persists seek medical advice.
- Eye contact: rinse, seek medical advice.

Spillage

- Clean contaminated area with lots of water, wash with detergent and water to avoid slippery floors. Do not absorb with combustible material.

Handling and storage

- Cool place away from direct sunlight, in a fire-resistant store.
- Fire: contents are flammable. In case of fire evacuate areas known to contain products and inform fire-fighters of their presence.

Your questions answered

What will happen if I don't check for contra-indications?
Infections of the hands and feet can be spread very easily – especially warts and verrucas.

Can I use a dark-coloured varnish on short or bitten nails?
Lighter colours will make the nails appear longer; a dark colour will draw attention to bitten and badly kept nails.

What happens if I don't keep the cuticle knife flat and wet?
Keeping the knife flat helps prevent cutting the skin, and wetting the knife prevents scratching the nail plate.

Why can't I use foam toe separators between the toes when painting the toenails?
Tissues are used because they are disposable. Foam separators may harbour germs and cause infections to be passed from client to client.

Test your knowledge

1   *How would you recognise a verucca?*

2   *Is athlete's foot a virus, fungus, or bacteria?*

3   *How should you cut toe nails?*

4   *What is the purpose of a hoof stick?*

5   *Why should a base coat be used before applying varnish?*

6   *What salon treatment could you recommend for a client with very dry skin or cuticles?*

7   *What is leuconychia?*

8   *Why do you bevel the nail when filing?*

9   *What are finger and toenails made from?*

10   *What nail shape suits most colours of varnish?*

11   *List five things that you should include in a consultation.*

12   *How should you store acetone?*

13   *If the nails have corrugations, what treatments could you offer to minimise this?*

Key skills Level 1 and NVQ Level 2 Customer Service

When completing tasks for your NVQ Level 2 Beauty therapy portfolio you will also be creating evidence that is suitable for your Key Skills portfolio and, if you take it, your NVQ Level 2 Customer Service.

The following is a guide to which evidence is most suitable for each and what is expected of that evidence. The Key Skills evidence is listed first, and the related Customer Service evidence follows.

Key Skills Level 1 Communication

C1.1 One-to-one discussion

This needs to be about different, straightforward subjects. Any of the following can be used as evidence.

- Practical units 5, 6, 7, 8 or 9 a treatment consultation with the client

The assessor who has observed your client interaction should sign the consultation sheet. The form must be neat and tidy, with clear writing, and no spelling mistakes. (See Unit 6, page 154.)

- Unit 3 One-to-one discussion for any tutorial interview with a subject or personal tutor

You and your tutor will decide on a clear pathway for your personal progression through the unit you are currently working on and you should both sign this. Any resulting action plan can contribute to Unit 3. (See Unit 3, page 76 – self-appraisal.)

- Units 2 and 3 – one-to-one discussion within your role as salon manager

If a discussion arises regarding the treatment page / treatments to do or jobs to be allocated, the discussion should be logged in your duty report form and signed by both parties. Your tutor will supply you with the appropriate paperwork.

- Units 2 and 3 – student discussion between two colleagues

Use a salon situation to discuss any practical issues that arise, and log it on the salon report sheet, or present the solution to a problem to your salon manager / assessor i.e. 'Joanna and I are going to cover the clients for Suzette, who is off sick – I will do XYZ and Joanna will do ABC'. (See Unit 3, page 76.)

C1.1 Group discussion

- Units 2 and 3 – class discussion between all class members

Suggestions on how to improve the salon / client set up – salon organisation, client rota or similar topic.

Class discussion on a straightforward subject linked to Beauty therapy e.g. cosmetic surgery or the use of Botox injections, permanent make-up or similar.

Do an evaluation sheet on the results of your discussion and remember to get signatures. Your tutor will provide the marking sheets.

Customer Service NVQ Level 2

If you complete the evidence for Key Skills Communication C1.1 One-to-one discussion, you have also achieved the following elements and units for NVQ Level 2 Customer Service.

Element 1.1 Questioning and listening techniques for services and products for example:

Finding out which products the client has been using or which treatments have been a success.

Element 5.3 Work with others to improve reliability of service

Produce evidence that you have worked with clients or colleagues to provide a more reliable salon service.

C1.2 Read 2 documents including an image

- Units 2, 3, 5, 6, 7, 8 and 9

Working as a salon manager and dealing with any health and safety instructions or manufacturer's instructions for anything relating to practical units 5–9.

- How to use the autoclave. (See Professional basics, page 29.)
- Fire evacuation procedures. (See Unit 1, page 47.)
- Client booking-in sheet – allocation of jobs. (See Professional basics, page 16.)
- Salon rules and regulations for professional attire and safe footwear. (See Professional basics, pages 12–13.)
- Also use information from Unit 1, health and safety for safe practices within the salon and spillage procedures. (See Unit 1, page 58.)

Customer Service NVQ Level 2

If you complete the evidence for Key Skills Communication C1.2 Read 2 documents including an image, you have also achieved the following elements and units in NVQ Level 2 Customer Service.

Element 1.1

Using products and services.
Following manufacturer's instructions.
Awareness of legal rights of customers.

C1.3 Write 2 documents including an image

- Unit 2 or Unit 5–9

Design a safety poster, which could be presented to the group, and a memo inviting students to attend the briefing. Also, a memo, inviting students to attend a salon manager meeting, could be sent. (See Unit 1, page 58.)

Design an aftercare leaflet for any practical unit 5–9: e.g. manicure, pedicure, waxing, facials (See Unit 7, pages 209 and 212.)

NVQ Level 2 Customer Service

If you complete the evidence for Key Skills Communication C1.3 Write 2 documents including an image, you have also achieved the following elements & units in NVQ Level 2 Customer Service.

Element 2.1

Design a client record card, bearing security of information in mind.

Element 5.3

Work with others to improve reliability of service.

Design a short questionnaire on the back of the record of evidence sheet, for customer evaluation of service or treatment, or sales to improve delivery of services.

Key Skills Application of Number Level 1

N1.1 Interpret information from 2 sources

- Unit 7

Refer to the waxing section, both the table and text, to work out how many minutes it would take to conduct a waxing treatment, which type of wax would be most successful, and how long setting up and finishing the treatment would take. (See Unit 7, pages 205 and 215.)

N1.2 Carry out calculations to do with amounts and sizes, scales and proportions, handling statistics

- Unit 7

  - Work out how many treatments you would realistically get from one wax pot, using the volume and division of number of wax used each time.
  - Calculate the cost of the wax to purchase, and the cost per treatment, remembering overheads. You should now be able to calculate the profit margin, per pot.

N1.3 Interpret results of calculations and present findings – must include 1 chart and 1 diagram

This lends itself very nicely to a bar chart, pie chart and / or line graph, to show profit margins and overhead costs. Your lecturer will help you, and provide the paperwork, as this can be used within the Key skills Level 1 IT, too.

NVQ Level 2 Customer Service

If you complete the evidence for Key Skills Application of Number N1.1 Interpret information from 2 sources, you have also achieved the following elements & units for NVQ Level 2 Customer service.

5.2 Using client feedback to improve service reliability

Design and conduct a short questionnaire on client preferences for type of wax used on different areas of the body, to include timings of preparation, actual treatment and finished results and reliability of each wax type. Give feedback to colleagues, based on the results, on the most popular choices and why.

Key Skills Level 1 Information and Computer Technology

You may need the help of your IT co-ordinator, because this Key Skill requires you to use ICT resources.

IT1.1 Find & explore and develop information – 2 different purposes; IT1.2 Present ×2 information for different purposes – including: ×1 text ×1 images, ×1 numbers

- Units 6 and 7

If you are creating client information sheets on, for example, waxing or facial treatments, you need to remember the following.

- Don't forget to check the spelling, punctuation and grammar.

- Keep a log detailing: how you found the information you required; the file names you used to save your work; your reasons for choosing or rejecting information.
- Keep **draft copies** of your work, and note on them why you decided to make changes.

(See also the suggestions below for Customer Service.)

NVQ Level 2 Customer Service

Unit 4 Solve problems for customers

Using a computer, design a short questionnaire to gather information on customer problems – it could be related to grumbles or praise the client has for hygiene procedures.

Or, you could relate your questionnaire to: Availability of stock, quality of products or services, Use of products or services, Organisation of systems, booking in etc.

Element 4.2

Analyse the results and discuss in a staff meeting with colleagues, the best way to solve the problem.

Design a poster explaining the new method of meeting the clients' problems. Include text, images and numbers.

It could be a timed booking-in system, with a fixed penalty for late clients or non-arrivals.

NB All of the above are suggested tasks only, with references to the book to help you identify where you may find evidence. Your lecturer may use other tasks, and give you guidance through your Key Skills and Customer Service activities.

Index